BODY FLUIDS

SECOND EDITION

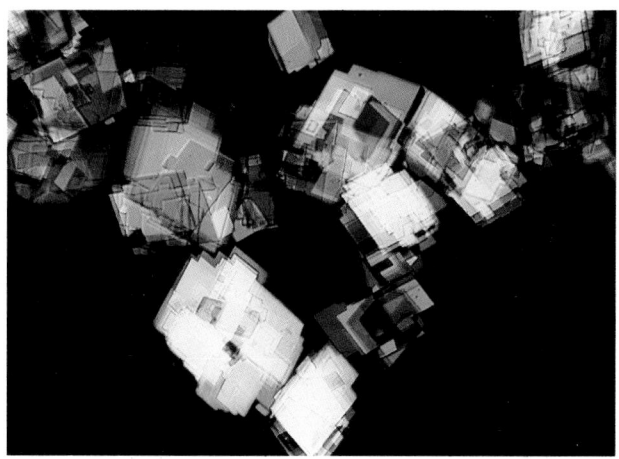

Body Fluids

Laboratory Examination of Amniotic,
Cerebrospinal, Seminal, Serous, & Synovial Fluids:
A Textbook Atlas

Carl R. Kjeldsberg, **MD**
Professor of Pathology and Medicine
Head, Anatomic Pathology
University of Utah School of Medicine, Salt Lake City
Executive Vice President, ARUP
(Associated Regional and University Pathologists, Inc.)

Joseph A. Knight, **MD**
Associate Professor of Pathology
Head, Clinical Pathology
University of Utah School of Medicine, Salt Lake City
Vice President, ARUP
(Associated Regional and University Pathologists, Inc.)

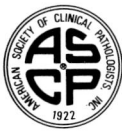

AMERICAN SOCIETY OF CLINICAL PATHOLOGISTS PRESS
Chicago

Cover *Figure 97: Vacuolated tumor cells in metastatic adenocarcinoma. Figure 110: Epithelial membrane antigen in tumor cells. Figure 116: Malignant cells in ascitic fluid.*

Notice

Trade names for equipment and supplies described herein are included as suggestions only. In no way does their inclusion constitute an endorsement or preference by the American Society of Clinical Pathologists. The ASCP did not test the equipment, supplies, or procedures and, therefore, urges all readers to read and follow all manufacturers' instructions and package insert warnings concerning the proper and safe use of products.

Library of Congress Cataloging-in-Publication Data

Kjeldsberg, Carl R., 1938–
  Body fluids.

  Includes bibliographies and index.
    1. Body fluids—Analysis. 2. Body fluids—Examination. 3. Body fluids—Examination—Atlases.
I. Knight, Joseph A., 1930–   . II. Title. [DNLM:
1. Body Fluids—analysis—atlases.   QY 17 K62b]
RB52.K56   1986   616.07'56   85-15086
ISBN 0-89189-201-X
ISBN 0-89189-202-8 (bk. & slides)

89 88 87 86   6 5 4 3 2 1

To our wives, Gillean and Pauline,
and our children, Tanya, Kristina, Leigh, and David

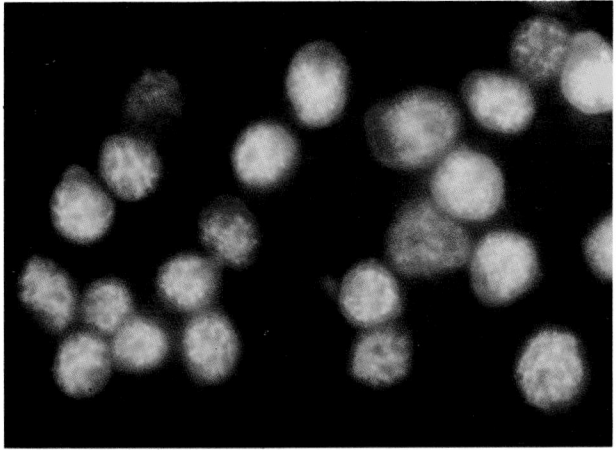

Contents

List of Illustrations

List of
Tables

Preface

The gratifying response to the first edition of *Body Fluids: Laboratory Examination of Cerebrospinal, Synovial, & Serous Fluids: A Textbook Atlas* has indicated to us that there is an ongoing need for a current text covering many aspects of the laboratory examination of body fluids. Hence, in this second edition, the text has been completely revised and updated, the illustrations have been significantly increased and updated, and two new chapters on amniotic and seminal fluid have been added.

Compared with the examination of serum and urine, the laboratory examination of other body fluids is still in its infancy. However, since the first edition, a wealth of new information has become available. Much of this is still in the experimental stage, but major advances have been made in many areas that are both diagnostically and prognostically useful in patient management. We have attempted to introduce the reader to new and interesting information while at the same time emphasizing those procedures that are clinically most useful.

The purpose of the book is to provide a narrative and pictorial description of cell morphology; methodology on how to collect, store, and examine specimens; and guidelines for selecting various tests according to their diagnostic significance. While cell morphology has been given considerable attention, this is not meant to be a cytology textbook. The majority of the illustrations show the morphologic features using a Romanovsky stain (Wright's stain) rather than the Papanicolaou stain. The former is the stain most commonly used for body fluids in hematology and microscopy laboratories and is also commonly used by cytologists in Europe. Hence a Wright's stain has been used unless otherwise indicated.

We are very grateful to the following individuals: Ronald Urry, PhD, Associate Professor of Surgery, Obstetrics and Gynecology, University of Utah School of Medicine, for writing the chapter on seminal fluid; Joe Marty, MS, MT (ASCP), for his assistance with the methodology section, the information on crystal examination, and his help with the photomicrography; Britt Adams, MT (ASCP), for assistance in writing the methodology section; Mary Perkins, MT (ASCP), and Kathy Hughes, MT (ASCP), for their work in developing a variety of techniques for tumor markers; Julian Maack, for assisting with the illustrations; and Irene Larson, for her patience in typing the manuscript many times.

Carl R. Kjeldsberg, MD
Joseph A. Knight, MD

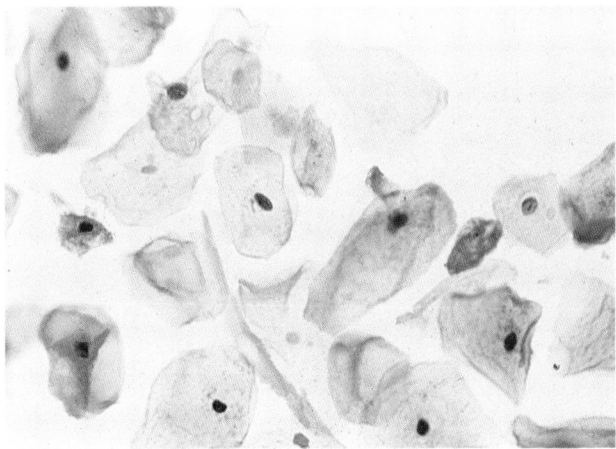

CHAPTER 1

Amniotic Fluid

Multiple perinatal disorders can be identified by examining the amniotic fluid. This field is, however, still in its infancy, and there is no uniform agreement as to which laboratory procedures are most clinically useful. There is also considerable controversy regarding the methodology used in many of the laboratory tests. We have emphasized the procedures that to date appear to be most reliable and clinically useful. In addition, we have briefly described other measurements, many of which are still experimental but in the future may be diagnostically useful.

ANATOMY AND PATHOPHYSIOLOGY

Approximately six days after ovulation, the fertilized ovum, which has differentiated to form the blastocyst, implants in the decidua of the uterus. The inner mass of the blastocyst then differentiates to form the embryonic disk. Subsequently, a cleft appears between the disk and the trophoblast and enlarges gradually to become the amniotic cavity. The amniotic cavity eventually surrounds the embryo and obliterates the chorionic space (Figure 1). The amnion, which is the inner membrane in contact with the amniotic fluid, has a single layer of cuboidal epithelial cells that lie on the basement membrane (Figure 2).

The regulation of amniotic fluid volume and its composition, particularly in the early part of pregnancy, are still poorly understood. It is thought that, during the second and third trimester, exchanges of water and solute take place between fluid and fetus by the following pathways: (1) fetal swallowing and reabsorption by intestine; (2) exchange with the respiratory tract where the alveolar capillary bed is perfused by amniotic fluid; and (3) fetal urination. In addition, there may be an exchange across the fetal skin of small, lipid-soluble compounds and a transfer of water and solute across the chorionic plate between the fetal circulatory system and the amniotic fluid.[1] The main site of water-exchange between mother and

FIGURE 1.   *Schematic drawing of the anatomic relationships of the fetus and the amniotic fluid.*

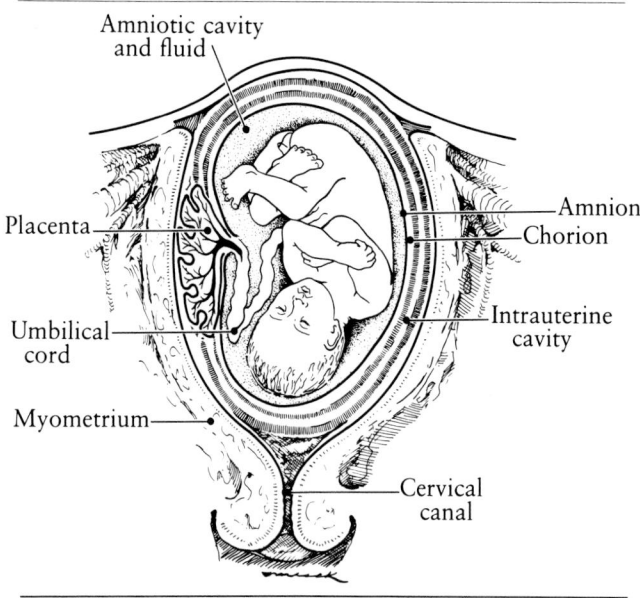

FIGURE 2.   *The amnion. A single layer of cuboidal cells lines the amniotic cavity (hematoxylin-eosin stain).*

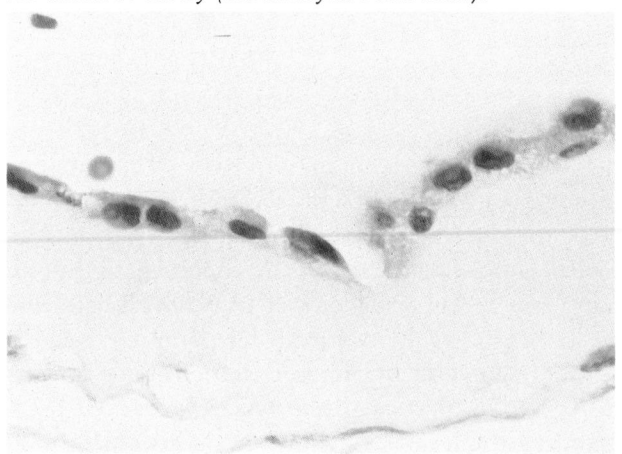

fetus is across the chorion frondosum of the placenta. Normally, water is exchanged between amniotic fluid and mother, between mother and fetus, and between fetus and fluid.

During pregnancy, there is a gradual increase in the volume of amniotic fluid, probably in response to the growth of the fetus. The mechanism for the control of this system is not known, but it is thought that the fetus itself may play a role in amniotic fluid volume homeostasis.[2] The fetus swallows between 200 and 500 mL of amniotic fluid per day, and increased swallowing has been observed when the mother carries larger-than-normal volumes of amniotic fluid.[3] Hydramnios (increased amniotic fluid volume) occurs when the fetus fails to swallow. This may be seen with such fetal malformations as anencephaly or esophageal atresia. Oligohydramnios (less than 300 mL of amniotic fluid) may develop when a chronically ill fetus swallows more fluid than is normal (eg, in placental insufficiency) and in cases of renal agenesis. The amniotic fluid volume increases during pregnancy from 35 mL at 12 weeks' gestation to 250 mL during the 18th week to 1,100 mL at term.[4] Markedly diminished volumes are associated with fetal insufficiency and fetal death; the largest volumes are seen with fetal anomalies.[5] The most direct and reliable method of estimating the amount of amniotic fluid is with ultrasound testing.

The functions of the amniotic fluid probably include (1) protecting the fetus, (2) allowing fetal movement and growth, (3) maintaining an even temperature, and (4) participating in fetal biochemical homeostasis.

SPECIMEN COLLECTION

Transabdominal amniocentesis is the preferred method for obtaining amniotic fluid. An adequate sample may also be collected with vaginal amniocentesis, but this method carries with it an increased rate of infection. It also complicates the analysis of the fluid because of contamination with vaginal bacteria, maternal vaginal cells, or both. The earliest time that amniocentesis can be performed safely is 16 weeks from the last menstrual period or the 14th week of gestation. The aim is to collect a clean sample under sterile conditions, avoiding damage to both the fetus and the placenta. Ultrasound examination is essential to localize the placenta and to assist the obstetrician in accurately directing the needle. In addition, ultrasound may be used to establish correct gestational age for optimal timing of the procedure. When performed by an experienced operator, amniocentesis is a safe procedure that can be performed on an outpatient basis.

As noted in Table 1-1, the indications for amniocentesis vary, depending on the gestational age. Amniocentesis is done during the 16th or 17th week of gestation to determine the karyotype of the fetus for possible genetic defects, to measure α_1-fetoprotein in order to detect neural tube defects, and to measure certain enzymes in patients with a high risk for enzyme deficiency (eg, patients with Tay-Sachs disease). Later in pregnancy, amniocentesis may be done to determine fetal lung maturity, to assess the severity of Rh isoimmunization, or to diagnose infection.

The amount of fluid required varies from 10 to 20 mL. No more than 20 mL should be removed because this may precipitate premature labor or spontaneous rupture of the membranes. The specimen should be processed soon after removal from the amniotic cavity to preserve the biochemical constituents (Figure 3). The appearance of the fluid before and after centrifugation of the specimen should be described, and any blood staining or discoloration should be noted. The cellular components should be separated by low-speed centrifugation (500 to 1,000g for five minutes).[6] The sediment and the supernatant can be stored for about 24 hours in the dark at 2° to 8 °C. The supernatant should be protected from light to preserve bilirubin if a diagnosis of hemolytic disease of the newborn is being considered.

Sometimes one has to determine whether a fluid specimen is maternal urine or amniotic fluid from rupture of fetal membranes. When the placenta and fetus are difficult to localize or when the infant is hydropic, the obstetrician may have technical problems obtaining fluid, and the specimen submitted to the laboratory may not be amniotic in origin. In such instances, a variety of tests may be performed to identify it. Creatinine levels in the amniotic fluid are similar to those in plasma, and values over 4 mg/dL indicate contamination of the amniotic fluid with urine. Protein measurements may also be used as indicators,

TABLE 1–1. Indications for Amniocentesis

INDICATION	WEEK OF GESTATION
Suspected chromosomal abnormality, metabolic disorder, or neural tube defect	16
Isoimmunization	20–28
Suspected fetal and pulmonary immaturity	34–42
Suspected chorioamnionitis	34–42

since little or no protein is normally present in the urine, while significant quantities are present in the amniotic fluid. A simple way to distinguish maternal urine from amniotic fluid is with a protein-glucose dipstick. Amniotic fluid will have a positive dipstick for both solutes, and urine will have a negative dipstick unless maternal diabetes or renal disease is present. These results should be confirmed by creatinine or urea analysis. If the amniotic fluid is contaminated with maternal urine, the interpretation may be very difficult.

For cytogenetic studies, the fluid must be collected in sterile syringes. The first milliliter of fluid, however, may be contaminated with maternal cells as the needle penetrates the abdomen of the mother. One way to prevent this is to run a stylet through the needle several times before withdrawing fluid and to collect the first few milliliters of fluid separately. The fluid should then be transferred to sterile tubes. Similar techniques are recommended for microbiologic studies.

GROSS EXAMINATION

The gross appearance of the fluid should be noted, as the color may be an indicator of fetal well-being (Table 1–2).

If meconium, which is a dark green mixture of secretions of the intestinal glands and amniotic fluid, stains the amniotic fluid, the fetus may be in distress or have hemolytic disease or some other condition. When large amounts of meconium are present, the fluid is turbid and dark green. When small quantities

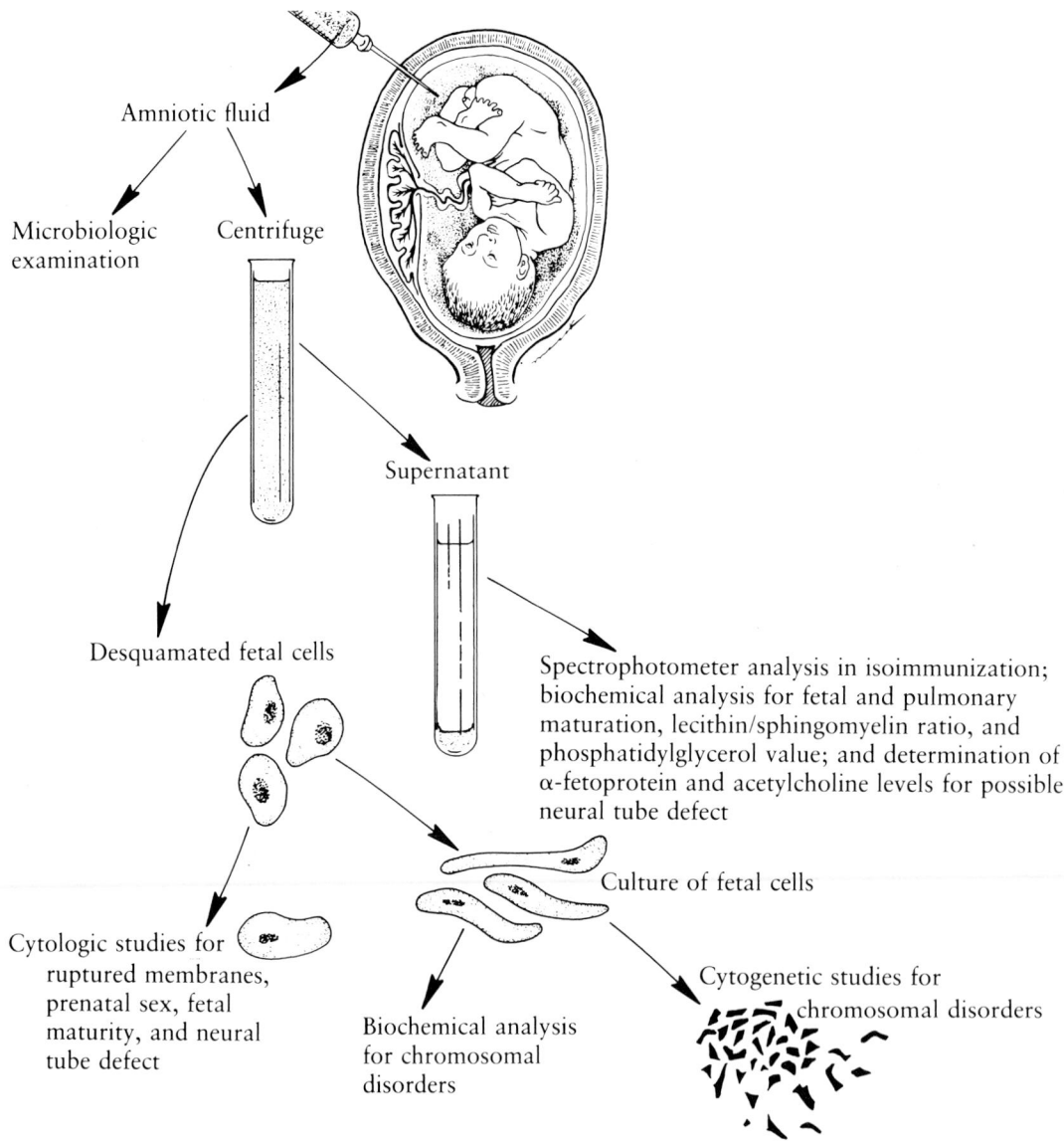

Amniotic fluid

Microbiologic examination

Centrifuge

Supernatant

Desquamated fetal cells

Spectrophotometer analysis in isoimmunization; biochemical analysis for fetal and pulmonary maturation, lecithin/sphingomyelin ratio, and phosphatidylglycerol value; and determination of α-fetoprotein and acetylcholine levels for possible neural tube defect

Culture of fetal cells

Cytologic studies for ruptured membranes, prenatal sex, fetal maturity, and neural tube defect

Biochemical analysis for chromosomal disorders

Cytogenetic studies for chromosomal disorders

are present, the fluid may be detected spectrophotometrically. In general, meconium staining early in pregnancy usually is not due to hemolytic disease and usually clears as term approaches. It is thought to represent a previous transient episode of fetal compromise and usually does not indicate a poor fetal outcome.[7]

MICROSCOPIC EXAMINATION

The cytologic examination of amniotic fluid may be of value for several purposes, including the diagnosis of ruptured membranes, the determination of fetal maturity, the determination of sex prenatally, and the detection of neural tube defects.

There have been several cytologic studies published, describing in great detail the various types of cells found in amniotic fluid; more than a dozen cell forms have been described.[8-11] There are two main sources of exfoliated cells in the amniotic fluid—the fetus and the amnion—and it should be noted that cells of different origin may be similar in appearance. The fetal squamous epithelial cells, believed to originate from fetal skin, oral mucosa, and the vagina, consist of anucleated squamous epithelial cells that are polygonal or ovoid in shape. Superficial and intermediate squamous epithelial cells may occur singly or in clumps. Occasional urothelial cells may also be found. The amnion or parabasal-like cells are frequently present. They are cuboidal or ovoid in shape and arranged in short chains or singly. The amniotic epithelial cells originate from the lining of the amniotic sac. Rarely, large multinucleated cells are seen, representing syncytial knots from the placenta (Figure 4). This may occur if the needle passes through the placenta.

For cytologic examination, smears may be made after centrifugation. However, cytologic filters or the cytocentrifuge method shows the morphologic characteristics more distinctly. The slides are usually stained with Papanicolaou's stain or with Nile blue dye.

CLINICAL CORRELATIONS

Several methods have been described for diagnosing *ruptured membranes*. The fern test for estrogen has been used for many years and is still used in many clinics because it is easy and quick to perform. The

TABLE 1–2. Amniotic Fluid Color and Associated Fetal Conditions

COLOR	ASSOCIATED CONDITION
Colorless to pale straw	Normal (appearance does not rule out erythroblastosis, however)
Yellow	Erythroblastosis
Greenish (meconium)	Fetal hypoxia (except during early pregnancy)
Dark red-brown	Fetal death

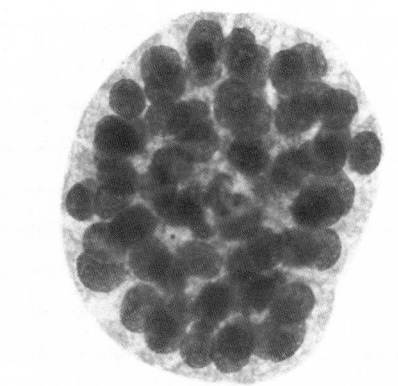

FIGURE 4. *Syncytial knot. These giant cells, rarely seen in amniotic fluid, originate from the placenta.*

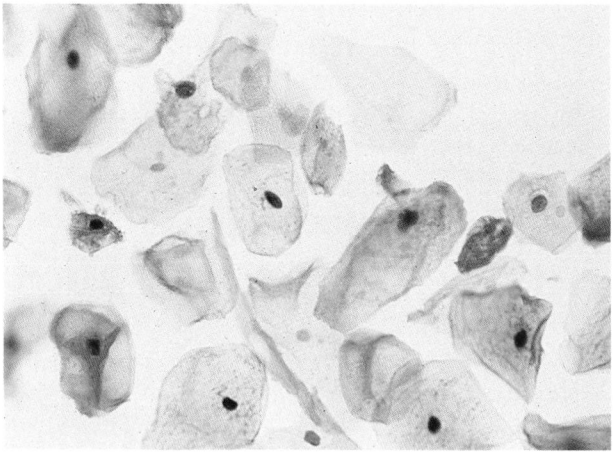

FIGURE 6. *Nile blue dye. Orange-yellow–staining cells are fetal epidermal cells.*

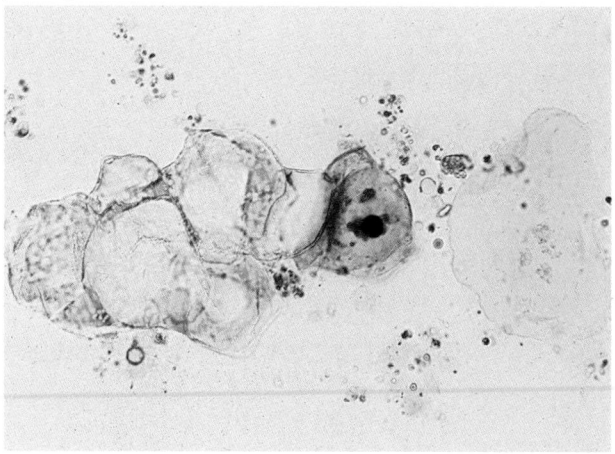

FIGURE 7. *Barr body (X-chromatin), identified as a small condensation of chromatin (arrow) along the nuclear membrane (Papanicolaou's stain).*

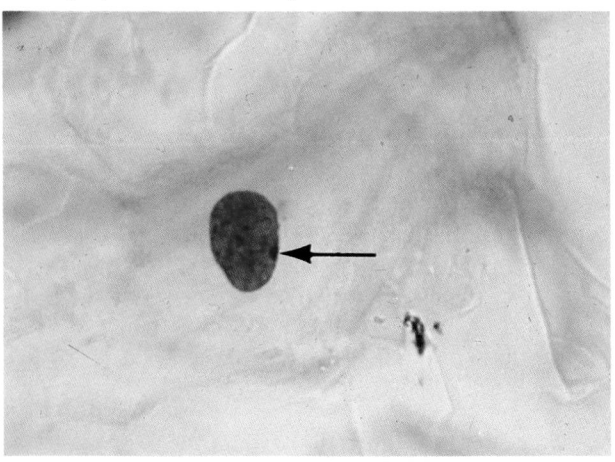

results, however, are inferior when compared with those of other tests, and false-positive results are common. A more reliable method is to identify amniotic fluid cells found in the vagina.[12] Vaginal fluid is obtained by scraping the vaginal wall or aspirating the posterior fornix. A Papanicolaou stain or Nile blue dye can then be used on the specimen. With the Papanicolaou stain, the fetal epidermal cells show a variable staining pattern, with colors ranging from emerald green to orange or pink (Figure 5). In contrast, the vaginal cells are uniformly green or bluish green. With the Nile blue dye, the fetal cells are orange-yellow and the vaginal cells are blue. The timing of cytologic studies depends on the stage of pregnancy, since fetal epidermal cells are not seen in significant numbers until the 36th week.

Cytologic examination, using the Nile blue dye, is a reliable assay for measuring *fetal maturity*, even in cases complicated by such fetal maternal diseases as Rh isoimmunization, hydramnios, or preeclamptic toxemia.[13–15] The Nile blue dye is a metachromatic fat stain (oxane sulfate) that stains neutral fat orange. Fetal epidermal cells stain orange-yellow due to the presence of lipid on the surface of the cells (vernix). The background of epidermal cells stains blue.

The Nile blue test consists of putting one drop of unspun agitated amniotic fluid on a slide and mixing it with one drop of a 0.1% aqueous solution of Nile blue dye. After a coverslip has been applied, the slide is gently heated to 50 °C to 60 °C for one or two minutes. The specimen is then examined with a light microscope under low power and the percentage of orange-yellow–staining cells is calculated (Figure 6). Brosens and Gordon[16] reported that less than 1% of cells stained orange-yellow at earlier than 34 weeks' gestation, while 1% to 10% stained at 34 to 38 weeks, 10% to 50% at 38 to 40 weeks, and more than 50% stained orange-yellow beyond term. Like several of the biochemical tests, Nile blue dye stain has a high predictive value for determining fetal and pulmonary maturity but is less accurate in predicting fetal and pulmonary immaturity.

While the Nile blue test is inexpensive and apparently simple to perform, the type of dye used appears to be very important for a reliable result.[17,18] The Nile blue hydrochloride appears to be preferable to the Nile blue A (sulfate).[18] However, the Food and Drug

Administration recently banned the use of one of the reagents (α-naphthylamine) used to prepare the Nile blue dye. This stain has therefore become very difficult to obtain in the United States, and the procedure has largely been replaced by biochemical tests (to be described).

Cytologic examination may be used as an ancillary method for detecting *neural tube defects*. When the fetus suffers failure of closure of the neural tube (as in anencephaly and spina bifida), the amniotic fluid may contain long bipolar cells, cells with multiple filamentous pseudopodia, and large, vacuolated cells with inclusions.[19–21] It has been noted that these cells adhere to tissue culture dishes within 24 hours of inoculation and resemble glial cells.[20] With a specific immunofluorescence assay, the presence of the glial protein S-100 can be detected.[21] Glial fibrillary acidic protein–specific staining of cytocentrifuged samples of amniotic fluid appears to be a rapid way to detect glial cells in fresh fluid and may aid in the prenatal diagnosis of neural tube defects.[22]

Fetal sex can be determined by calculating the percentage of cells in which the nucleus contains an X-chromatin mass (Barr body) (Figure 7). The latter is a condensation of chromatin along the nuclear membrane and represents one of the two X chromosomes present in female cells. A variety of nuclear stains may be used for the identification of the X-chromatin mass, including hematoxylin-eosin, Papanicolaou, and orcein stains, the Feulgen method, and carbol-fuchsin. One hundred cells with an unwrinkled interphase nucleus are counted, and the percentage of X-chromatin–positive nuclei is determined. An X-chromatin–positive count of greater than 10% indicates a female genotype.[23] When an adequate number of cells is present, an accuracy of greater than 90% can be obtained.

The accuracy can be even greater with the identification of the Y chromosome, which is technically much simpler than identification of the X-chromatin mass. The distal end of the Y chromosome shows a brilliant fluorescence with quinacrine dihydrochloride and is easily identified as a single fluorescent spot between the center and periphery of the nucleus. A male phenotype is determined by a Y-positive count of greater than 50%. In a small percentage of male infants, the Y chromosome may be small or deleted and thus not detectable. It is recommended that the fathers also undergo Y-chromosome determination when X-chromatin–mass and Y-chromosome identification are used for fetal sex determination.[23] When determining fetal sex for genetic counseling purposes, chromosomal karyotyping should be used, along with the procedures just described. Another method used is based on the fact that testosterone concentrations in amniotic fluid are higher with male fetuses than with female fetuses.[24]

CHEMICAL ANALYSIS

As with other body fluids, the chemical makeup of amniotic fluid is complex (Table 1–3), and its composition varies considerably as gestation proceeds. In the very early stages of pregnancy, the composition mimics that of serum. As pregnancy progresses, the concentration of some analytes (protein, sodium, chloride, and bilirubin) decreases, while that of others (creatinine, uric acid, amylase, alkaline phosphatase, and various lipids) progressively increases.

Although studies of the chemical composition of amniotic fluid were first performed about 50 years ago,[25,26] it is only in the last ten years or so that these studies have become widely available for use in clinical diagnosis and management.

Protein

The concentration of amniotic fluid total protein steadily decreases with gestation. Initial studies showed that fluid specimens collected at seven to nine months' gestation had a mean protein concentration of 0.53 g/dL and a range of 0 to 1.5 g/dL.[26] More recent measurements showed a range of about 0.38 to 0.83 g/dL at 28 weeks' gestation and 0.15 to 0.35 g/dL at 38 weeks.[27] Although some variations exist in different reports, these early findings are generally consistent with more recent ones.[28,29] Amniotic fluid albumin concentration also decreases as pregnancy progresses. Reported mean values are 0.4 g/dL during the second trimester and 0.05 g/dL at term.[28]

Fibrinogen is absent in amniotic fluid. Immunoglobulins IgG, IgA, and IgD increase toward midpregnancy and thereafter decrease to term. The immunoglobulin IgM remains relatively constant through

TABLE 1–3. Normal Values for Amniotic Fluid Components

COMPONENT	VALUE	SI UNITS
Appearance	Colorless to pale straw or clear	
Epithelial cells		
Immature	<10% keratinized squames	NA
Equivocal	10%–20% keratinized squames	NA
Mature	>20% keratinized squames	NA
α-Fetoprotein level		
14 weeks	<50 mg/L (mean + 3 SD)	<0.050 g/L
22 weeks	<30 mg/L (mean + 3 SD)	<0.030 g/L
Bilirubin level		
28–30 weeks	Δ A450 < 0.06; < 0.075 mg/dL	<1.28 μmole/L
40 weeks (term)	Δ A450 < 0.02; < 0.025 mg/dL	<0.43 μmole/L
Bilirubin-to-total-protein ratio		
No HDN	<0.35	NA
Moderate HDN	0.35–0.55	NA
Severe HDN	>0.55	NA
Creatinine level		
Immature	<1.5 mg/dL	<132.6 μmole/L
Equivocal	1.5–2.0 mg/dL	132.6–176.8 μmole/L
Mature	>2.0 mg/dL	>176.8 μmole/L
L/S ratio (acetone precipitation)		
Immature	<2.0	NA
Mature	>2.0	NA
Phosphatidylglycerol		
Immature	Absent	NA
Mature	Present	NA
Total protein concentration		
28 weeks	0.38–0.83 g/dL	3.8–8.3 g/L
38 weeks	0.15–0.35 g/dL	1.5–3.5 g/L
Urea nitrogen		
Immature	<25 mg/dL	<8.93 mmole/L
Equivocal	25–30 mg/dL	8.93–10.71 mmole/L
Mature	>30 mg/dL	>10.71 mmole/L
Uric acid level		
Immature	<7.6 mg/dL	<452.05 μmole/L
Mature	>7.6 mg/dL	>452.05 μmole/L

Note: See text for analytes not listed (sodium, potassium, lactate dehydrogenase, etc).

Abbreviations: HDN = hemolytic disease of the newborn, L/S = lecithin/sphingomyelin ratio, NA = not applicable.

the 35th week of gestation but thereafter increases to term.[30] Comparative studies of amniotic fluid and maternal and cord serum samples by disk electrophoresis show that the major protein components of amniotic fluid are IgG, transferrin, postalbumin proteins, and albumin.[31,32]

Nonprotein Nitrogen Compounds

Urea, uric acid, and creatinine concentrations all increase with the progression of gestation, with mean levels at term of about two to three times the corresponding maternal serum values.[28,29,33] Both uric acid and creatinine measurements have predictive value for fetal maturity, as will be discussed in a later section.

Uric acid and urea concentrations are reported to be higher than normal in amniotic fluids of pregnant women with diabetes.[34] However, the maternal serum levels are elevated proportionately, suggesting increased fetal urinary excretion of these compounds, possibly caused by elevated fetal serum values.[34]

Enzymes

A variety of enzymes has been measured in amniotic fluid, including lactate dehydrogenase (LD), aspartate aminotransferase (AST or GOT), alkaline phosphatase (ALP), γ-glutamyltransferase (GGT), creatine kinase (CK), and amylase. To date, their measurements have limited clinical value.

Lactate dehydrogenase activity in amniotic fluid changes little during gestation and is normally a little lower than that in maternal serum.[28,29] However, greatly increased LD values are usually noted in association with fetal death. Aspartate aminotransferase levels increase slightly as pregnancy progresses.[28] This increase may be caused by increased numbers of AST-containing epithelial cells in the fluid as gestation progresses.[28] Amylase levels increase with gestation and have been suggested as a measure of fetal maturity, as will be discussed in a later section.[35]

Creatine kinase activity is higher in maternal serum than in amniotic fluid, the former having a mean value of about twice the latter (86.4 units/L).[29] Creatine kinase–BB is the major isoenzyme in amniotic fluid and is increased in cases of fetal teratoma, gastroschisis, and anencephaly.[36,37] Between the 14th and 36th weeks of gestation there appears to be no relationship between total CK levels and gestational age.[36,37]

An early study of amniotic fluid ALP showed a mean activity at term of about three times the mean value detected during the second trimester.[28] However, the results were found to vary so much during the second and third trimesters that the measurement of ALP has no clinical use. These results may be explained by the observation that the amniotic fluid ALP level initially peaks at about 19 to 21 weeks' gestation, decreases to a nadir at 28 to 30 weeks, and then rapidly rises to its highest point at 39 to 40 weeks.[38] Alkaline phosphatase isoenzyme studies indicate that between 31 weeks' gestation and term, the heat-stable (placental) fraction increases only slightly, while the heat-labile fraction increases sevenfold during the same period.[39]

Both γ-glutamyltransferase and 5'-nucleotidase levels are greatly elevated in amniotic fluid at 13 to 15 weeks' gestation, only to fall rapidly by 25 to 27 weeks. Both remain low throughout the remainder of gestation.[38,40]

Inorganic Ions

Amniotic fluid becomes progressively hypotonic as pregnancy proceeds. This is due primarily to a decrease in sodium and chloride concentrations.[41–43] The mean amniotic fluid sodium level at term is about 125 to 130 mmole/L.[41,43] Potassium levels remain relatively constant throughout pregnancy, averaging 4.0 to 4.5 mmole/L. Amniotic fluid sodium ion concentration is normal in patients with preeclampsia and eclampsia, while potassium levels are lower than in normotensive patients.

A variety of other inorganic substances, including phosphate, bicarbonate, calcium, magnesium, copper, and iron, have all been measured in amniotic fluid.[28,29,33,44] At this point in time, their measurement has no apparent clinical value.

Miscellaneous Biochemical Measurements

A wide variety of other substances have been measured in amniotic fluid, including 5-hydroxyindoleacetic acid, estriol, prostaglandins, bilirubin, squalene, cholesterol, and other lipids. A few of these, especially bilirubin and certain lipids, will be discussed in more detail as they relate to hemolytic disease of the newborn and fetal maturity.

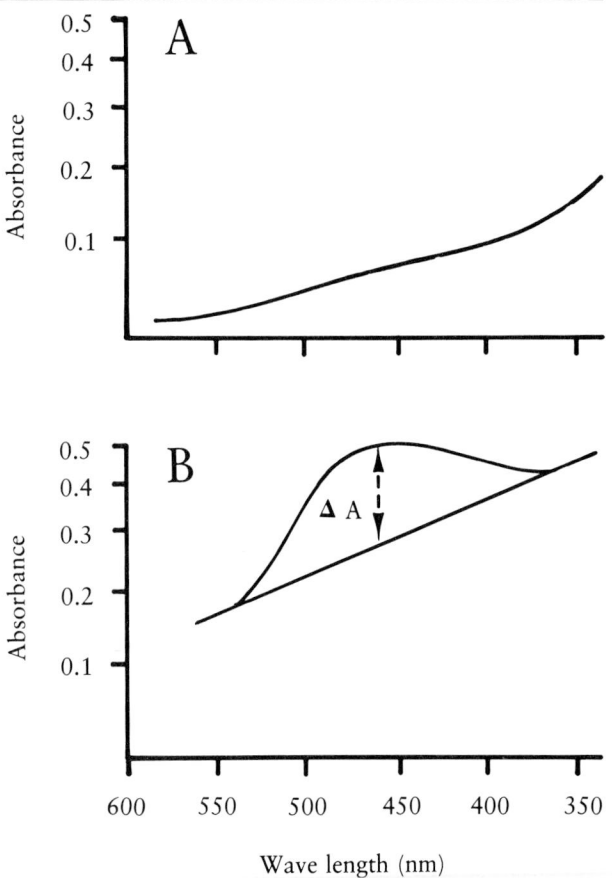

HEMOLYTIC DISEASE OF THE NEWBORN

In erythroblastosis fetalis (hemolytic disease of the newborn, or HDN), the fetus possesses an erythrocyte antigen that the mother lacks. If the antigen gains access to the maternal circulation, antibody production may be stimulated in the mother. Hemolytic disease of the newborn results when these maternal antibodies are returned to the fetus via the placenta, where they interact with fetal RBCs, causing hemolysis.

One of the clinician's challenges in managing the Rh-isoimmunized patient is to predict accurately the degree of fetal involvement so that clinical management is optimal under these difficult conditions. Until the analysis of amniotic fluid became routine, the assessment of the fetal state was based largely on the indirect Coombs' titer of the maternal serum and the outcome of previous pregnancies. However, neither of these methods is reliable.[45] Currently, the most decisive means for evaluating the condition of these fetuses in utero is by periodic examination of the amniotic fluid throughout gestation.

Bevis[46] initially noted that the amniotic fluid from some Rh-sensitized pregnancies was yellow-green. Since this fluid was nonreactive with Fouchet's reagent and van den Bergh's reaction, it was initially assumed that bile pigments were absent.[46] However, it was noted that the measurement of both urobilinogen and nonhematin iron were valuable in predicting HDN.[46,47] Bevis[48,49] later showed that by estimating the bilirubin and oxyhemoglobin content of amniotic fluid, either spectrophotometrically or biochemically, it was possible to detect those cases in which kernicterus was likely to develop.

Several years later, Liley[50,51] correlated the clinical course of the disease with *spectral absorption curves* of the amniotic fluid and showed that this technique was a highly reliable guide in predicting the outcome of the involved pregnancy. The concentration of bilirubin-like pigments in amniotic fluid decreases with the progression of normal pregnancies. Thus, when the absorbance of normal amniotic fluid at term is measured continuously at 350 to 650 nm, the curve is essentially a straight line. However, bilirubin absorbs maximally at 450 nm, thereby producing increased absorbance (A) at this wavelength when present (Figure 8). As normal gestation progresses, the net absorbance at 450 nm (ΔA_{450}) decreases. Thus, in a normal or minimally affected fetus with HDN, the ΔA_{450} is less than 0.06 at 28 weeks and less than 0.02 at 40 weeks.

Liley[51] found that when the ΔA_{450} is plotted against gestational age on a semilogarithmic graph, three zones can be delineated, from which the severity of the fetal hemolytic disease can be predicted (Figure 9). The lower zone (C) includes unaffected or only mildly affected fetuses. If the absorbance value is within this zone, the fetus is usually delivered at term. The central zone (B) absorbance values are associated with a moderate degree of hemolytic anemia. These fetuses are candidates for elective premature delivery, usually at 35 to 38 weeks' gestation. The upper zone (A) represents levels usually associated with severe hemolytic disease; fetuses in this category usually die. However, they are usually candidates for fetal blood transfusion and, if the transfusion is successful, eventual elective delivery by cesarean section.

Several other measurements have been suggested in an attempt to improve the in utero diagnostic accuracy in HDN. Amniotic fluid total protein concentration normally decreases steadily between 28 and 40 weeks' gestation; hydropic fetuses, however, usually have higher-than-normal amniotic fluid total protein levels.[29,52,53] Of possible greater diagnostic value is the *bilirubin-to-protein ratio*.[29,52] When appropriately calculated, ratios of less than 0.35 suggest mild to no disease and ratios of 0.35 to 0.55 suggest moderate involvement; ratios greater than 0.55 indicate severe disease.[29,52]

Many attempts, beginning with that of Bevis,[46] have also been made to relate the bilirubin concentration in amniotic fluid to the severity of hemolytic disease. The major problems with these investigations, however, involved the technical difficulties of accurately measuring the low bilirubin levels present in amniotic fluid, along with the clinical difficulty of determining exact gestational age when bilirubin concentrations were measured. Yet when carefully performed, a reliable correlation can be drawn between the chemically measured bilirubin (in milligrams per deciliter) and bilirubin absorbance measured by the ΔA_{450} method.[54,55] However, the advantages of the ΔA_{450} method include (1) the extensive experience and confidence of most physicians with the technique; (2) the high

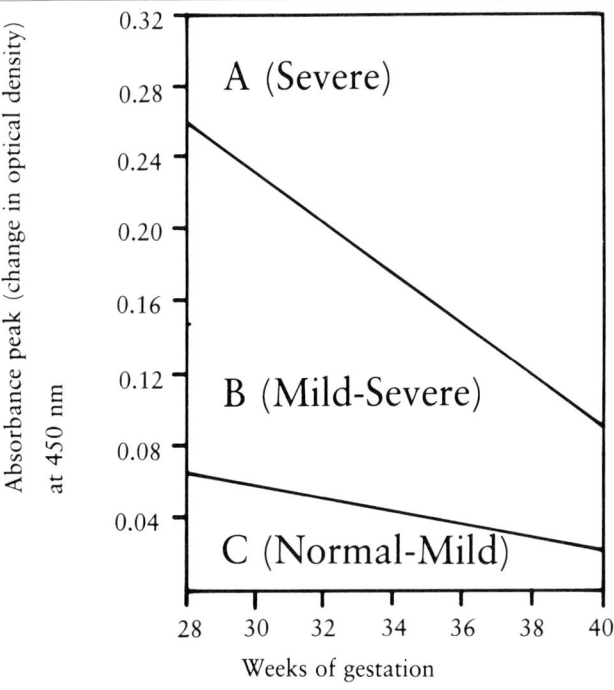

FIGURE 9. *Hemolytic disease of the newborn—prediction of severity. Zones (A, B, and C) indicate varying severity of disease when ΔA_{450} is plotted against gestational age.*

sensitivity of spectral measurement at 450 nm in measuring very small amounts of pigment; and (3) the lesser sensitivity and precision of chemical methods in measuring bilirubin at very low concentrations (less than 0.1 to 0.2 mg/dL). The technique for the measurement of the ΔA_{450} scan of amniotic fluid is described in detail elsewhere.[55]

It is important to recognize that there are several potential sources of error in the estimation of amniotic fluid bilirubin levels, regardless of the method employed. They include the following: (1) bilirubin light sensitivity: false low values may be reported if the amniotic fluid is either not analyzed immediately or not protected from light; (2) contamination with maternal blood: the specimen should be centrifuged immediately to remove any erythrocytes present; (3) fetal blood contamination: this causes significant bilirubin elevation since serum levels exceed amniotic fluid values by a factor of 10 to 100; (4) meconium-contaminated fluid: this adds to the absorbance at 450 nm and thereby elevates the reported bilirubin value; (5) polyhydramnios: this decreases the bilirubin level by dilution, giving a falsely low value; (6) elevated amniotic fluid bilirubin levels: they will be present if the mother is hyperbilirubinemic (eg, maternal hepatitis and sickle cell disease); and (7) the occasional drawing of maternal urine rather than amniotic fluid for submission to the laboratory; this is best prevented by having the mother empty her bladder before amniocentesis.

ESTIMATION OF FETAL MATURITY, GESTATIONAL AGE, AND PULMONARY MATURITY

Erythroblastosis fetalis, toxemia of pregnancy, maternal diabetes, and a growing list of other conditions that may complicate pregnancy, delivery, or both are indications for delivery before term. However, unless the fetus can be expected to do better outside the uterus, there is little to justify early elective delivery. Unexpected prematurity is the major factor in perinatal mortality after elective induction of labor. Therefore, accurate assessment of the maturity of the unborn fetus is essential. Serious errors can be made if the gestational age is estimated on the basis of calculation and palpation alone. Amniotic fluid tests for

fetal maturity are indicated (1) before induction of labor for abnormal pregnancy states, (2) in the differential diagnosis of prematurity vs dysmaturity, and (3) before elective cesarean section or induction when gestational age is in doubt.

Tests for Estimating Overall Maturity

There is no one test available to assess all aspects of maturity, and no single test is 100% reliable. Therefore, a combination of clinical and laboratory studies should be used. Most fetal maturity tests have been related to pulmonary maturity. In a preterm situation, the best time to deliver is usually decided on the basis of fetal pulmonary maturity. There may be a discrepancy, however, between the state of maturity of fetal lungs and that of other tissues. Thus a functionally immature infant may have mature lungs.

Of the many tests described, the most reliable methods for assessing fetal maturity appear to be cytologic examination with Nile blue dye, determination of the creatinine concentration and the lecithin/sphingomyelin (L/S) ratio, and testing for the presence of phosphatidylglycerol. Determination of the L/S ratio was introduced primarily as a test for pulmonary maturity but is also valuable in assessing overall fetal maturity. The cytologic test, as mentioned earlier, is now seldom used in the United States.

The fetal renal contribution to amniotic fluid is particularly evident in the latter half of pregnancy, when the fetal urine excretion significantly adds to the composition and volume of amniotic fluid. It has been shown that the creatinine concentration remains relatively constant at about 1.0 to 1.5 mg/dL from the 20th to the 34th week of gestation. At 34 weeks, however, it begins to rise sharply so that at 37 weeks, levels measure 2 mg/dL or higher, signifying fetal maturity.[56] Although far from ideal, this measurement, often combined with the cytologic test, was extremely helpful during the earlier days of amniotic fluid analysis and still has some value when used in conjunction with the more specific analyses. Low creatinine values at term, in the presence of a mature L/S ratio, may indicate fetal malformations.

Uric acid is also present in amniotic fluid, arriving primarily via the renal route. It increases in concentration with pregnancy and has been shown to correlate with fetal maturity. However, its concentration is more variable than that of creatinine. In general, mature fetuses have amniotic fluid uric acid concentrations in excess of 7.7 mg/dL.[28,57]

The activity of several *enzymes* in amniotic fluid has been proposed as an aid in establishing fetal maturity. Amylase determination has been recommended as a reliable screening test for maturity.[58] In a study by De Grandi et al,[58] when the amniotic fluid amylase activity exceeded 300 units/L, the L/S ratio was greater than 2.0 in 94% of cases; when it was less than 200 units/L, the L/S ratio was less than 2.0 in 85% of cases.[58] There was no consistent correlation between the L/S ratio and amylase activity when the latter was 200 to 300 units/L.[58] Determination of an L/S ratio was necessary only when the amylase activity was in the equivocal range (200 to 300 units/L). More recent studies, however, indicate that amniotic fluid amylase levels may not be reliably used as a screening test for deciding the need for an L/S ratio determination.

Alkaline phosphatase activity, according to one study,[38] follows a biphasic pattern, peaking at about 16 to 18 weeks, falling to a low at 28 to 30 weeks, and then rising to a second peak at term. This study suggested that a total alkaline phosphatase measurement of 0.36 kat/L (21.6 units/L) or greater at 30 °C, or an alkaline phosphatase–to–γ-glutamyltransferase ratio greater than 2.0, indicates pulmonary maturity. It was concluded in the study that any fluid with obvious meconium contamination cannot be evaluated for alkaline phosphatase, since meconium is rich in this enzyme.

Ultrasonography provides an additional tool in assessing gestational age. In fetuses at high risk for the development of respiratory distress syndrome (RDS), it may be useful to confirm gestational age by ultrasonic cephalometry.

Tests for Estimating Pulmonary Maturity

The major problem with preterm delivery is the possibility of fetal immaturity, especially lung immaturity. Respiratory distress syndrome (hyaline membrane disease) is currently responsible for approximately one third of all neonatal deaths (about 25,000) in this country each year, making it the single most common cause of death in the newborn. In addition, the need in many cases for a timely interrup-

tion of pregnancy—as soon as fetal lungs are mature—has prompted the investigation of numerous methods to assess pulmonary maturity.

During expiration, pulmonary alveoli decrease in diameter. According to the law of Laplace ($P = 2T/R$, where P is the distending pressure across a curved gas-liquid interface, T is the wall tension, and R is the radius), the decreased alveolar radius causes an increased tension of the alveolar wall. Unless this increased alveolar surface tension is negated, the alveoli will collapse, resulting in pulmonary atelectasis. In the normally functioning lung, the type II alveolar pneumocyte synthesizes and secretes lipid compounds ("surfactant") that act as surface-active agents (biologic detergents), thereby lowering surface tension and preventing alveolar collapse during expiration. The surfactant is stored in lamellar bodies (symmetric layers of protein and lipid) within the alveolar pneumocyte. Premature infants who cannot synthesize adequate quantities of surfactant develop RDS and frequently die. At autopsy, those who died within a few hours after birth are found to have pulmonary atelectasis, while those who lived for several hours usually are found to have pulmonary hyaline membranes (Figure 10).

Analysis of pulmonary surfactant shows that it is composed primarily of the phospholipid dipalmitoyl lecithin (phosphatidylcholine). Two major biosynthetic pathways of lecithin have been shown to exist and are summarized in Table 1–4[60].

Pulmonary lecithin production increases with gestation and is manifested by the increasing concentration of lecithin in amniotic fluid. In 1971, Gluck et al[61] made the significant observation that the amniotic fluid concentrations of the phospholipids sphingomyelin and lecithin are essentially equal to each other from 18 to 33 weeks' gestation, at which time the sphingomyelin concentration slowly decreases and the lecithin concentration abruptly increases. At 35 to 36 weeks' gestation, the *lecithin-to-sphingomyelin (L/S) ratio* is 2.0 or greater, signifying fetal lung maturity (Figure 11). The measurement of the L/S ratio as developed by Gluck et al[61] involves thin-layer chromatography of amniotic fluid that has been extracted with methanol and chloroform and then precipitated with cold acetone. The ratio is then interpreted by visual estimation, planimetry, or densitometry. It is

FIGURE 10. *Hyaline membrane disease. Histologic section of lung showing air spaces lined by pink hyaline membranes with adjacent atelectasis (hematoxylin-eosin stain).*

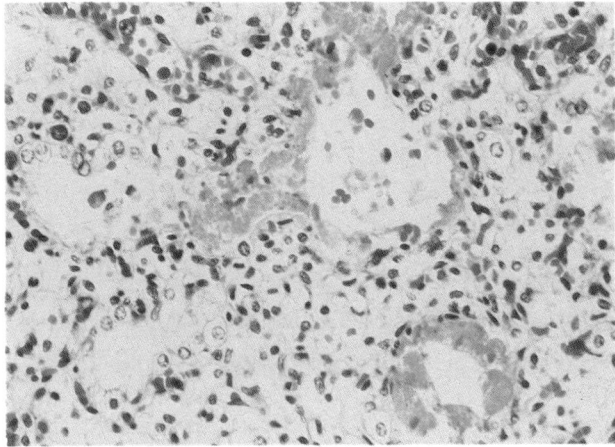

TABLE 1–4. Two Major Biosynthetic Pathways of Lecithin

1. Choline incorporation pathway (phosphocholine transferase reaction):

   Cytidine diphosphate choline (CDP-choline)
   $+ \alpha,\beta$-diglycerides $\rightarrow$ lecithin

2. Methylation pathway (methyl transferase reaction):

   Phosphatidylethanolamine $+ 3$ CH$_3$* $\rightarrow$ lecithin

*Methyl groups derived from S-adenosyl-L-methionine.

considered the standard against which all other methods are compared. In this regard, it should be emphasized that Gluck's original method involves an acetone precipitation step, a variation often lacking in more recent methodologies.[62] As a result, the L/S ratio calculated by different techniques may not be comparable.[63]

When the L/S ratio is greater than 2.0, RDS will not occur in 95% of cases. However, the value of a low L/S ratio (L/S < 2.0) in predicting an immature fetus is not as good.[64] With an L/S ratio of 1.0, there is an 85% to 90% certainty that RDS will develop in the newborn. However, with L/S ratios of 1.5 to 2.0, RDS may only occur 60% to 70% of the time.[64] It should be noted that the presence of meconium or blood in the fluid interferes with the test, making it unreliable.

More recent studies have shown the presence of other phospholipids in amniotic fluid,[65] including phosphatidylglycerol (PG), phosphatidylinositol, phosphatidylethanolamine, and phosphatidylserine. Phosphatidylglycerol measurement has been shown to be a particularly useful adjunct to the determination of the L/S ratio in the assessment of fetal lung maturity. Phosphatidylglycerol is normally undetectable in amniotic fluid before about 35 weeks' gestation, at which time it appears and rapidly increases to make up about 10% of the total lipid content at term. Its mere presence signifies maturity with a high degree of reliability. When reported routinely with the L/S ratio, the accuracy of prediction is significantly enhanced.[65] The PG level and L/S ratio can be determined simultaneously (a "lung profile") using two-dimensional thin-layer chromatography.[66–68]

Phosphatidylglycerol measurement has the added advantage of not being affected by the presence of blood or meconium, and it may eliminate the confusion caused by a false mature L/S ratio in diabetic pregnancies.[69,70] In maternal diabetes and possibly in other complicated pregnancies where the L/S ratio may be greater than 2.0, RDS still might develop in the infant. Phosphatidylglycerol is often absent in these cases,[71] however, suggesting that the L/S ratio greater than 2.0 may represent inadequate surfactant activity. On the other hand, in a diabetic pregnancy of any class, the infant can safely be delivered free of

RDS after PG is detected.[71,72] Phosphatidylglycerol may also be useful in identifying other respiratory dysfunctions such as transient tachypnea, symptomatic pneumothorax, and persistence of fetal circulation.[73]

In addition to the "classic" L/S ratio determination and PG measurement as determined by thin-layer chromatography, several other techniques that measure phospholipids directly or indirectly have been suggested. One of the first to be proposed is the relatively rapid and simple "foam" or "shake" test, which approximates the *total surfactant concentration*.[74] In this test, amniotic fluid is diluted with 95% alcohol, shaken for 15 seconds, left undisturbed for 15 minutes, and observed for foam stability. If there is a continuum of bubbles around the circumference of the liquid surface, the fetus is considered to be mature; if not, it is immature. As initially performed, the test presented numerous problems, and false-negative results were reported in up to 40%.[75] More recently, following methodologic changes, the test has been reported to compare more favorably with the standard L/S ratio determination.[76-78] The test is now available in a commercial kit. Although some investigators[79,80] have found it to be quite reliable, our evaluation[81] of this method is less favorable. We recommend that this method only be used as a screening test in those institutions that do not have access to the more standard techniques.

A variety of other tests have been suggested, including fluorescence polarization,[82] enzymatic assays for lecithin[83] and other phospholipids,[84] tests for lamellar body phospholipid content,[85,86] specific methods for measuring disaturated phosphatidylcholine,[87] and absorbance readings at 650 nm.[79] Of these, fluorescence polarization has received the most attention.[89-93]

The physical basis of *fluorescence polarization* stems from the empirically observed relationship between viscosity and the surface tension of fluids. These physical properties are both determined by the intermolecular forces of the fluid, so that the surface tension of the pulmonary surfactant can be translated into intrinsic viscosity, which may be expressed in terms of "microviscosity."[82] The microviscosity, as measured by the fluorescence polarization of 1,6-diphenyl-1,3,5-hexatriene (DPH), is an excellent in-

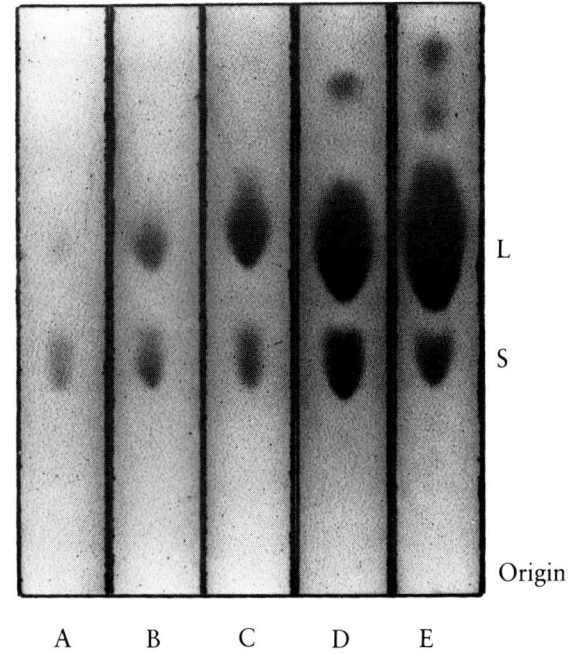

FIGURE 11. *Estimation of pulmonary maturity. Varying lecithin/sphingomyelin (L/S) ratios are shown in this thin-layer chromatographic scan of amniotic fluid. A, 0.4; B, 1.0; C, 2.5; D, 3.5; and E, 5.0.*

dicator of the relative amounts of lecithin and sphingomyelin in lipid-prepared dispersions. The major disadvantage of this technique is that it requires an expensive specialized instrument.

Recently, a rapid, technically simple, semiquantitative immunologic *slide agglutination assay for PG* has been developed.[93] The initial clinical data suggest that this test may serve as a screening procedure for fetal lung maturity in laboratories where L/S ratio determination and PG measurement are not readily available. This test is now commercially available in kit form (Amniostat-FLM, Hana Biologics, Inc). Our studies, however, indicate that the slide agglutination assay is considerably less sensitive than either the L/S ratio determination or PG measurement as determined by thin-layer chromatography.[94] When the test result is clearly positive, it appears to be a reliable indicator of fetal lung maturity. On the other hand, a negative value does not necessarily indicate immaturity. Hence all negative results given by this test should be rechecked by the standard tests for L/S ratio and PG measurement.

The subject of amniotic fluid surfactant measurements and fetal maturity has been recently reviewed.[95,96]

It has been known for several years that *cortisol* plays an important role in fetal lung maturation. In one study that used a specific assay for unconjugated cortisol, it was shown that, after an initial rise in amniotic fluid cortisol at about 20 weeks' gestation, there is a plateau until about 35 weeks, followed by a rapid rise, particularly in the two weeks immediately before the onset of labor.[97] Although there is a positive relationship between the progress of gestation and amniotic fluid cortisol levels, the latter apparently cannot be used with confidence to predict lung maturity.[98] More recent studies have shown a high correlation between fetal maturity and amniotic fluid activated partial thromboplastin time[99] and catecholamine level.[100]

Although numerous tests are available to evaluate fetal lung maturity, simultaneous L/S ratio determination and PG measurement, as performed by thin-layer chromatography, are the current reference methods and are the procedures of choice whenever possible.

OTHER CLINICAL CONDITIONS

Although the examination of amniotic fluid is not the primary method for diagnosing the following conditions, the measurement of certain substances in the amniotic fluid may be very useful.

Intrauterine Growth Retardation

When the diagnosis of intrauterine growth retardation (IUGR) is secure, based on confirmed dates and serial ultrasound examinations, determination of fetal lung maturity is helpful in deciding the time of delivery. If growth retardation is not severe and fetal signs are normal, delivery may be safely delayed until the test results indicate "maturity." Since pulmonary maturity in these cases is often accelerated, a mature L/S ratio and the presence of PG may be seen as early as at 35 weeks' gestation—or even one to two weeks earlier if retardation is severe.

The minimum clinical criteria necessary for the inclusion of a newborn in the dysmature or small-for-gestational-age group are (1) evidence of decreased subcutaneous fat, (2) inappropriate weight for length, (3) morphologic evidence of placental insufficiency, and (4) meconium staining of amniotic fluid, membranes, and the umbilical cord.[101] The prenatal diagnosis of this condition may be difficult, especially if the fetus is not in any apparent distress. The physician, knowing the date of the last menstrual period, may suspect IUGR on the basis of fetal size, position, or movement. At the time IUGR is suspected, the examination of amniotic fluid may show meconium staining (greenish grey fluid), suggesting chronic fetal hypoxia. The presence of meconium in the amniotic fluid in the face of apparent IUGR may be an indication for early elective delivery, providing the tests for lung maturity are supportive.

If the fetus is subject to caloric deficiency because of placental dysfunction, it might be expected to use its fat stores, with consequent hyperlipidemia and hyperketonemia. In such situations, the concentration of amniotic fluid β-hydroxybutyrate will be elevated and predictive of a dysmature fetus,[102] with the β-hydroxybutyrate levels exceeding 0.5 mmole/L.[102] Values below this level should indicate a normal infant. More recent studies have suggested that the measurement of amniotic fluid catecholamines, their metabolites, or both could be used in assessing IUGR.

The metabolites that appear to be particularly useful are 4-hydroxy-3-methoxyphenylglycol (MHPG) or the MHPG/VMA (vanillylmandelic acid) ratio,[103] and 3,4-dihydroxyphenylglycol.[104]

Acute Fetal Distress

The measurement of amniotic fluid pH and other acid-base quantities has been studied in cases of both acute and chronic intrauterine hypoxia.[105] However, these determinations are not considered clinically useful. Currently, the evaluation of acute fetal distress relies on the external monitoring of heart rate (using the non-stress test and contraction stress test). Nevertheless, laboratory examinations are useful in some cases.

In addition to the studies used to diagnose hemolytic disease of the newborn, the examination of both maternal serum and urine for estriol (or total estrogens, since estriol makes up about 90% of the total) may be of value in detecting fetal distress. Although only rarely measured, the amniotic fluid estriol concentration has been shown to correlate well with maternal urinary estriol as an indicator of acute fetal distress.[106] More recent studies, however, have indicated that amniotic fluid estriol concentration is a poor reflection of fetal condition in IUGR pregnancies.[107]

Fetal Death

In utero fetal death may, at times, be difficult to diagnose. The usual indicators include (1) absence of fetal movement, (2) absence of fetal heart sounds and a "flat" fetal ECG, (3) various roentgenographic signs, and (4) pertinent results of Doppler ultrasound testing. However, as errors may occur with all of these indicators, a relatively simple and reliable laboratory technique is needed as an adjunct to them. Currently, the most sensitive and specific technique for diagnosing fetal death is real-time ultrasonography. This technique is not available in all hospitals, however. A second technique, the measurement of amniotic fluid creatine kinase (CK) levels, has been suggested as a reliable way to diagnose fetal death.[108] In a study analyzing 91 normal amniotic fluid samples, the CK activity was 0 to 3 Sigma units/mL. In samples from 17 cases of fetal death, however, the amniotic fluid CK activity varied from 5,000 to 9,800 Sigma units/mL;

in most, the CK activity was in excess of 200 Sigma units/mL.

Postdates Pregnancy

The decision whether to deliver an infant if a pregnancy has lasted more than 42 weeks is based on many factors, including fetal heart-rate testing (non-stress test and contraction stress test), the condition of the cervix, and amniotic fluid maturity studies. Although testing for surfactant activity may prevent premature delivery up to the 37th week of gestation, it is impossible to discriminate between 38 and 42 weeks' gestation. Under these circumstances, the measurement of amniotic fluid creatinine levels and a cytologic evaluation may be quite helpful. A creatinine level higher than 2.5 mg/dL and a keratinized squamous cell count ("orange" cells) higher than 50% indicate that the patient is beyond term.

It has been recently reported that levels of *squalene*, a hydrocarbon originating in fetal sebaceous glands, markedly increase in the amniotic fluid when pregnancy reaches 39 to 40 weeks' gestation.[109] The squalene-to-cholesterol ratio progressively increases near and after term. These findings have been recently verified[110]: the ratio before the 40th week is 0.40; at the 40th week and later, the ratio exceeds 0.40. Moreover, in the few cases exceeding 42 weeks where fluid was available for study, the squalene-to-cholesterol ratio was greater than 1.0.[110] Although contamination of amniotic fluid does not affect this ratio, meconium staining lowered it, as it (meconium) is rich in cholesterol.[110] Therefore, meconium staining leads to false-negative results.

Neural Tube Defects

A defect in the closure of the embryonic neural tube (anencephaly, exencephaly, encephalocele, meningocele, or meningomyelocele) occurs in approximately one of every 500 live-born infants in the United States. A married couple who has previously had a child with a neural tube defect (NTD) has a 10- to 20-fold increase in risk for having another similarly affected child.

In 1972, Brock and Sutcliffe[111] first noted the association of an elevated amniotic fluid α-*fetoprotein* (AFP) level with an open leaking NTD. Since that time, extensive experience has confirmed that the

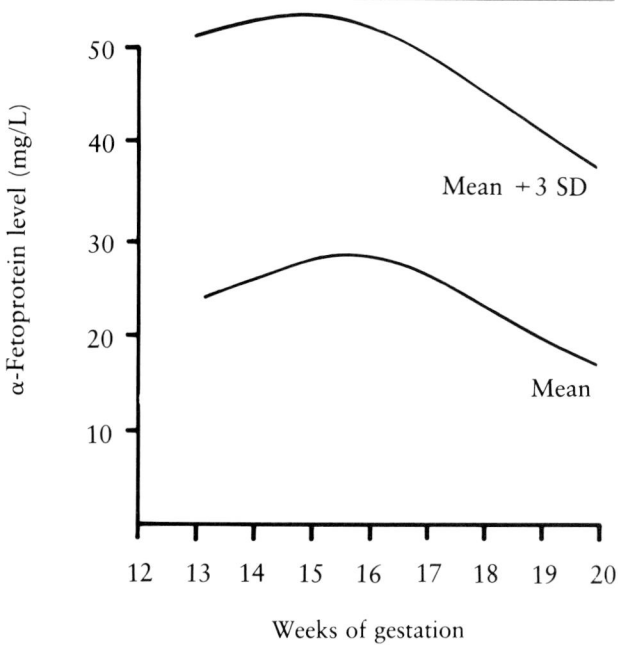

FIGURE 12. *α-Fetoprotein levels in amniotic fluid during gestation. (From Johansson et al.[116] Used by permission.)*

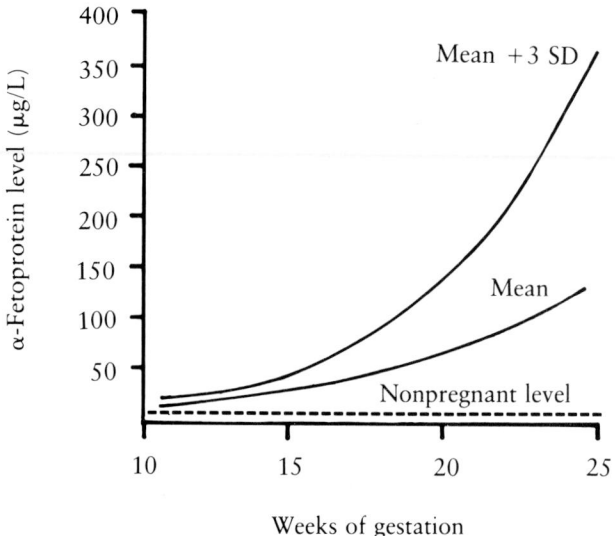

FIGURE 13. *α-Fetoprotein levels in maternal serum during gestation. (From Johansson, et al.[116] Used by permission.)*

measurement of AFP in amniotic fluid is an extremely valuable and efficient tool in the prenatal detection of NTDs.[112] The measurement of amniotic fluid AFP should be suggested to any woman who has previously had a child with an NTD, to any woman who is or whose mate is the survivor of an NTD, and to siblings of the parents of an affected child.[113] An extensive US study on NTDs was recently published that involved 20,000 pregnancies.[112] The false-positive rate for this test was well below 1% (0.06%), mainly because the amniotic fluid was contaminated with fetal blood (fetal serum concentrations average 100 to 150 times the amniotic fluid level).[112] A larger study from the United Kingdom reported a false-positive rate of 0.3%.[114] The sensitivity of AFP testing was 98% (2% false-negative). Definitive action, however, should never be taken on the basis of a single elevated amniotic fluid AFP measurement.[115] Elevated levels of AFP should be confirmed by repeated amniocentesis, ultrasound testing, and possibly other diagnostic procedures such as measurement of amniotic fluid acetylcholinesterase activity.

α-Fetoprotein is a glycoprotein (64,000 daltons) that is first synthesized in the embryonic yolk sac and later in the fetal liver. It begins to appear in the fetal serum by the sixth week of gestation and peaks between 12 and 15 weeks at a mean level of 300 mg/L (3.0 g/L), after which it rapidly declines to term (10 to 150 mg/L).[115] It is thought to escape from the fetal circulation into the surrounding compartments (to maternal circulation via the placenta and into the amniotic fluid from the fetal urine). The peak amniotic fluid level at 14 to 15 weeks (mean +3 SD) is about 50 to 52 mg/L. This upper reference level drops rapidly to about 30 mg/L (mean +3 SD) at 20 weeks (Figure 12).[116]

Because fetal AFP enters the mother's circulation, maternal serum may also be used to screen for fetal NTDs, although measurements of *serum AFP* are much less reliable than those of amniotic fluid AFP. This is due primarily to a wide serum reference interval (upper limit, 43.2 μg/L at 14 weeks, mean +3 SDs; upper limit, 141 μg/L at 20 weeks, mean +3 SD)[116] and the occasional fetomaternal transfusion (Figure 13). The maternal serum levels are also elevated in twinning. The optimal time for maternal AFP testing is from 14 to 18 weeks. Amniotic fluid and maternal serum levels of AFP may be prominently elevated in several other types of fetal maldevelopment, including congenital nephrosis, omphalocele, duodenal and esophageal atresia, hemolytic disease of the newborn secondary to Rh isoimmunization, and hydrocephalus.[117] There is also evidence that raised maternal serum AFP levels in the absence of a fetal NTD are associated with a higher perinatal morbidity and mortality and a high risk of low birth weight.[118] High levels are also seen in cases of intrauterine death.

α-Fetoprotein in amniotic fluid may be reliably measured using either radial immunodiffusion[119] or rocket immunoelectrophoresis.[120] Serum AFP must be measured by a sensitive radioimmunoassay technique.[121] However, the utility of routine assays continues to be basically limited by the lack of readily available standard reference material.[122]

The measurement of the enzyme *acetylcholinesterase* (AChE) is a useful adjunct to AFP measurement for the detection of NTDs.[123] Acetylcholinesterase is considered to be fetospecific and to originate in the brain or spinal cord. Several reports have substantiated the high correlation between AChE and AFP levels in NTD detection.[124–130] In addition, there is considerable advantage in AChE measurement since it is not affected by the presence of fetal blood and is less dependent on fetal age. In a recent report, 200 pregnancies were selected for study because of known fetal abnormalities or difficulties in prenatal diagnosis.[125] High AFP and AChE levels were detected in all 66 cases of open NTDs. Correct reclassification was possible in 89% of normal pregnancies with spuriously elevated AFP but normal AChE levels. In nine of these difficult cases, both AFP and AChE levels were elevated despite a normal outcome.

In most studies, AChE activity has been determined qualitatively by polyacrylamide gel electrophoresis. In normal pregnancies, the electrophoretic pattern shows the presence of a single band of nonspecific cholinesterase. In affected fetuses there are two bands, nonspecific cholinesterase and AChE. Several studies have reported using spectrophotometric assays for measurement of total cholinesterase activity[126] and AChE activity after chemical inhibition of nonspecific cholinesterase,[127,128] or immunoassay for measurement of AChE.[129] All have shown good correlation with AFP measurement in prenatal NTD detection. Qualitative gel electrophoresis is the current method of choice, primarily because there has been extensive experience with it. The measurement of amniotic fluid AChE should be used as an adjunct to AFP measurement. It is especially useful in difficult cases and in those in which the presence of fetal blood might affect AFP measurement.

A recent study compared five biochemical tests that have been proposed as adjuncts to the measurement of amniotic fluid AFP, namely, the measurement of the AFP component that is nonreactive with concanavalin A, the measurements of AChE activity, total cholinesterase activity, and α_2-macroglobulin, and the electrophoretic identification of AChE.[130] Measurement of the AFP component that is nonreactive with concanavalin A was considered ineffective in differentiating between normal and abnormal fetuses. The other four measurements, however, were all considered effective in differentiating normal fetuses from those with NTDs. Measurement of total cholinesterase activity was particularly effective in differentiating between the two fetus groups and can be done rapidly. On the other hand, identification of AChE by electrophoresis was considered to be the most specific test and that least affected by blood contamination. It should be emphasized that, as with AFP, elevation of acetylcholinesterase levels is not specific for NTD and has been seen in omphalocele, extrophy of the cloaca, fetal death, Turner's syndrome, and fetus papyraceous.

PRENATAL DIAGNOSIS OF GENETIC DISORDERS

The prenatal detection of genetic disorders by the examination of amniotic fluid during the second trimester of pregnancy has added a new dimension to genetic counseling. However, the highly specialized resources needed to analyze amniotic fluid appropriately in these complex cases limit these services to the high-risk population.[131] In addition, very few medical centers are able to analyze the fluid fully for all diagnostic possibilities. It should be kept in mind that chromosomal disorders and inborn errors of metabolism are quite rare. The indications for prenatal genetic studies can be grouped into four categories of sus-

TABLE **1–5**. Indications for Prenatal Chromosome Studies

In Mother
    Aged 35 years or older
    History of three or more spontaneous abortions
    High amniotic fluid α-fetoprotein value

In Either Parent
    Chromosome abnormality
    Previous child with a chromosome abnormality, multiple
        congenital malformations, or neural tube defect
    Identification as a carrier of an X-linked disorder
    Family history of Down's syndrome

pected abnormalities: (1) chromosomal disorders, (2) sex-linked disorders, (3) inherited metabolic disorders, and (4) congenital malformations (Table 1–5).

Amniocentesis should be performed in the 14th week of gestation (abortion should be considered, if at all, before the 20th week). A sonogram should be done routinely, immediately before the procedure, to assess fetal and placental status and gestational age. Twelve to 24 mL of fluid is extracted for cell and fluid analysis and placed in sterile tubes. Fluid must be sampled from each amniotic cavity if multiple pregnancies are present. The cells are karyotyped using the Giemsa banding method, and biochemical assays can be performed on the supernatant fluid. Approximately 24 days are required for karyotyping and 35 days for the biochemical assays on cultured cells. As described in the next section, some biochemical determinations can be performed directly on the fluid. Occasionally the cells fail to grow and another amniocentesis is necessary. Discolored (usually greenish brown) amniotic fluid is not diagnostic of fetal abnormalities but warrants further investigation. The discoloration is caused by aged blood pigments.[132] Amniotic fluid specimens can be successfully sent by mail to centers specializing in the diagnosis of prenatal genetic disorders.[133]

Chromosomal Disorders

The largest group that should be tested is composed of those at risk for chromosomal abnormalities (Table 1–6). Approximately 4,000 new cases of Down's syndrome are diagnosed in this country each year, and about half of these occur in fetuses of mothers older than 35 years. More specifically, data from several sources suggest that the risk of having chromosomally defective offspring is 2.2% for women aged 35 to 39 years. This increases to 3.4% for women aged 40 years and rises sharply to about 10% at age 45 years.[134]

Next to maternal age, the identification of a parent as a carrier of chromosomal translocation is the second most appropriate indication for chromosomal study of amniotic fluid. The risk of a chromosome disorder occurring in each offspring approaches 9% if the mother is such a carrier and is about 4% when the father is the carrier.[134] The third major indication for chromosomal study is a woman having previously given birth to a child with Down's syndrome (trisomy 21). The risk for recurrence in women younger than 35 years is about 1% to 2%.[134]

Sex-Linked Disorders

The ability to determine fetal sex by the presence of nuclear chromatin bodies in amniotic fluid cells was described previously. This technique, and the more recent and specific chromosomal analysis, has practical application for the identification of male fetuses in women who are known carriers of X-linked recessive disorders, such as hemophilia, Hunter's syndrome, and muscular dystrophy.

Recent advances in ultrasound imagery permit sex determination during the second trimester.[135] This method has the advantage of being inexpensive, quick, and noninvasive. Sex can also be determined in the first trimester with karyotyping through chorionic biopsy. The latter is, however, still an unsafe procedure, with a 12% rate of fetal loss.[136]

Male fetuses born to mothers who are carriers of X-linked recessive disorders have a 50% probability of disease expression. Of the sex-linked disorders, however, only Hunter's syndrome, Menkes' syndrome, Fabry's disease, and the Lesch-Nyhan syndrome can be specifically diagnosed by amniotic fluid analysis. Sex prediction is the only current option left for the approximately 150 remaining sex-linked disorders, which are particularly difficult to manage. Selective abortion may be indicated with fetuses in this category, provided the carrier status of the mother is known. Abortion is only a partially adequate solution,

TABLE 1-6. Chromosomal Abnormalities Detectable Prenatally

SYNDROME	ABNORMALITY	INCIDENCE
Down's (trisomy 21)	47,XX or 47,XY	1 in 500 live births (94% of all cases of the syndrome)
Translocation	Variable	3% of all cases
Mosaicism	Variable	3% of all cases
Turner's	45,XO	1 in 3,000 live births
Klinefelter's	47,XXY	1 in 500 live male births
Patau's (D trisomy)	47,XY, +D or 47,XX +D	1 in 5,000 live births
Edwards' (E trisomy)	47,XY +E or 47,XX +E	0.3 in 1,000 live births
Others (eg, cri du chat syndrome)	Multiple X and/or Y chromosomes, etc	

however, as sex prediction does not distinguish between normal and affected fetuses.

Inherited Metabolic Disorders

The number of inborn errors of metabolism that currently (or potentially) can be diagnosed by amniocentesis has increased dramatically over the past several years (Table 1–7). The diagnostic laboratory techniques used for these disorders usually require tissue culture of the amniotic fluid cells and subsequent specific analysis for the enzyme marker. Since the number of cultured cells is invariably limited and the enzyme analyses are complex and costly, prior heterozygote (carrier) detection is the first step in prenatal diagnosis. Ideally, carrier detection takes place before pregnancy.

The amniotic fluid supernatant may also be analyzed directly for abnormal metabolites or, in some cases, for enzyme activity. The measurement of galacticol, using gas-liquid chromatography, may provide a prenatal diagnosis of galactosemia without time-consuming tissue culture.[137] In propionic acidemia, excess methylcitrate is present in the fluid supernatant.[138] In addition, direct analysis for the enzyme N-acetyl-β-D-hexosaminidase A, which is greatly reduced in Tay-Sachs disease, is a reliable procedure. Intrauterine detection of cystic fibrosis, the most common neonatal recessive disorder (one case per 200 live births), may be possible with measurements of methylumbelliferylguanidinobenzoate-reac-

tive proteases in amniotic fluid.[139] Preliminary enzymatic studies on amniotic fluid supernatant for the enzymes arginine esterase[140] and trypsin[141] suggest that these enzymes might form the basis of antenatal testing for the presence of fetal cystic fibrosis.

The new technique of fetoscopy has proven helpful in the antenatal diagnosis of a few disorders and will prove to be even more valuable in the future. This procedure allows tiny amounts of fetal blood (10 to 50 μL) to be collected in the second trimester of pregnancy. This approach has already led to the prenatal diagnosis of β-thalassemia and sickle-cell anemia.[134,142,143]

Congenital Malformations

Fetoscopy will also ultimately be very valuable in the antenatal diagnosis of various syndromes involving gross physical defects, of which at least 60 are associated with mental retardation.[144] Currently, the major malformations that can be detected by amniotic fluid analysis are the NTDs discussed previously.

HLA typing of cultured amniotic fluid cells has been used to diagnose prenatally such diseases as congenital adrenal hyperplasia and complement C4 deficiency (when the gene is linked to the HLA complex), to identify the origin of triploidy, and to determine paternity prenatally. This type of testing is not widely used, however, because of its many unsolved technical problems.[145]

TABLE 1–7.   Inherited Disorders Identifiable by Amniocentesis

CATEGORY	SELECTED DISORDERS
Amino acid and related disorders	Argininosuccinicaciduria Citrullinemia Cystinosis Hyperammonemia, type II Maple syrup urine disease Methylmalonic aciduria Propionic acidemia
Carbohydrate metabolism	Galactosemia Glycogen storage diseases Glucose-6-phosphate dehydrogenase deficiency Mannosidosis
Lipid metabolism	Fabry's disease Gaucher's disease GM gangliosidosis Niemann-Pick disease Sandhoff's disease Tay-Sachs disease Wolman's disease
Mucopolysaccharidoses	Hurler's syndrome Hunter's syndrome Sanfilippo's disease I-cell disease
Miscellaneous	Adrenogenital syndrome Congenital erythropoietic porphyria Lesch-Nyhan syndrome Orotic aciduria

MICROBIOLOGIC EXAMINATION

Chorioamnionitis

Chorioamnionitis is defined as an inflammatory reaction of the fetal membranes, a diagnosis generally considered possible only by histologic examination of the placenta following delivery (Figure 14). Clinically, amniotic fluid infection exists when there is, in the absence of other infection, maternal and fetal tachycardia with a maternal temperature of greater than 38° C; uterine tenderness, irritability, or both; or a foul-smelling vaginal discharge. Unfortunately, most of these criteria are late signs. As a result, clinical and pathologic correlation is frequently poor, especially in early or mild cases. As might be expected, the bacteria known to cause chorioamnionitis are primarily those normally found in the cervix and include both aerobic and anaerobic organisms. The major bacteria include group B streptococci, α-hemolytic streptococci, enterococci, *Escherichia coli*, *Klebsiella pneumoniae*, and various species of *Bacteroides, Peptococcus, Peptostreptococcus,* and *Clostridium*, among others.

Several factors have been identified as influences on bacterial colonization of amniotic fluid, including premature delivery, prolonged labor, and premature rupture of membranes. With regard to the last, there is increasing evidence that amniotic fluid infections may be the cause rather than the result of the premature rupture of fetal membranes.[146,147] In one study, an increased number of vaginal examinations were correlated with increased colonization of amniotic fluid,[148] but this study has not been substantiated.[149–151] The association of poor maternal weight gain and intrauterine growth retardation with in utero infections and increased perinatal death has also been reported.[152]

Under normal conditions, the fetus matures in a germ-free environment that is safeguarded by a variety of mechanisms. However, bacterial invasion, through either intact or ruptured placental membranes near the cervical os, is apparently a common event. It is also now well accepted that amniotic fluid contains several substances that inhibit bacterial growth, including lysozyme, β-lysin, transferrin, peroxidase, metal-mediated systems, cationic peptides, immunoglobulins, and polymorphonuclear leukocytes.[153–155] Perhaps the most thoroughly studied bacterial inhibitor is a zinc-peptide system that is reversed by phosphate.[156] The specific peptide has a molecular weight of 630 daltons and consists of three molecules of glutamine–glutamic acid, two glycines, and a single lysine amino acid.[157] These naturally occurring agents inhibit both aerobic and anaerobic bacteria,[158] an effect that increases as the fetus matures.[159] As a result, third-trimester is more inhibitory than second-trimester fluid, and second-trimester is more inhibitory than first-trimester fluid. This antibacterial property is not decreased in polyhydramnios.[160]

Chorioamnionitis is, however, a relatively common event and leads to significant neonatal and maternal mortality and morbidity. The exact incidence is unknown, but various observations suggest that it is greater than is currently recognized, since some infants dying of sepsis are incorrectly diagnosed as having respiratory distress syndrome.[146,161,162]

Since the clinical criteria for the early diagnosis of chorioamnionitis are neither sensitive nor specific and when present usually indicate severe and long-standing infection, many studies on maternal blood and amniotic fluid have been carried out in an attempt to improve the diagnostic accuracy for this condition. The detection of maternal leukocytosis is of little help, if any, and does not signify infection since normal patients in labor may have leukocyte counts of $20 \times 10^3/\mu L$ or more.[163]

Recently, the maternal serum *C-reactive protein* has received some interest in the differentiation between inflammatory and noninflammatory gynecologic pathologic conditions, as well as in the prediction of an infectious process in cases of premature membrane rupture.[164,165] In the latter study, an elevated maternal serum C-reactive protein level accurately separated patients with evidence of infectious morbidity from those without. In 109 patients, there were 11 false-negative test results but no false-positives.[165] In 14 of 20 patients followed up serially and in whom infection developed, the C-reactive protein level became elevated at least 12 hours before any other entity measured (leukocyte count, differential WBC count, and temperature course).[165] Studies currently under way at our institution support the value of the maternal serum C-reactive protein determination as an early and reliable predictor of infectious morbidity.[166]

The examination of amniotic fluid obtained by as- piration through an intrauterine pressure catheter has received considerable attention.[151,167,168] The results have been confusing, however, with some investigators reporting that the presence of bacteria will probably be associated with maternal or neonatal infection but that the presence of leukocytes in the amniotic fluid probably will not (Figure 15).[169] Others have found that the presence of amniotic fluid neutrophils correlates better with the likelihood of infection than does the presence of bacteria on Gram's stain. Still others find that the presence of neither bacteria nor neutrophilic leukocytes correlates with the incidence of intrapartum or postpartum infection. It is highly probable that this lack of agreement may be related to the fact that in many intrapartum studies, the amniotic fluid was obtained transcervically, introducing the possibility of contamination.[169]

As one might expect, studies on fluid obtained by amniocentesis or needle amniotomy may be more consistent and reliable. Bobitt and Ledger,[146] using an intrauterine catheter, reported that quantitative amniotic fluid cultures with bacterial counts of less than 10^3 microorganisms per milliliter showed no subsequent clinical infection. On the other hand, 13 (81%) of 16 patients with colony counts higher than 10^3 microorganisms per milliliter subsequently experienced maternal infection, premature delivery, neonatal sepsis, or a combination of these conditions.[146] Transabdominal amniocentesis has been used successfully for bacteriologic evaluation of the amniotic fluid in patients suspected of being infected with or at high risk for chorioamnionitis (eg, those with premature rupture of membranes).[170] Bacterial growth of greater than 10^2 colony-forming units per milliliter of amniotic fluid has been associated with clinical chorioamnionitis.[171,172] Colonization was also observed in five afebrile patients, four of whom were in premature labor.[172] In the last study, the method used to collect the fluid (catheter, amniocentesis, or during cesarean section) did not appear to influence the culture results. Bacteria seen on Gram's stain in fluid obtained during cesarean section appear to correlate with postpartum endometritis.[171,172] Wallace and Herrick[173] have, however, pointed out that amniocentesis performed solely for the diagnosis of asymptomatic amnionitis in the patient in premature labor may be of questionable value because of the possible risk of spontaneous rup-

FIGURE 14. *Chorioamnionitis. Band of polymorphonuclear leukocytes is seen below the chorionic plate (arrows) (hematoxylin-eosin stain).*

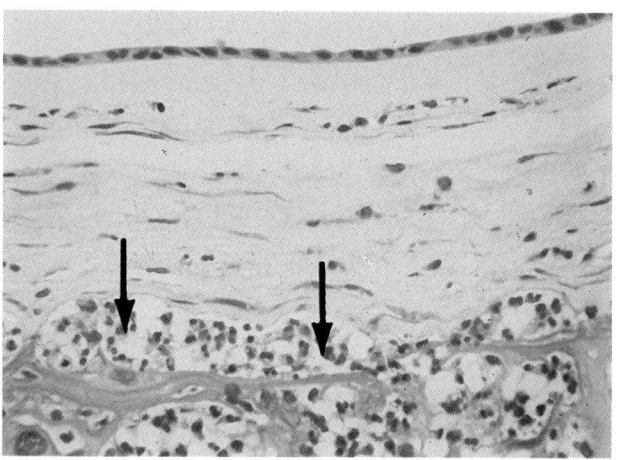

FIGURE 15. *Chorioamnionitis. The significance of this neutrophilic leukocytosis in the amniotic fluid is controversial.*

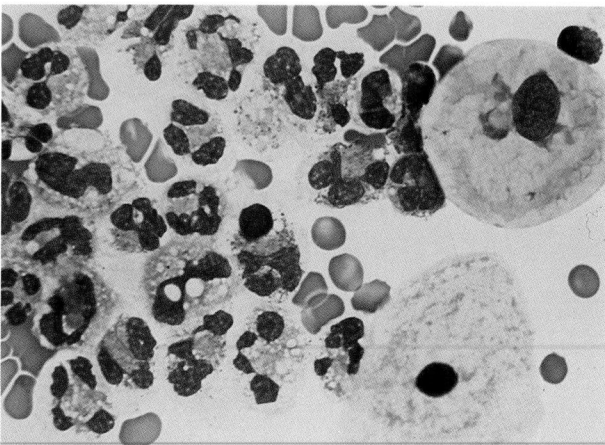

ture of the membranes after the procedure.

In addition to the more traditional methods of bacterial diagnosis, a method for the rapid diagnosis of amniotic fluid infection by gas-liquid chromatography has been reported.[174] In one study, an abnormal chromatographic pattern of organic acids was found in 15 of 16 patients with proven infection but in only one of 22 patients who were free of infection.[174] Lactate was present in all amniotic fluids, but acetate, succinate, butyrate, and oxaloacetate were identified, with some individual variation, only in the infected fluids.[174] Even though an amniotic fluid culture must be done to identify the type of organism, the gas-liquid chromatography method of identifying bacterial metabolites is rapid and sensitive. It may prove to be a valuable test for patients in whom amniotic fluid infection is suspected.

Of the protozoan infections, toxoplasmosis should be mentioned. Congenital toxoplasmosis occurs through transmission to the fetus from the mother.[175] Toxoplasma, its antigens, or both may be demonstrated in the amniotic fluid.[176]

Immunoglobulins have also been measured in amniotic fluid in an attempt to improve the clinical diagnosis of chorioamnionitis.[177,178] At present, this method has little diagnostic value in the clinical laboratory.

Viral Infections

As documented previously, amniotic fluid has the capacity to inhibit the growth of various bacteria. Its antiviral properties are, however, less well understood. Specific viral antibodies have been identified in amniotic fluids, especially those against herpes simplex virus and cytomegalovirus.[179,180] To date, the diagnosis of three cases of severe fetal cytomegalovirus infection from amniotic fluid has been reported.[181] It is anticipated that this area of research will enlarge considerably in the future.

REFERENCES

1. Seeds AE: Current concepts of amniotic fluid dynamics. *Am J Obstet Gynecol* 138:575–586, 1980

2. Hutchinson DL, Gray MJ, Plentl AA, et al: The role of the fetus in the water exchange of amniotic fluid of normal and hydramniotic patients. *J Clin Invest* 38:971, 1959

3. Pritchard JA: Deglutition by normal and anencephalic fetuses. *Obstet Gynecol* 25:289–297, 1965

4. Queenan JT, Thompson W, Whitfield CR, et al: Amniotic fluid volumes in normal pregnancies. *Am J Obstet Gynecol* 114:34–38, 1972

5. Gadd RL: The volume of the liquor amnii in normal and abnormal pregnancies. *J Obstet Gynaecol Br Commonw* 73:11–23, 1966

6. van Voorst tot Voorst EJGM: Effects of centrifugation, storage, and contamination of amniotic fluid on its total phospholipid content. *Clin Chem* 26:232–234, 1980

7. Svigos JM, Stewart-Rattray SF: Meconium stained liquor at second trimester amniocentesis: Is it significant? *Aust NZ J Obstet Gynecol* 21:5–6, 1981

8. Huisjes HJ: Cytology of the amniotic fluid and its clinical applications, in Fairweather DVI, Eskes TKAB (eds): *Amniotic Fluid-Research and Clinical Applications,* revised ed 2. Amsterdam, Excerpta Medica, 1978, pp 93-128

9. Morris HHH, Bennett MJ: The classification and origin of amniotic fluid cells. *Acta Cytol* 18:149–154, 1974

10. Casadei R, D'Ablaing G, Kaplan BJ, et al: A cytologic study of amniotic fluid. *Acta Cytol* 17:289–298, 1973

11. Schrage R, Bogelspacher HR, Wurster KG: Amniotic fluid cells in the second trimester of pregnancy. *Acta Cytol* 26:407–416, 1982

12. Braseus I, Gordon H: The cytological diagnosis of ruptured membranes using Nile Blue sulphate staining. *J Obstet Gynaecol Br Commonw* 73:342–346, 1965

13. Morrison JC, Whybrew WD, Bucarez ET, et al: Nile Blue and fetal maturity. *Obstet Gynecol* 49:38–42, 1977

14. Doran TA, Ford JA, Allar LC, et al: Amniotic fluid lecithin/sphingomyelin ratio, palmitic acid, palmitic/stearic acid ratio, total cortisol, creatinine percentage of lipid-positive cells in assessment of fetal maturity and fetal pulmonary maturity: A comparison. *Am J Obstet Gynecol* 133:302–307, 1979

15. Tydein O, Bergstrom S, Lindmark G: A comparison of the amniotic fluid cytology, lecithin/sphingomyelin ratio and creatinine in predicting fetal maturity. *Acta Obstet Gynecol Scand* 60:63–69, 1981

16. Brosens IA, Gordon H: The estimation of maturity by cytological examination of the liquor amnii. *J Obstet Gynaecol Br Commonw* 73:88–90, 1966

17. Morrison JC, Morrison FA, Lovett FA, et al: Nile Blue staining of cells in amniotic fluid for fetal maturity: I. A reappraisal. *Obstet Gynecol* 44:355–361, 1974

18. Morrison JC, Whybrew WD, Bucovaz ET, et al: Nile Blue and fetal maturity: Further investigations. *Obstet Gynecol* 49:38–42, 1977

19. Bobrow M, Evans CJ, Noble J, et al: Cellular content of amniotic fluid as a predictor of central nervous system malformation. *J Med Genet* 15:97–100, 1978

20. Gosden CM, Brock DJD: Morphology of rapidly adhering amniotic fluid cells as an aid to the diagnosis of neural tube defects. *Lancet* 1:919–922, 1977

21. Sartar S, Chang HC, Porreco RP, et al: Neural origin of cells in amniotic fluid. *Am J Obstet Gynecol* 136:67–72, 1980

22. von Koskull H: Rapid identification of glial cells in human amniotic fluid with indirect immunofluorescence. *Acta Cytol* 28:393–400, 1984

23. Adams C, Kilpatrick B, Kabacy G, et al: Fetal sex determination. *Acta Cytol* 17:233–236, 1973

24. Giles HR, Lox CD, Heine MV, et al: Intrauterine sex determination by radioimmune assay of amniotic fluid testosterone. *Gynecol Invest* 5:317–321, 1974

25. Makepeace AW, Fremont-Smith M, Dailet M, et al: The nature of the amniotic fluid: A comparative study of human amniotic fluid and maternal serum. *Surg Gynecol Obstet* 53:635–644, 1931

26. Cantarow A, Stuckert H, Davis RC: The chemical composition of amniotic fluid. *Surg Gynecol Obstet* 57:63–70, 1933

27. Cherry SH: Amniotic fluid analysis as an index of fetal health in utero. *Med Times* 95:713–717, 1967

28. Wolf PL, Bloch D, Tsudaka T: Biochemical profile of amniotic fluid to assess fetal maturity. *Clin Chem* 16:843–844, 1970

29. Weissberg HF: Clinical chemical analysis of sixty-two amniotic fluids from women in early pregnancy, in Natelson S, Scommegna A, Epstein MB (eds): *Amniotic Fluid: Physiology, Biochemistry, and Clinical Chemistry.* New York, John Wiley & Sons Inc, 1974, pp 47–71

30. Cederguist LL, Ewool LC, Bonsnes RW, et al: Detectability pattern of immunoglobulin in normal amniotic fluid throughout gestation. *Am J Obstet Gynecol* 130:220–224, 1978

31. Usategui-Gomez M, Morgan DF, Toolan HW: A comparative study of amniotic fluid, maternal sera and cord sera by disc electrophoresis. *Proc Soc Exp Biol Med* 123:547–557, 1966

32. Usategui-Gomez M: Immunoglobulins and other protein constituents of amniotic fluid, in Natelson S, Scommegna A, Epstein MB (eds): *Amniotic Fluid: Physiology, Biochemistry, and Clinical Chemistry.* New York, John Wiley & Sons Inc, 1974, pp 111–124

33. Ogunbode O, Onifade A: Amniotic fluid electrolytes, urea and creatinine in normal pregnancy and cholera during pregnancy. *Obstet Gynecol* 39:441–445, 1972

34. Cherry SH, Dolger H, Rosenfield RE, et al: Amniotic fluid urea nitrogen, uric acid, and creatinine in diabetic pregnancies. *Bull NY Acad Med* 45:46–52, 1969

35. De Grandi P, Ramzin M, Luthi A, et al: Relationship between amylase concentration, L/S ratio, and lecithin concentrations in amniotic fluid. *Gynecol Obstet Invest* 10:23–31, 1979

36. Delahunty TJ, Foreback CC: Creatine kinase isoenzyme BB in human amniotic fluid. *Clin Chem* 26:1756, 1980

37. Hall M, Silverman LM, Chapman JF, et al: Creatine kinase BB in human amniotic fluid. *Clin Chem* 28:558–559, 1982

38. Brocklehurst D, Wilde CE: Amniotic fluid alkaline phosphatase, gammaglutamyltransferase, and 5′-nucleotidase activity from 13–40 weeks gestation, and alkaline phosphatase as an index of fetal lung maturity. *Clin Chem* 26:588–591, 1980

39. Beckman G, Beckman L, Lofstrand T: Acid and alkaline phosphatase in amniotic fluid in normal and complicated pregnancy. *Acta Obstet Gynecol Scand* 57:1–5, 1978

40. Piedra C, Jerez E: Glutamyltransferase activity during pregnancy. *Clin Chem* 26:1514, 1980

41. Battaglia F, Prystowsky H, Smisson C, et al: On the changes in total osmotic pressure and sodium and potassium concentrations of amniotic fluid during the course of human gestation. *Surg Gynecol Obstet* 109:509–512, 1959

42. Howard WF: An analysis of amniotic fluid electrolytes in toxemia of pregnancy. *Am J Obstet Gynecol* 86:245–248, 1963

43. Doran TA, Bjerre S, Porter CJ: Creatinine, uric acid, and electrolytes in amniotic fluid. *Am J Obstet Gynecol* 106:325–332, 1970

44. Nusbaum MJ, Zettner A: The content of calcium, magnesium, copper, iron, sodium, and potassium in amniotic fluid from eleven to nineteen weeks' gestation. *Am J Obstet Gynecol* 115:219–226, 1973

45. Misenhimer HR: Role of amniotic fluid studies (ΔA_{450}) in the management of RH immunization, in Natelson S, Scommegna A, Epstein MB (eds): *Amniotic Fluid: Physiology, Biochemistry, and Clinical Chemistry.* New York, John Wiley & Sons Inc, 1974, pp 171–178

46. Bevis DCA: Composition of liquor amnii in hemolytic disease of newborn. *Lancet* 2:443, 1950

47. Bevis DCA: The antenatal prediction of hemolytic disease of the newborn. *Lancet* 1:395–398, 1952

48. Bevis DCA: The composition of liquor amnii in haemolytic disease of the newborn. *J Obstet Gynaecol Br Emp* 60:244–251, 1953

49. Bevis DCA: Blood pigments in hemolytic disease of the newborn. *J Obstet Gynaecol Br Emp* 63:68–75, 1956

50. Liley AW: Liquor amnii analysis in the management of the pregnancy complicated by rhesus sensitization. *Am J Obstet Gynecol* 82:1359–1370, 1961

51. Liley AW: Errors in the assessment of hemolytic disease from amniotic fluid. *Am J Obstet Gynecol* 86:485–494, 1963

52. Cherry SH, Kochwa S, Rosenfield RE: Bilirubin-protein ratio in amniotic fluid as an index of the severity of erythroblastosis fetalis. *Obstet Gynecol* 26:826–832, 1965

53. Usategui-Gomez M, Hopkins MS, DeCastro AF: Serum proteins in amniotic fluids in erythroblastosis fetalis. *Obstet Gynecol* 36:865–374, 1970

54. Gambino SR, Freda VJ: The measurement of amniotic fluid bilirubin by the method of Jendrassik and Grof. *Am J Clin Pathol* 46:198–203, 1966

55. Fiereck EA: Amniotic fluid, in Tietz N (ed): *Fundamentals of Clinical Chemistry*, ed 2. Philadelphia, WB Saunders Co, 1976, pp 1163–1176

56. Pitkin RM, Zwirek SJ: Amniotic fluid creatinine. *Am J Obstet Gynecol* 98:1135–1139, 1967

57. Glasser L, Finley PR: Amniotic fluid and the quality of life. *Sigan Med* Sept./Oct.: 31–52, 1981

58. De Grandi P, Ramzin M, Luthi A, et al: Relationship between amylase concentration, L/S ratio, and lecithin concentrations in amniotic fluid. *Gynecol Obstet Invest* 10:23–31, 1979

59. Williams LH, Gilbert R, Mailhot EA, et al: Correlation of amylase and lecithin sphingomyelin ratios in amniotic fluid samples. *Am J Clin Pathol* 78:85–89, 1982

60. Gluck L: Surfactant: 1972. *Pediatr Clin North Am* 19:325–330, 1972

61. Gluck L, Kulovich MV, Borer RC, et al: Diagnosis of the respiratory distress syndrome by amniocentesis. *Am J Obstet Gynecol* 109:440–445, 1971

62. Brown LM, Duck-Chong CG, Hensley WJ: Improved procedure for lecithin/sphingomyelin ratio in amniotic fluid reduces false predictions of lung maturity. *Clin Chem* 28:344–348, 1982

63. Gebhardt DOE: The acetone precipitation step is needed in determining the lecithin/sphingomyelin (L/S) ratio of amniotic fluid. *Clin Chem* 29:214, 1983

64. Gluck L: Diagnosis of fetal lung maturity, in Young BK (ed): *Perinatal Medicine Today.* New York, Alan R Liss Inc, 1980, pp 189–203

65. Hallman M, Gluck L: Phosphatidylglycerol in lung surfactant: III. Possible modifier of surfactant function. *J Lipid Res* 17:257–262, 1976

66. Gotelli GR, Stanfill RE, Kabra PM, et al: Simultaneous determination of phosphatidylglycerol and lecithin/sphingomyelin ratio in amniotic fluid. *Clin Chem* 24:1144–1146, 1978

67. Painter PC: Simultaneous measurement of lecithin, sphingomyelin, phosphatidylglycerol, phosphatidylinositol, phosphatidylethanolamine, and phosphatidylserine in amniotic fluid. *Clin Chem* 26:1147–1151, 1980

68. Tsai MY, Marshall JG: Phosphatidylglycerol in 261 samples of amniotic fluid from normal and diabetic pregnancies, as measured by one-dimensional thin-layer chromatography. *Clin Chem* 25:682–685, 1979

69. Hallman M, Kulovich M, Sugarman RG, et al: Phosphatidylinositol and phosphatidylglycerol in amniotic fluid: Indices of lung maturity. *Am J Obstet Gynecol* 125:613–617, 1976

70. Tsai MY: Relative merits of one- and two-dimensional TLC of phospholipids in amniotic fluid. *Clin Chem* 27:1957–1958, 1981

71. Cunningham MD, Desai NS, Thompson SA, et al: Amniotic fluid phosphatidylglycerol in diabetic pregnancies. *Am J Obstet Gynecol* 131:719–724, 1978

72. Kulovich MV, Gluck L: The lung profile: II. Complicated pregnancy. *Am J Obstet Gynecol* 135:64–70, 1979

73. Hallman M, Teramo K: Measurement of the lecithin/sphingomyelin ratio and phosphatidylglycerol in amniotic fluid: An accurate method for the assessment of fetal lung maturity. *Br J Obstet Gynecol* 88:806–813, 1981

74. Clements JA, Platzker CG, Tierney DF, et al: Assessment of the risk of the respiratory-distress syndrome by a rapid test for surfactant in amniotic fluid. *N Engl J Med* 286:1077–1081, 1972

75. Keniston BJ: A prospective evaluation of the lecithin/sphingomyelin ratio surfactant test in relation to fetal pulmonary maturity. *Am J Obstet Gynecol* 121:324–332, 1975

76. Freer DE, Statland BE, Sher G: Rational basis for foam-stability assay of amniotic fluid surfactant. *Clin Chem* 24:1980–1984, 1978

77. Statland BE, Sher G, Freer DE, et al: Evaluation of a modified foam stability (FS-50) test. *Am J Clin Pathol* 69:514–519, 1978

78. Amenta JS, Silverman JA: Amniotic fluid lecithin, phosphatidylglycerol, L/S ratio, and foam stability test in predicting respiratory distress in the newborn. *Am J Clin Pathol* 79:52–64, 1983

79. Sher G, Statland BE: Assessment of fetal pulmonary maturity by the Lumadex foam stability index test. *Obstet Gynecol* 61:444–449, 1983

80. Lipshitz J, Anderson GD, Whybrew WD: Accelerated pulmonary maturity as measured by the Lumadex foam stability index test. *Obstet Gynecol* 62:31–36, 1983

81. Bryson M: Oral communication, 1983

82. Shinitzky M, Goldfisher A, Bruck A, et al: A new method for assessment of fetal lung maturity. *Br J Obstet Gynaecol* 83:838–844, 1976

83. Anaokar J, Garry PJ, Standefer JC: Enzymic assay for lecithin in amniotic fluid. *Clin Chem* 25:103–107, 1978

84. Siegel R, Walker SI, Robin NI: An enzymic radiochemical method for determining phosphatidylglycerol in amniotic fluid. *Clin Chem* 29:782–785, 1983

85. Duck-Chong CG, Gupta JM, Storey GNB, et al: Lamellar body phospholipid content of amniotic fluid and L/S ratio compared in assessing fetal lung maturity. *Clin Chem* 26:766–769, 1980

86. Duck-Chong CG, Brown LM, Hensley WJ: Sedimentation of lung-derived phospholipid during low-speed centrifugation of amniotic fluid. *Clin Chem* 27:1424–1426, 1981

87. Mason RJ, Nellenbogen J, Clements JA: Isolation of disaturated phosphatidylcholine with osmium tetroxide. *J Lipid Res* 17:281–284, 1976

88. Cetrulo CL, Sharra AJ, Selvaraj RJ, et al: Amniotic fluid optical density and neonatal respiratory outcome. *Obstet Gynecol* 55:262–264, 1980

89. Blumenfeld TA, Cheskin HS, Shinitsky M: Microviscosity of amniotic fluid phospholipids, and its importance in determining fetal lung maturity. *Clin Chem* 25:64–67, 1979

90. Golde SH, Mosley GH: A blind comparison study of the lung phospholipid profile, fluorescence microviscosimetry, and the lecithin/sphingomyelin ratio. *Am J Obstet Gynecol* 136:222–227, 1980

91. Simon NV, Hohman WA, Elser RC, et al: Fetal lung maturity in complicated pregnancy, as predicted from microviscosity of amniotic fluid. *Clin Chem* 28:1754–1757, 1982

92. Cox KH, Ross JBA, Peterson AP, et al: Fetal lung maturity assessed by fluorescence polarization: Evaluation of predictive value correction for endogenous fluorescence, and comparison with L/S ratio. *Clin Chem* 29:346–349, 1983

93. Garite TJ, Yabusaki KK, Moberg LJ, et al: A new rapid slide agglutination test for amniotic fluid phosphatidylglycerol: Laboratory and clinical correlation. *Am J Obstet Gynecol* 147:681–686, 1983

94. Knight JA, Miya T, Wu JT: Standard lecithin/sphingomyelin and phosphatidylglycerol techniques compared with immunologic slide test. *Obstet Gynecol* 65:840–843, 1985

95. Freer DE, Statland BE: Measurement of amniotic fluid surfactant. *Clin Chem* 27:1629–1641, 1981

96. Depp R: Present status of the assessment of fetal maturity. *Semin Perinatol* 4:229–247, 1980

97. Murphy BEP, Patrick J, Denton RL: Cortisol in amniotic fluid during human gestation. *J Clin Endocrinol Metab* 40:164–167, 1975

98. Sharp-Cageorge SM, Blicker BM, Gordon ER, et al: Amniotic fluid cortisol and human fetal lung maturation. *N Engl J Med* 296:89–92, 1977

99. Weiner CP, Brandt J: A modified activated partial thromboplastin time with the use of amniotic fluid. *Am J Obstet Gynecol* 144:234–240, 1982

100. Divers WA, Babaknia A, Hopper BR, et al: Fetal lung maturation: Amniotic fluid catecholamines, phospholipids, and cortisol. *Am J Obstet Gynecol* 142:440–444, 1982

101. Clifford SH: Postmaturity—with placental dysfunction. *J Pediatr* 44:1–13, 1954

102. Smith AL, Scanlon J: Amniotic fluid D(-)-β-hydroxybutyrate and the dysmature newborn infant. *Am J Obstet Gynecol* 115:569–574, 1973

103. Lagercrantz H, Sjoquist B, Bremme K, et al: Catecholamine metabolites in amniotic fluid as indicators of intrauterine distress. *Am J Obstet Gynecol* 136:1067–1070, 1980

104. Divers WA, Wilkes MM, Babaknia A, et al: Amniotic fluid catecholamines and metabolites in intrauterine growth retardation. *Am J Obstet Gynecol* 141:608–610, 1981

105. Seeds AE, Hellegers AE: Acid-base determinations in human amniotic fluid throughout pregnancy. *Am J Obstet Gynecol* 101:257–260, 1968

106. Bolognese RJ, Corson SL, Touchstone JC, et al: Correlation of amniotic fluid estriol with fetal age and well-being. *Obstet Gynecol* 37:437–441, 1971

107. Laatikainen TJ, Peltonen JI: Amniotic fluid estriol, estriol precursors, and pregnanediol in intrauterine growth retardation. *J Steroid Biochem* 13:265–269, 1980

108. Stempel LE, Lott JA: Diagnosis of fetal death in utero with amniotic fluid creatine kinase. *Am J Obstet Gynecol* 138:1173–1176, 1980

109. Wysocki SJ, Hahnel R, Millward MJ, et al: Amniotic fluid squalene and fetal maturity. *Br J Obstet Gynaecol* 86:854–860, 1979

110. Messeri G, Billi D: Amniotic fluid squalene and gestational age. *Clin Chem* 28:1810–1811, 1982

111. Brock DTH, Sutcliffe RG: Alpha-fetoprotein in the antenatal diagnosis of anencephaly and spina bifida. *Lancet* 2:197–199, 1972

112. Milunsky A: Prenatal detection of neural tube defects. *JAMA* 244:2731–2735, 1980

113. Lippman-Hand A, Fraser FC, Biddle CJC: Indications for prenatal diagnosis in relatives of patients with neural crest defects. *Obstet Gynecol* 51:72–76, 1978

114. Wald NJ, Cuckle HS: Amniotic fluid alpha-fetoprotein measurement in antenatal diagnosis of anencephaly and open spina bifida in early pregnancy: Second report of UK collaborative study on AFP in relation to neural tube defects. *Lancet* 2:651–661, 1979

115. Kjessler B, Johansson SGO: Monitoring of the development of early pregnancy by determination of alpha-fetoprotein in maternal serum and amniotic fluid samples. *Acta Obstet Gynecol Scand* 69(suppl):5–14, 1977

116. Johansson SGO, Kjessler B, Sherman MS, et al: Alpha-fetoprotein (AFP) levels in maternal serum and amniotic fluid in singleton pregnant women in their 10th-25th week post last menstrual period. *Acta Obstet Gynecol Scand* 69(suppl):20–24, 1977

117. Yachnin S: The clinical significance of human alpha-fetoprotein. *Ann Clin Lab Sci* 8:84–90, 1978

118. Stirrat GM, Gough JD, Wald NJ, et al: Raised maternal serum AFP, oligohydramnios and poor fetal outcome. *Br J Obstet Gynaecol* 88:231–235, 1981

119. Wald NJ, Cuckle HS: Amniotic fluid alpha-fetoprotein measurement in antenatal diagnosis of anencephaly and open spina bifida in early pregnancy. *Lancet* 2:651–661, 1979

120. Brock DJH, Sutcliffe RG: Alpha-fetoprotein in the antenatal diagnosis of anencephaly and spina bifida. *Lancet* 2:197–199, 1972

121. Wu JT, Book L, Sudar K: Serum alpha-fetoprotein (AFP) levels in normal infants. *Pediatr Res* 15:50–52, 1981

122. Goldberg ML: Alpha-fetoprotein and the need for a reference preparation. *Pathologist* 37:846–847, 1983

123. Smith AD, Wald NJ, Cuckle HS, et al: Amniotic fluid acetylcholinesterase as a possible diagnostic test for neural tube defects in early pregnancy. *Lancet* 1:685–688, 1979

124. Wald NJ, Cuckle HS: Report of the collaborative acetylcholinesterase study, amniotic fluid acetylcholinesterase electrophoresis as a secondary test in the diagnosis of anencephaly and open spina bifida in early pregnancy. *Lancet* 2:321–327, 1981

125. Milunsky A, Sapirstein VS: Prenatal diagnosis of open neural tube defects using the amniotic fluid acetylcholinesterase assay. *Obstet Gynecol* 59:1–5, 1982

126. Smith AF: Amniotic fluid acetylcholinesterase assay and the antenatal detection of neural tube defects. *Clin Chem Acta* 123:1–9, 1982

127. Milunsky A, Blusztain JK, Zensel S: Amniotic fluid total cholinesterase and neural tube defects. *Lancet* 2:36, 1979

128. Hay DL, Ibrahim GF, Horacek I: Rapid acetylcholinesterase screening test for neural tube defect. *Clin Chem* 29:1065–1069, 1983

129. Norgaard-Pedersen B, Hangaard J, Bjerrum OJ: Quantitative enzyme antigen immunoassay of acetylcholinesterase in amniotic fluid. *Clin Chem* 29:1061–1064, 1983

130. Coombes EJ, Wood PJ, Spencer K, et al: Improved discrimination in the detection of neural tube defects: Five biochemical tests compared. *Clin Chem Acta* 122:249–259, 1982

131. Bell JA, Ansford AJ: Prenatal diagnosis of chromosome abnormalities: Analysis of 1,000 consecutive amniotic fluids. *Aust NZ J Obstet Gynecol* 21:207–210, 1981

132. Golbus MS: The current scope of antenatal diagnosis. *Hosp Pract* 17:179–186, 1982

133. Squire JA, Nouth L, Ridler MAC, et al: Prenatal diagnosis and outcome of pregnancy in 2,036 women investigated by amniocentesis. *Hum Genet* 61:215–222, 1982

134. Milunsky A: Current concepts in genetics. *N Engl J Med* 295:377–380, 1976

135. Birnholz JC: Determination of fetal sex. *N Engl J Med* 309:942–944, 1983

136. Hobbius JC: Determination of sex in early pregnancy. *N Engl J Med* 309:979–980, 1983

137. Allen JT, Holton JB, Gillett MG: Gas-liquid chromatographic determination of galacticol in amniotic fluid for possible use in prenatal diagnosis of galactosemia. *Clin Chem Acta* 110:59–63, 1981

138. Sweetman L, Weyler W, Shafai T, et al: Prenatal diagnosis of propionic acidemia. *JAMA* 242:1048–1052, 1979

139. Nadler HL, Walsh MMJ: Intrauterine detection of cystic fibrosis. *Pediatrics* 66:690–692, 1980

140. Dann LG, Blau K: Amniotic fluid arginine esterases as a marker for cystic fibrosis. *Lancet* 1:619, 1982

141. Pocknee RC, Abramovich DR: Origin and levels of trypsin in amniotic fluid throughout pregnancy. *Br J Obstet Gynaecol* 89:142–144, 1982

142. Kan YW, Golbus MS, Trecartin R, et al: Prenatal diagnosis of homozygous β-thalassemia. *Lancet* 2:790–791, 1975

143. Alter BP: Intrauterine diagnosis of hemoglobinopathies. *Semin Perinatol* 4:189–198, 1980

144. Milunsky A: *The Prevention of Genetic Disease and Mental Retardation*. Philadelphia, WB Saunders Co, 1975

145. Whitsett CF, Priest JH, Priest RE: HLA typing of cultured amniotic fluid cells. *Am J Clin Pathol* 79:186–194, 1983

146. Bobitt JR, Ledger WJ: Amniotic fluid analysis: Its role in maternal and neonatal infection. *Obstet Gynecol* 51:56–62, 1978

147. Naeye RL, Peters EC: Causes and consequences of premature rupture of fetal membranes. *Lancet* 1:192–194, 1980

148. Harris JW, Brown JH: The bacterial content of the uterus at caesarian section. *Am J Obstet Gynecol* 73:133–143, 1927

149. Fara FJ, Steward M, Stendard J: Use of unlimited nonsterile vaginal examinations in conduct of labor. *Am J Obstet Gynecol* 72:1–11, 1956

150. Slotnick IJ, Stellute M, Prystowsky H: Microbiology of the female genital tract: II. Comparative investigation of cervical flora of parturients receiving either rectal or vaginal examinations. *Am J Obstet Gynecol* 85:519–526, 1963

151. Miller JM, Hill GB, Welt SI: Bacterial colonization of amniotic fluid in the presence of ruptured membranes. *Am J Obstet Gynecol* 137:451–458, 1980

152. Naeye RL, Peters EC: Amniotic fluid infections with intact membranes leading to perinatal death: A prospective study. *Pediatrics* 61:171–177, 1978

153. Galask RP, Snyder IS: Bacterial inhibition by amniotic fluid: I. In vitro evidence for bacterial growth inhibiting activity. *Am J Obstet Gynecol* 102:949–955, 1968

154. Bergman N, Bercovici B, Sacks T: Antibacterial activity of human amniotic fluid. *Am J Obstet Gynecol* 114:520–523, 1972

155. Schlievert P, Johnson W, Galask RP: Bacterial growth inhibition by amniotic fluid: IV. Evidence for a zinc-peptide antibacterial system. *Am J Obstet Gynecol* 125:906–910, 1976

156. Larsen B, Snyder IS, Galask RP: Bacterial growth inhibition by amniotic fluid: II. Reversal of amniotic fluid bacterial growth inhibition by addition of a chemically defined medium. *Am J Obstet Gynecol* 119:497–501, 1974

157. Schlievert P, Johnson W, Galask RP: Isolation of a low-molecular-weight antibacterial system from human amniotic fluid. *Infect Immunol* 14:1156–1166, 1976

158. Thadepalli H, Appleman MD, Maidman JE: Antimicrobial effect of amniotic fluid against anaerobic bacteria. *Am J Obstet Gynecol* 127:250–254, 1977

159. Thadepalli H, Bach VT, Davidson EC: Antimicrobiologic effect of amniotic fluid. *Obstet Gynecol* 52:198–204, 1978

160. Larsen B, Klinzman DV, Galask RP: Bacterial growth inhibiting activity in polyhydramnios. *Obstet Gynecol* 59:162–166, 1982

161. Ablow RC, Driscoll SG, Effman EL, et al: A comparison of early-onset group B streptococcal neonatal infection and the respiratory distress syndrome of the newborn. *N Engl J Med* 294:65–70, 1976

162. Jacob J, Edwards D, Gluck L: Early onset sepsis and pneumonia observed as respiratory distress syndrome. *AJDC* 134:766–768, 1980

163. Schreiber J, Benedetti T: Conservative management of preterm premature rupture of the fetal membranes in a low socioeconomic population. *Am J Obstet Gynecol* 136:92–96, 1980

164. Hajj SN, Angerman NS, Evans MI, et al: C-reactive protein in the differential diagnosis of gynecologic pathology. *J Reprod Med* 23:284–287, 1979

165. Evans MI, Hajj SN, Devoe LD, et al: C-reactive protein as a predictor of infectious morbidity with premature rupture of membranes. *Am J Obstet Gynecol* 138:648–652, 1980

166. Rote N, Thurnau G, Kochenour N: Oral communication, August 1983

167. Larsen JW: Can amniotic fluid analyses predict infection? *Contemp Ob/Gyn* 14:53–62, 1979

168. Gibbs RS, Blanco JD, St Clair PJ, et al: Quantitative bacteriology of amniotic fluid from women with clinical intraamniotic infection at term. *J Infect Dis* 145:1–8, 1982

169. Mead PB: Management of the patient with premature rupture of the membranes. *Clin Perinatol* 7: 243–255, 1980

170. Garite TJ, Freeman RK, Linzay EM: The use of amniocentesis in patients with premature rupture of membranes. *Obstet Gynecol* 54:226–230, 1979

171. Miller JM, Pupkin MJ, Hill GB: Bacterial colonization of amniotic fluid from intact fetal membranes. *Am J Obstet Gynecol* 136:796–804, 1980

172. Miller JM, Hill GB, Welt SI, et al: Bacterial colonization of amniotic fluid in the presence of ruptured membranes. *Am J Obstet Gynecol* 137:451–458, 1980

173. Wallace RL, Herrick CN: Amniocentesis in the evaluation of premature labor. *Obstet Gynecol* 57: 483–486, 1981

174. Gravett MG, Eschenbach DA, Speigel-Brown CA, et al: Rapid diagnosis of amniotic fluid infection by gas-liquid chromatography. *N Engl J Med* 306:725–728, 1982

175. Desmonts G, Courreur J: Congenital toxoplasmosis: A prospective study of 378 pregnancies. *N Engl J Med* 290:1110–1116, 1974

176. Tentsch SM, Sulzer AJ, Ramsey JE: Toxoplasma gondii isolated from amniotic fluid. *Obstet Gynecol* 55(suppl):25–45, 1980

177. Curl CW: Immunoglobulin levels in amniotic fluid. *Am J Obstet Gynecol* 109:408–410, 1971

178. Cederqvist LL, Francis LC, Zervoudakis IA, et al: Fetal immune response following prematurely ruptured membranes. *Am J Obstet Gynecol* 126:321–327, 1976

179. Cesario T, Goldstein A, Lindsey M, et al: Antiviral activities in amniotic fluid. *Proc Soc Exp Biol Med* 168:403–407, 1981

180. Cox D, Hawkins SL, Hartley CE, et al: Antibody activity against herpes simplex virus in human amniotic fluid. *Br J Obstet Gynaecol* 89:226–230, 1982

181. Huikeshoven FJM, Wallenburg HCS, Jahoda MGJ: Diagnosis of severe fetal cytomegalovirus infection from amniotic fluid in the third trimester of pregnancy. *Am J Obstet Gynecol* 142:1053–1054, 1982

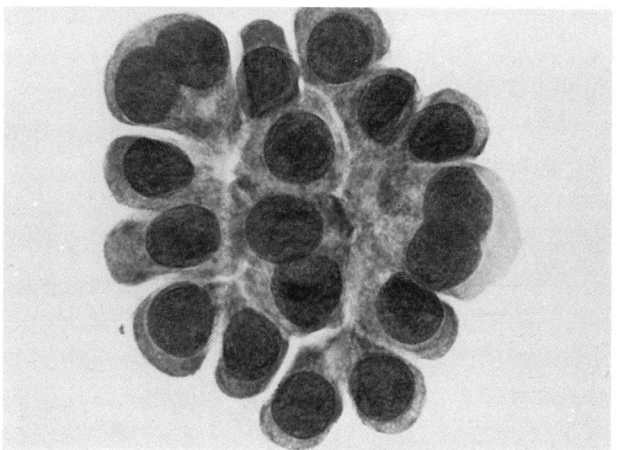

CHAPTER 2

Cerebrospinal Fluids

ANATOMY AND PHYSIOLOGY

The brain and spinal cord are covered by three meningeal membranes, which are as follows from the outside inward: dura mater, arachnoid mater, and pia mater. Cerebrospinal fluid (CSF) is present in the subarachnoid space between the arachnoid mater and the pia mater and circulates over the cerebral hemispheres and downward over the spinal cord (Figure 16). Most of the CSF is formed by the choroid plexuses through ultrafiltration and active secretion. Extrachoroidal sites such as the ependymal lining of the ventricles and the cerebral subarachnoid space are other sites of CSF formation. Absorption of the CSF occurs through the arachnoid villi.

The total CSF volumes are 90 to 150 mL in adults and 10 to 60 mL in neonates. There is a constant turnover of CSF of approximately 150 mL/hr.[1]

The CSF acts as a protective cushion for the underlying central nervous tissue. Other functions of the CSF include collection of wastes, circulation of nutrients, and lubrication of the CNS.

The choroid plexus epithelium and the endothelium of capillaries in contact with CSF make up the anatomic structure of the blood-CSF barrier. The endothelium of these capillaries regulates the passage of various substances into the CSF from the blood. Reference values for the normal components of CSF are presented in Table 2–1.

LUMBAR PUNCTURE

Most CSF studies are performed on a lumbar puncture specimen, which is obtained by a relatively simple procedure. However, since complications may occur, lumbar puncture should only be performed for specific diagnostic or therapeutic purposes (Table 2–2). Before the spinal puncture is performed, a careful clinical history and physical examination should be

TABLE 2–1. Reference Values for Cerebrospinal Fluid

COMPONENT*	CONVENTIONAL UNITS	SI UNITS
Albumin	10–30 mg/dL	100–300 mg/L
Calcium	2.1–2.7 mEq/L	1.05–1.35 mmole/L
Chloride	115–130 mEq/L	115–130 mmole/L
Glucose	50–80 mg/dL	2.75–4.40 mmole/L
Lactate	9–26 mg/dL	1.13–3.23 mmole/L
Lactate dehydrogenase	0–25 U/L at 37 °C	NA
Leukocyte count		
Adults	0–5 mononuclear cells/μL	$0–0.005 \times 10^9$/L
Neonates	0–30 mononuclear cells/μL	$0–0.030 \times 10^9$/L
Leukocyte differential count		
Adults		
Lymphocytes	60% ± 20%	NA
Monocytes	30% ± 15%	NA
Neutrophils	2% ± 4%	NA
Neonates		
Lymphocytes	20% ± 15%	NA
Monocytes	70% ± 20%	NA
Neutrophils	4% ± 4%	NA
Total Protein	15–45 mg/dL	150–450 mg/L
Adults older than 60 years	15–60 mg/dL	150–600 mg/L
Neonates	15–100 mg/dL	150–1,000 mg/L

Notes: Data partially adapted from Krieg.[2] Used by permission. Except where noted, reference values apply to adults. NA = not applicable.

*Reliable values for most enzymes have not yet been established.

completed. The optic fundi should be examined for evidence of increased intracranial pressure. If increased pressure is present, great care must be taken when removing fluid, as herniation of the uncus through the tentorium cerebelli or of the cerebellar tonsils through the foramen magnum may occur. When a spinal puncture is performed in the presence of increased intracranial pressure, a neurosurgeon should be consulted. The lumbar puncture skin site must be thoroughly cleansed to reduce the possibility of contamination by bacteria normally present on the skin. As will be discussed under "Microbiology," α-hemolytic *(viridans)* streptococci can pose a special problem.

A spinal puncture is contraindicated if there is infection at the proposed puncture site, as puncture may result in the spread of the infection into the meninges. Septicemia and general systemic infection also can be contraindications because spinal puncture may result in meningitis.

After the puncture is performed and before any fluid is withdrawn, a manometer is attached to record the opening pressure of the CSF. The normal pressure is 50 to 180 mm Hg when the patient is in a lateral position but slightly higher with the patient in a sitting position. Small transient changes in the pressure are noted with respiration, coughing, or straining. These changes are normal and indicate patency of the channels through which the CSF flows. The CSF pressure may be decreased or increased in a variety of disorders[1] (Table 2–3). If the pressure is normal, up to 20 mL of CSF can be removed without danger. If the initial pressure is greater than 200 mm Hg, not more than 2 mL of fluid should be removed. Ideally, the specimen should be divided into three samples and placed in sterile tubes, which are labeled sequentially. Tube 1 should be used for chemical and immunologic studies, tube 2 for microbiologic examination, and tube 3 for total cell count and differential cell count. Before the spinal puncture needle is removed, the closing pressure should be recorded.

GROSS EXAMINATION

The CSF is normally clear and colorless. If a disease is present, however, the fluid may appear cloudy, turbid, or bloody. Cloudy or turbid fluid may be due to pleocytosis (leukocyte count greater than 200/μL), the presence of microorganisms or RBCs (more than 400/μL), or an increased protein level. Following injection of radiographic contrast medium, the CSF may have an oily appearance. A fat embolism in the brain may be associated with fat globules of varying sizes in the CSF.

When the CSF is pinkish red, this usually indicates the presence of blood, a condition that may have resulted from subarachnoid hemorrhage, intracerebral hemorrhage, infarct, or traumatic tap. It is, of course, extremely important to differentiate traumatic tap from pathologic bleeding. Traumatic taps are more common in infants. If a child squirms during performance of a puncture, several punctures may be required before the dura is successfully entered. The following observations are useful in differentiating between the two types of bleeding: (1) A traumatic tap shows a maximum amount of blood in the first sample, with a progressive decrease in subsequent samples. In subarachnoid hemorrhage, the blood is generally evenly mixed in the three tubes. The presence of crenated RBCs is not useful in differentiating traumatic tap from pathologic bleeding. (2) After the CSF is centrifuged, the supernatant fluid is clear with a traumatic tap but xanthochromic (pink or yellow due to breakdown of hemoglobin) with a subarachnoid hemorrhage. (3) A clot may be seen in the CSF when there is a very bloody traumatic tap, while subarachnoid hemorrhage per se is usually not associated with clot formation. It should be noted, however, that traumatic and subarachnoid bleeding may be concurrent and that the supernatant fluid may be clear for the first three hours after the onset of subarachnoid hemorrhage. In addition, a very traumatic tap may be associated with the persistence of blood and

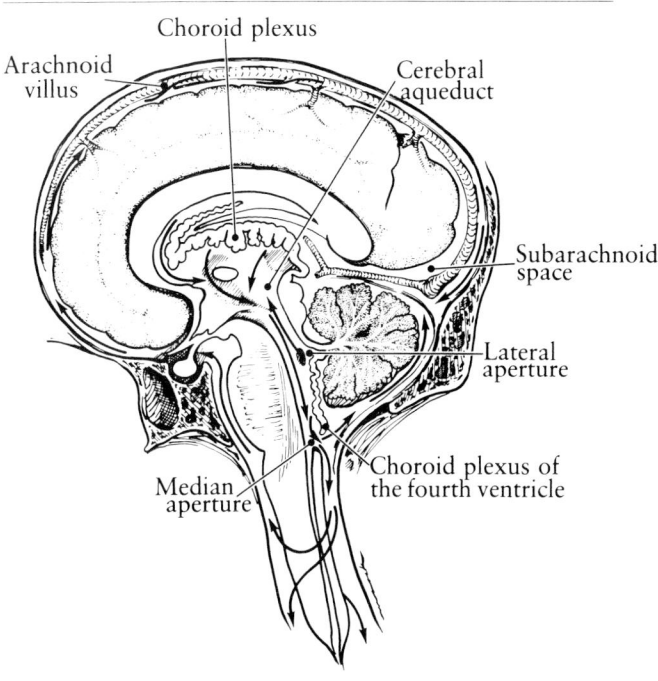

FIGURE 16. *Schematic drawing illustrating the circulation of the CSF.*

TABLE 2–2. Indications for Lumbar Puncture

Suspected Conditions
    Meningitis, encephalitis, syphilis, brain abscess
    Subarachnoid and intracerebral hemorrhage
    Multiple sclerosis, Guillain-Barré syndrome
    Acute leukemia and lymphoma with CNS involvement
    Spinal cord and brain tumor

Therapy
    Chemotherapy for leukemia and lymphoma
    Introduction of anesthetics, radiographic contrast media
    Amphotericin therapy in fungal meningitis

TABLE 2–3. Causes of CSF Pressure Changes

Increased Pressure
  Congestive heart failure
  Meningitis
  Thrombosis of venous sinuses
  Superior vena cava obstruction
  Cerebral edema
  Mass lesion (abscess, tumor, cerebral hemorrhage)
  Hypo-osmolality
  Impairment of CSF absorption

Decreased Pressure
  Spinal-subarachnoid block
  Dehydration
  Circulatory collapse
  CSF leakage

TABLE 2–4. Causes of Xanthochromia

Subarachnoid and intracerebral hemorrhage
Traumatic tap
Jaundice
Elevated protein level (>150 mg/dL)
Premature birth
Hypercarotenemia
Meningeal melanoma

---

xanthochromia of the CSF two to five days after the initial puncture.

Xanthochromia of the CSF refers to a pink, orange, or yellow color of the supernatant after the CSF has been centrifuged. Two to four hours after a subarachnoid hemorrhage, lysis of the RBCs occurs. This gives a pale orange color to the supernatant due to the release of oxyhemoglobin. Within 24 hours, hemoglobin is converted to bilirubin, giving a yellowish tint to the supernatant. Bilirhachia usually reaches a peak in about 36 hours and may persist for several weeks. There are other causes of xanthochromia in addition to subarachnoid hemorrhage, as shown in Table 2–4.[2]

Normal CSF does not clot; however, clotting may be seen when the CSF protein content is sharply elevated, as with Froin's syndrome and with a very bloody traumatic tap.

CELL COUNTS

The cell counts are performed in a counting chamber with undiluted CSF. Electronic cell counters should not be used for the CSF, as their precision is poor in the normal ranges. The normal mononuclear leukocyte counts are 0 to $5/\mu L$ in adults, 0 to $30/\mu L$ in children younger than 1 year of age, 0 to $20/\mu L$ in children 1 to 4 years of age, and 0 to $10/\mu L$ in children 5 years of age to puberty.[2,3] It should be pointed out, however, that there is no absolute agreement on the normal values for children.[4] In our experience, the upper limits of these figures for children are high. In a series of 153 specimens taken from children aged 6 months to 4 years, 95% had a leukocyte count of less than $6/\mu L$. For obvious reasons, it is difficult to arrive at a reliable set of normal CSF leukocyte values for children.

If a traumatic tap is suspected, a count of RBCs in the CSF may be used to correct CSF leukocyte counts or CSF protein determinations. This correction, however, is valid only if the cell count and the total protein concentration are determined for the same tube of CSF.[2] In addition, it should be noted that this correction is an approximation and is limited by any imprecision of the CSF RBC count. The following formula may be used:

$$W = WBC_f - \frac{WBC_b \times RBC_f}{RBC_b}$$

where:

  W = CSF leukocyte count before the blood was added

  WBC_f = total CSF leukocyte count

  RBC_f = total CSF RBC count

  RBC_b = RBC count in the blood

  WBC_b = leukocyte count in the blood

In general, with a normal peripheral blood cell count, this correction amounts to approximately 1 to 2 leukocytes per 1,000 RBCs.[2] Recent studies, however, suggest that both calculation and estimation methods for the correction of WBC counts in blood-contaminated CSF specimens usually overcorrect the counts.[5] Hence concern has been expressed that overreliance on the accuracy of such formulas may obscure an infectious process, and it has been recommended that all blood-contaminated CSF specimens be cultured as well.[6]

Similarly, a calculation of the true CSF protein content can be made in a traumatic tap by using a correction factor of 1 mg/dL for every 1,200 RBCs per microliter.[2] This is assuming, however, that the patient has a normal hematocrit reading and a normal serum protein level.

In recent in vitro studies, it was suggested that if the CSF specimen is not examined promptly after withdrawal, WBC lysis will give a false impression of the number of WBCs present.[7] When homologous blood was added to acellular samples of CSF in the same studies, it was found that 40% of the WBCs had lysed after two hours at room temperature.[7] At 4 °C, 15% of the WBCs had lysed. No significant lysis was seen of the RBCs. It is therefore recommended that cell counts be performed as soon as possible. If a delay is anticipated, the specimen should be refrigerated.

MICROSCOPIC EXAMINATION

Differential Count

A differential cell count should be performed on a stained smear made from the CSF. A "chamber differential" (performed in a counting chamber) is unsatisfactory, as one cannot be certain of the cell types present in a wet preparation. Furthermore, concentration of the CSF sample on a smear will provide a larger number of cells for study, and proper staining will allow an accurate identification of the cell types present. Recently many new techniques have been introduced to increase the cellular yield and provide satisfactory visualization of cell structure. These include filter techniques, sedimentation methods, and cytocentrifugation (all are discussed in Appendix A). It is recommended that stained smears be made for all CSF specimens even when the total cell count is within normal limits. When 0.5 mL of normal CSF is used, approximately 30 to 50 cells are obtained by the cytocentrifuge or sedimentation method.[8,9] Normal values are provided in Table 2–5.

Normal Cytology

A few RBCs are frequently found in the CSF due to contamination by blood from vessels injured during

TABLE 2–5. Normal CSF Differential Cell Count

CELL TYPE	ADULTS	NEONATES
Lymphocytes	60% ± 20%	20% ± 15%
Monocytes	30% ± 15%	70% ± 20%
Neutrophils	2% ± 4%	4% ± 4%*
Neuroectodermal cells	Rare	Rare

Note: Sedimentation or cytocentrifuge methods used. Data adapted from Krieg[2] and Sheth.[8] Used by permission.

*In high-risk neonates without meningitis, the CSF may have ± 60% neutrophils. Data from Sarff et al.[3]

the lumbar puncture. This finding is particularly common in infants. The CSF normally contains a small number of *lymphocytes* and *monocytes* (Figures 17 and 18). There is some disagreement, however, regarding the normal ratio of lymphocytes to monocytes, probably because of the different methods used in preparing the smears. Recent literature cites an approximate ratio of lymphocytes to monocytes of 70:30.[10] In young children, the CSF has a higher percentage of monocytes, and up to 80% may be a normal finding.[11] Reticulomonocytes, meningeal histiocytoid cells, and pia-arachnoid mesothelial cells are other terms used for monocytes in CSF. The origin of lymphocytes and monocytes in CSF is uncertain. Some researchers believe they originate from leptomeningeal stem cells, while others suspect that they originate from the blood.[10] Recent studies in animals indicate that lymphocytes and monocytes are capable of leaving the peripheral blood and appearing in the CSF.[12]

There is also disagreement as to whether *polymorphonuclear leukocytes* (PMNs) occur in normal CSF (Figure 19). The older literature indicates that any PMNs in the CSF are indicative of disease. However, since the introduction of new techniques for concentrating CSF specimens, there have been reports that a small number of PMNs may be present in normal CSF.[8] Our experience confirms this. Using the cytocentrifuge, a neutrophil count of up to 10% has been described as normal by one investigator.[5] The same investigator believes that the presence of PMNs is clinically significant only if the total leukocyte count exceeds 10/μL. It is possible that the neutrophils in CSF result from contamination by peripheral blood through a traumatic tap. In general, it is recommended

FIGURE 17. *Normal CSF with small, normal-appearing lymphocytes.*

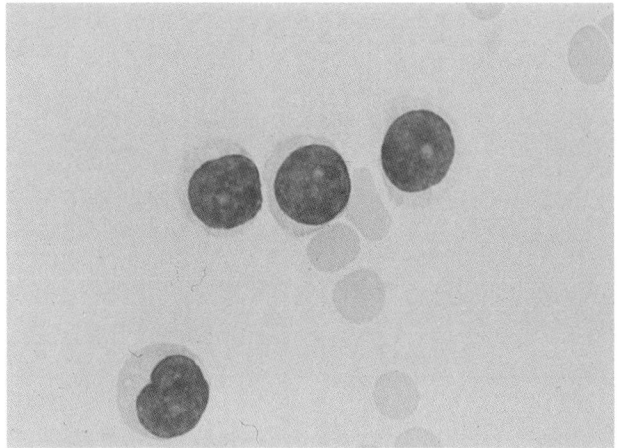

FIGURE 18. *Monocytes in CSF from a newborn.*

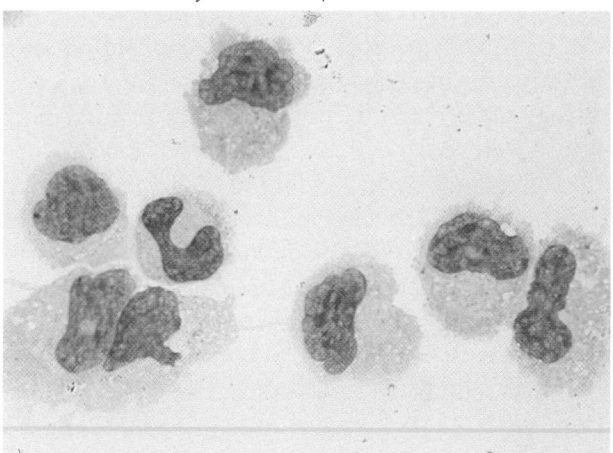

FIGURE 19. *Occasional polymorphonuclear leukocytes in a "normal" CSF specimen.*

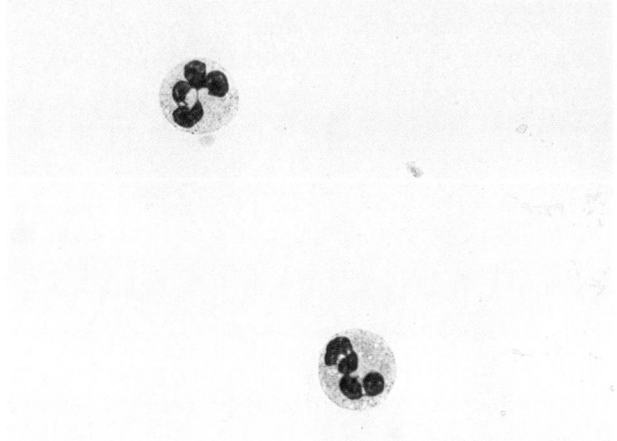

that one consider the presence of a small number of PMNs in the context of the clinical situation and the results of other laboratory tests.[2]

Ependymal cells from the ventricular lining and *choroid plexus cells* may occasionally be seen in both normal and abnormal CSF. From a cytologic viewpoint, it is difficult to differentiate between ependymal and choroid plexus cells.[10] Both are usually seen in clusters and are uniform in size, shape, and appearance. The nuclei are the size of small lymphocytes, while the cytoplasm is abundant, cloudy, and gray-blue. The nuclear chromatin is delicate (Figures 20 and 21). The ependymal and choroid plexus cells are more frequently seen in CSF obtained by cisternal or ventricular puncture than in CSF obtained by a lumbar puncture. They may be seen following trauma, surgery, pneumoencephalography, myelography, or ischemic infarction of the brain. It is important to be able to recognize these cells because they may be mistaken for malignant cells, but their presence is of little diagnostic value.[10,13]

Additional cell types that may be found in the normal CSF include *cartilage cells* and *bone marrow cells* (Figure 22).[12] The presence of such cells has no diagnostic significance and is the result of accidental puncture of the vertebral body. Bone marrow contamination of CSF is seen particularly in infants and in patients with vertebral bone abnormalities such as osteoporosis and kyphoscoliosis.[14] In rare cases, *squamous epithelial cells* from the skin and endothelial cells may be observed.

Abnormal Cytology

Lymphocytes in the CSF have a similar appearance to their counterparts in the blood and become transformed in a similar fashion when confronted by an antigen. Thus, a spectrum of lymphoid cells may be seen, including lymphocytes of varying sizes (Figure 23), plasmacytoid lymphocytes (Figure 24), plasma cells, immunoblasts, and lymphoblasts.[10,13] It may be difficult to identify the cells as lymphocytes when marked reactive changes occur. The stimulated, atypical, reactive, or transformed lymphocyte (immunocyte or immunoblast) is large and has basophilic cytoplasm and moderately coarse chromatin with one or more nucleoli (Figures 25 through 27). Atypical, reactive, or transformed lymphocytes are commonly

FIGURE 20.   *A cluster of choroid plexus cells in CSF.*

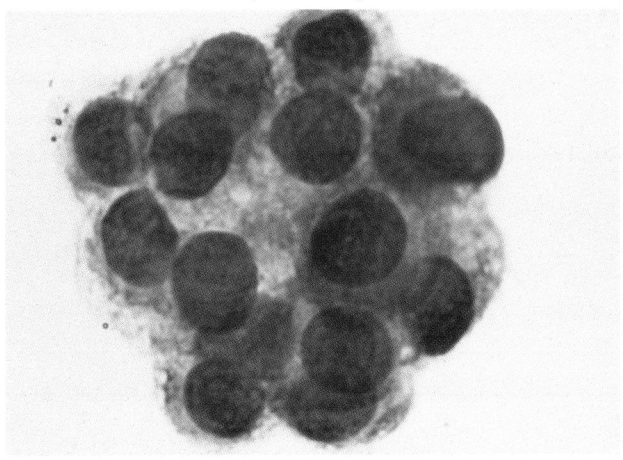

FIGURE 21.   *A cluster of ependymal cells in CSF.*

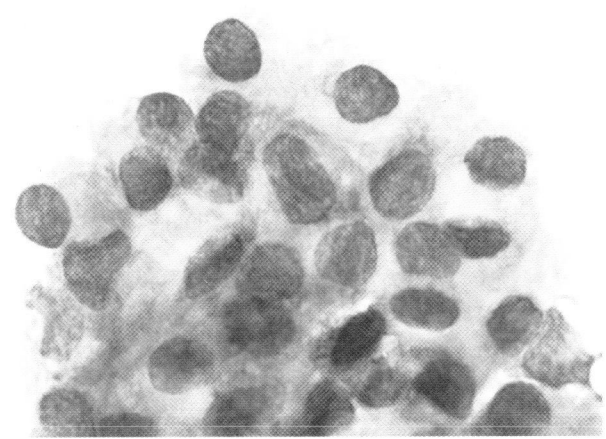

FIGURE 22.   *Normal bone marrow cells in CSF resulting from accidental puncture of a vertebral body.*

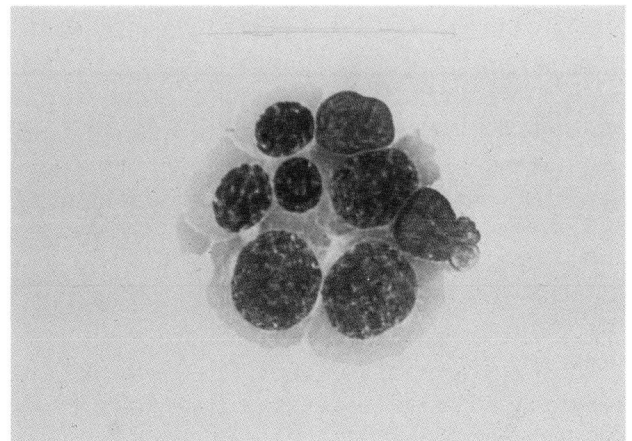

FIGURE 23.   *CSF lymphocytosis in viral meningitis.*

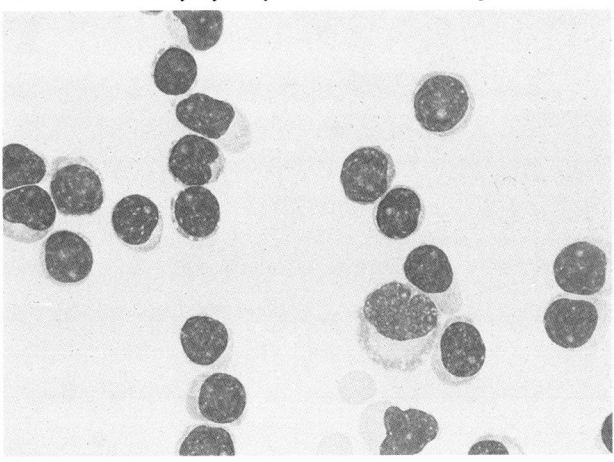

FIGURE 24.   *Lymphocytes and plasmacytoid lymphocytes in the CSF from a patient with multiple sclerosis.*

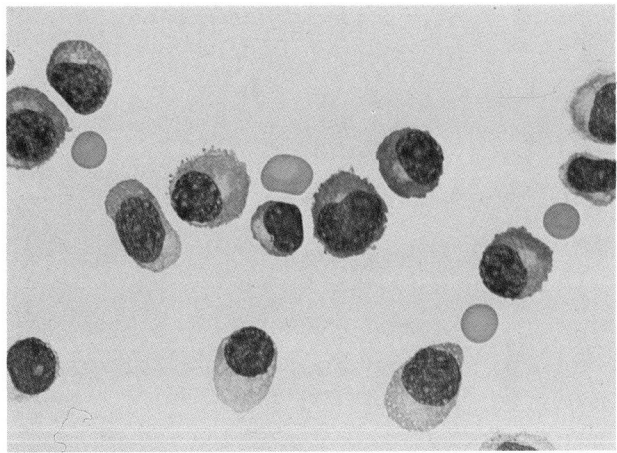

FIGURE 25.   *Transformed (atypical) lymphocyte in CSF.*

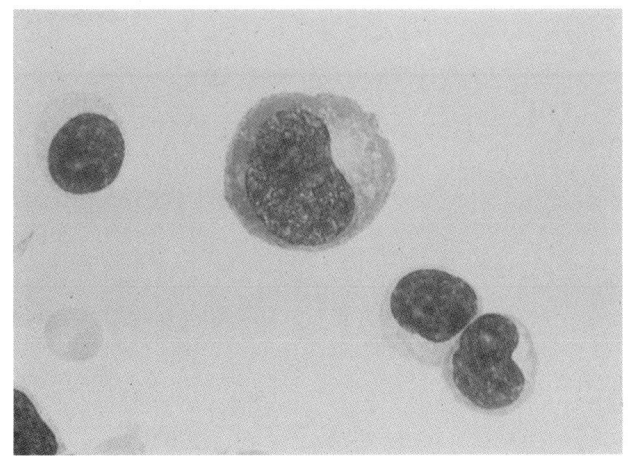

FIGURE 26. *CSF lymphocytosis in a partially treated case of bacterial meningitis. The large mononuclear cell (arrow) is a transformed lymphocyte or an immunoblast.*

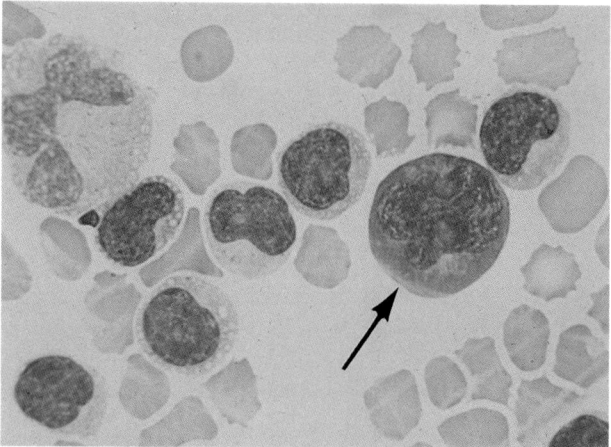

FIGURE 27. *Immunoblast in CSF.*

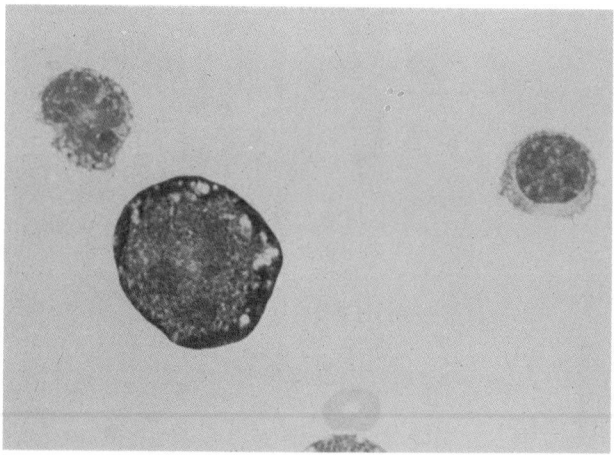

FIGURE 28. *Cluster of blast-like lymphocytes in CSF from a newborn.*

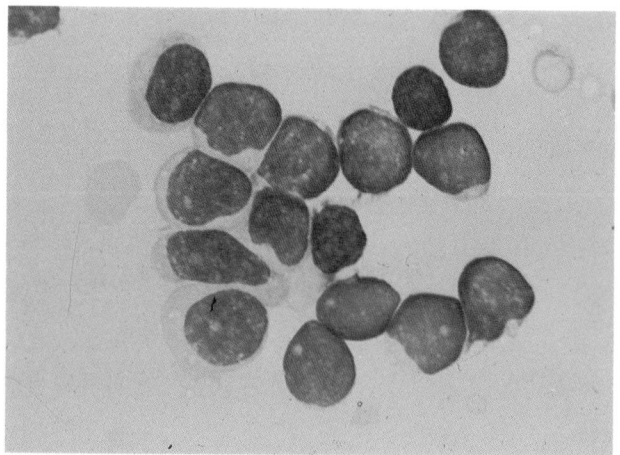

seen in patients with viral meningitis. The immature-appearing lymphocyte or lymphoblast has scant cytoplasm, a delicate chromatin pattern, and nucleoli that may or may not be prominent. Lymphoblasts may be noted in the CSF of newborns and neonates and should not be mistaken for leukemic cells (Figure 28). The most helpful feature in differentiating between benign lymphoid cells and malignant cells is the mixture of small, large, and transformed lymphocytes that is usually present in benign cases; malignant cells are more uniform. Lymphocytosis of the CSF is seen in a variety of infectious and noninfectious diseases (Table 2–6).[2] Cell surface-marker studies have shown that the lymphocyte populations (B and T cells) in the CSF parallel those seen in the peripheral blood. In inflammatory diseases, the CSF lymphocytes are primarily T-lymphocytes.[15–17]

Plasma cells are not seen in CSF specimens from normal patients, and their presence suggests an inflammatory process (Figure 29). They are seen particularly in patients with acute viral diseases and certain chronic inflammatory conditions such as tuberculosis, syphilis, sarcoidosis, subacute sclerosing panencephalitis, and multiple sclerosis.[10,13]

Monocytes, together with neutrophils and lymphocytes, are usually present in increased numbers in a variety of disorders (Table 2–7).[2,13] Such a mixed cell reaction is the usual presentation, while a pure monocytosis in the CSF is rarely seen.

Macrophages in CSF are thought to develop from pluripotent stem cells in the reticuloendothelial tissue of the leptomeninges and from monocytes.[10] Macrophages may be seen to phagocytose RBCs, leukocytes, other macrophages, microorganisms, pigments, and lipids.[13] The material that has been phagocytosed is acted upon by enzymes. Material that cannot be utilized by the macrophage is often stored in the cytoplasm in the form of vacuoles, which may fuse and push the nucleus to the periphery, forming a so-called signet ring cell (Figure 30). Such cells may measure up to 100 μm in diameter.[13]

Hemorrhage is associated with the appearance of neutrophils and many macrophages; the latter phagocytose RBCs within a few hours (Figure 31).

The phagocytosed RBCs rapidly lose their color and appear as empty vacuoles in the cytoplasm of the macrophages (Figure 32). After approximately four

TABLE 2–6. Causes of CSF Lymphocytic Pleocytosis

Viral meningoencephalitis
Aseptic meningitis
Tuberculous meningoencephalitis (mixed-cell reaction)
Partially treated bacterial meningitis
Syphilitic meningoencephalitis
Leptospiral meningitis (often mixed-cell reaction)
Fungal meningitis (mixed-cell reaction)
Parasitic disease
Multiple sclerosis
Guillain-Barré syndrome
Polyneuritis
Sarcoidosis of meninges

Note: Data adapted from Krieg.[2] Used by permission.

TABLE 2–7. Causes of CSF Monocytic Pleocytosis*

Chronic bacterial meningitis
Partially treated bacterial meningitis
Syphilitic meningoencephalitis
Viral meningoencephalitis
Fungal meningitis
Leptospiral meningitis
Amebic encephalomyelitis
CNS hemorrhage
Cerebral infarct
Multiple sclerosis
Reaction to foreign material
CNS malignant conditions

Note: Data adapted from Krieg.[2] Used by permission.

*Monocytic pleocytosis is usually associated with mixed-cell reactions.

FIGURE 29. *Plasma cells in CSF sample from a patient with syphilis.*

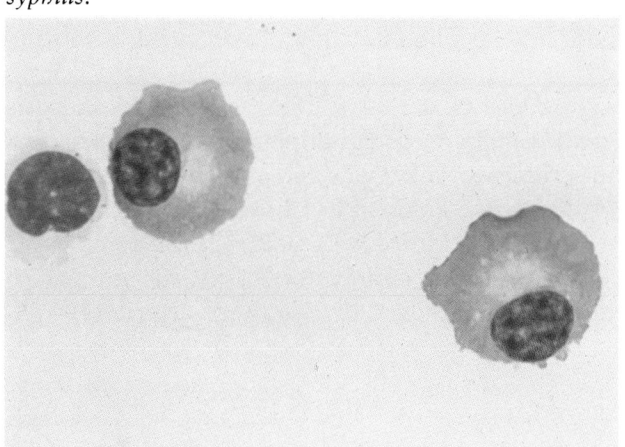

FIGURE 30. *Signet-ring cell macrophage in CSF.*

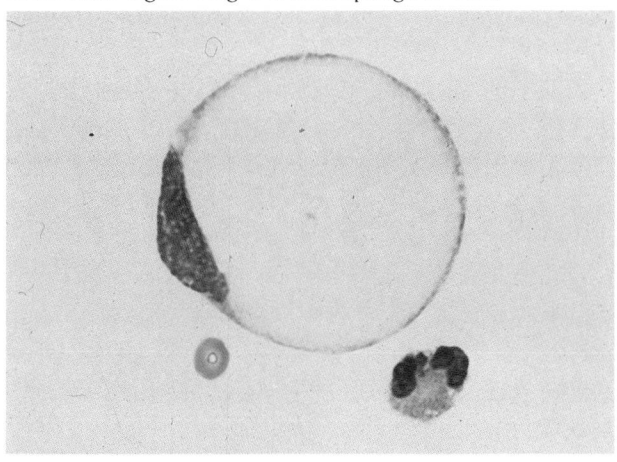

FIGURE 31. *Erythrophagocytosis by macrophage in CSF.*

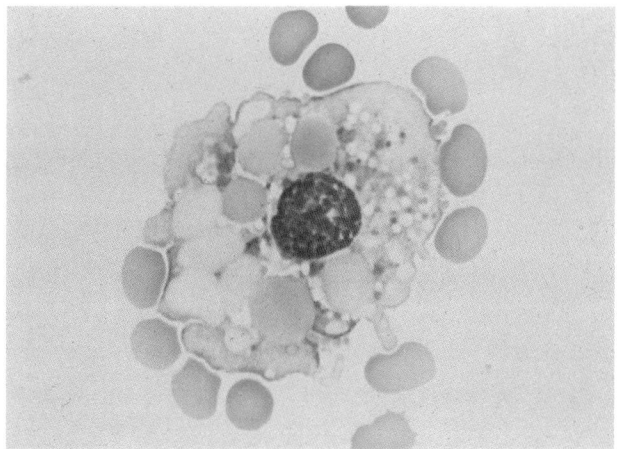

FIGURE 32. *Macrophage in CSF with phagocytosed RBCs appearing as empty holes, and hemosiderin pigment.*

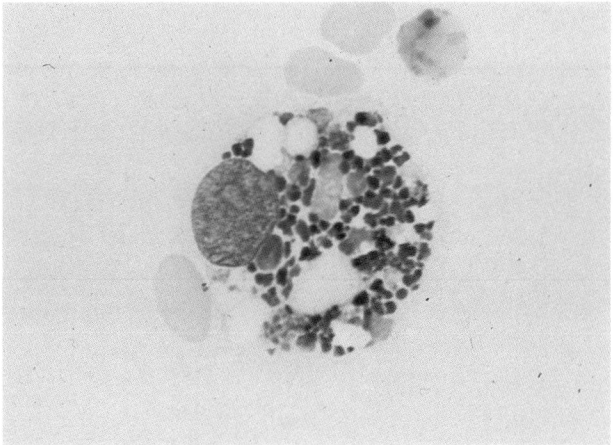

FIGURE 33. *Macrophage in CSF with hemosiderin (bluish-black) pigment and hematoidin pigment (yellow crystals).*

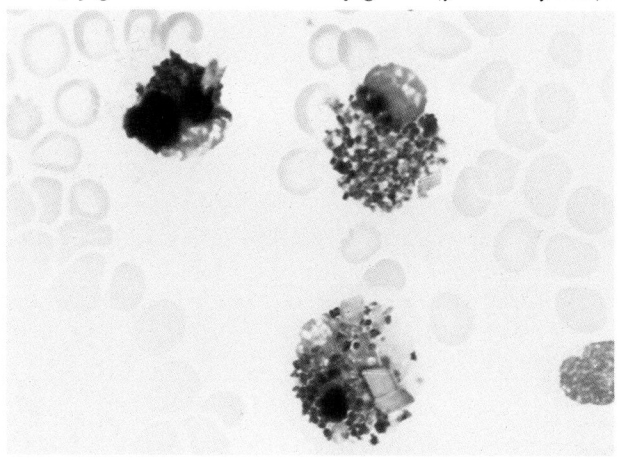

FIGURE 34. *Macrophage in CSF containing hemosiderin (siderophage) as demonstrated with an iron stain.*

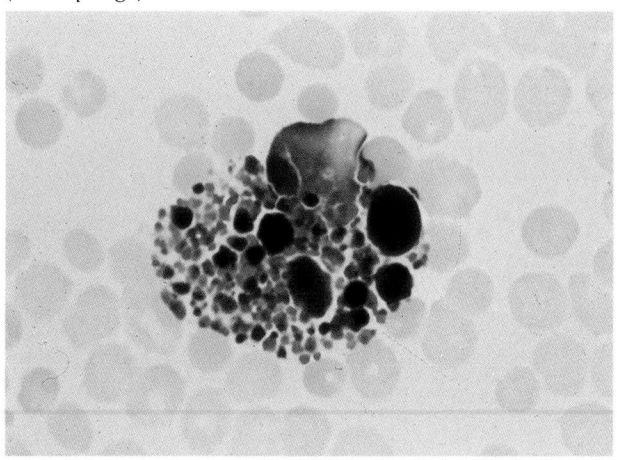

FIGURE 35. *Several siderophages in CSF sample from a patient with repeated intracerebral hemorrhages.*

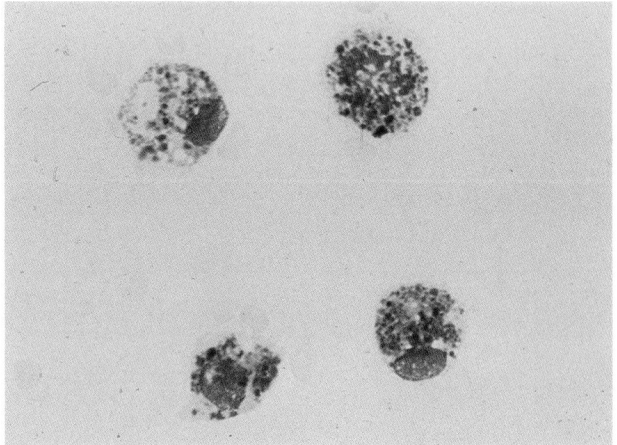

days, hemosiderin is seen as dark brown or black granules (Figure 32).[10,13] Later, hematoidin pigment may be seen as brownish yellow or sometimes red crystals (Figure 33). The presence of iron within a macrophage (siderophage) may be demonstrated with an iron stain (Figure 34). The presence of several such siderophages is usually a good indication that hemorrhage has occurred (Figure 35). Siderophages may still be present several months after hemorrhage occurred.[13] The presence of a single macrophage showing erythrophagocytosis is not an absolute indicator of hemorrhage. Erythrophagocytosis may also occur in vitro or may be caused by blood contamination of the CSF from a puncture repeated eight to 12 hours following the initial lumbar puncture.[13] However, large numbers of macrophages showing erythrophagocytosis and several siderophages are good evidence that pathologic hemorrhage has occurred. Furthermore, the presence of erythrophagocytosis and siderophages in the CSF specimen taken a week or more after the initial hemorrhage is highly suggestive of recurrent hemorrhage.[13] The changes in CSF following hemorrhage are summarized in Table 2–8.

Lipophages or macrophages containing fat may be seen in traumatic or liquefaction necrosis associated with cerebral infarcts and following myelography (Figure 36). Macrophages may also be observed in the CSF following pneumoencephalography, intrathecal therapy, and irradiation of the brain.[13]

Neutrophils may be seen in increased numbers in a variety of infectious and noninfectious disorders of the CNS (Table 2–9). The cytoplasmic granules of the PMNs are often less prominent than in the blood and show rapid disintegration upon standing (Figures 37 and 38).[10,13] The latter may result in an inaccurate differential cell count.

Eosinophils are rarely seen in normal CSF. Increased numbers of eosinophils have been described in a variety of infectious and noninfectious disorders (Table 2–10, Figure 39).[18] In our experience, eosinophils are associated with malfunctioning shunts. So-called idiopathic eosinophilic meningitis without evidence of a pathogen has also been described.[19]

Basophils are not seen in normal CSF but may be found in small numbers in a variety of abnormal conditions (Figure 39). Such conditions include inflammatory diseases, foreign body reactions, parasitic

TABLE 2–8. Changes in CSF Following Hemorrhage

Gross Examination

2–12 hours	Pink to orange xanthochromia
12–24 hours	Yellow xanthochromia (disappears in 2–4 weeks)

Microscopic Examination

2–24 hours	Erythrocytes, neutrophilic granulocytes (30% to 60%), mononuclear phagocytes, lymphocytes
12–48 hours	Mononuclear phagocytes, erythrophagocytosis, lymphocytes
48 hours	Mononuclear phagocytes, erythrophagocytosis, siderophages (may persist for 2–8 weeks)

Note: Data adapted from Oehmichen.[13] Used by permission.

TABLE 2–9. Causes of CSF Neutrophilic Pleocytosis

Bacterial meningitis
Early viral meningoencephalitis
Early tuberculous and mycotic meningitis
Amebic encephalomyelitis
Aseptic meningitis
Cerebral abscess, subdural empyema
CNS hemorrhage
Cerebral infarct
Malignant conditions
Previous lumbar puncture
Myelography, pneumoencephalography
Intrathecal injection of drugs

Note: Data adapted from Krieg.[2] Used by permission.

TABLE 2–10. Causes of CSF Eosinophilic Pleocytosis

Common Causes
Parasitic infections
Fungal infections
Idiopathic eosinophilic meningitis
Reaction to foreign material in CNS (drugs, shunts)
Acute polyneuritis

Rare Causes
Bacterial meningitis
Tuberculous meningoencephalitis
Viral meningitis
Leukemia, lymphoma
Primary brain tumors

Note: Data adapted from Krieg.[2] Used by permission.

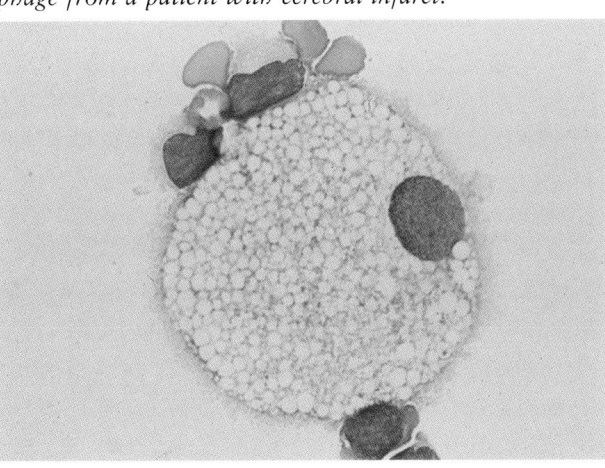

FIGURE 36. *Macrophage in CSF sample containing lipophage from a patient with cerebral infarct.*

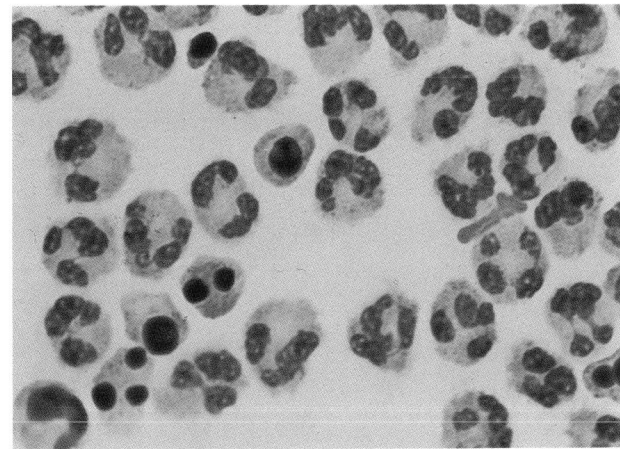

FIGURE 37. *Neutrophils in CSF sample from a patient with bacterial meningitis. Degenerating cells with pyknotic nuclei may be mistaken for nucleated RBCs.*

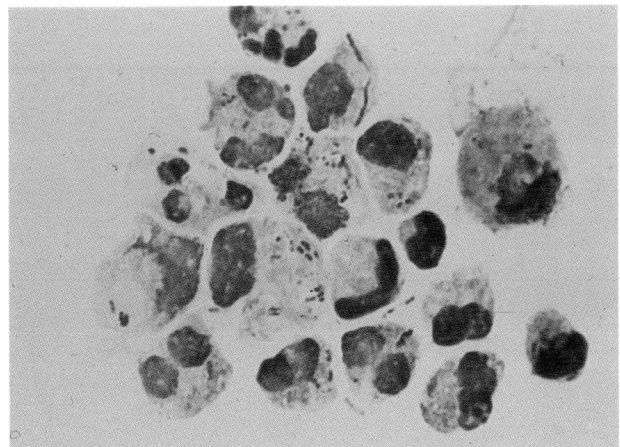

FIGURE 38. *Degenerating neutrophils in the CSF, with intracellular bacteria, showing poor staining characteristics.*

FIGURE 39. *Eosinophils and two basophils in CSF sample from a patient with malfunctioning intracranial shunt.*

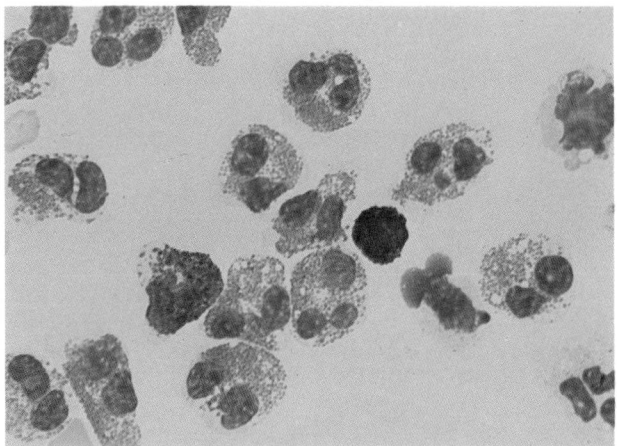

FIGURE 40. *Numerous neutrophils in CSF sample from a patient with bacterial meningitis.*

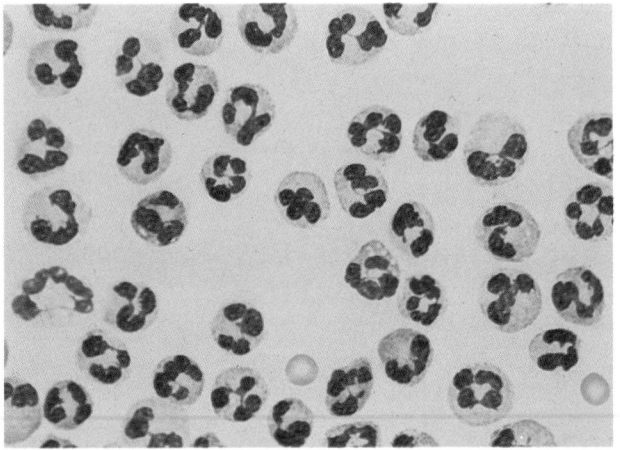

FIGURE 41. *Gram's stain showing intracellular gram-negative bacteria in CSF from a patient with* Hemophilus influenzae *meningitis.*

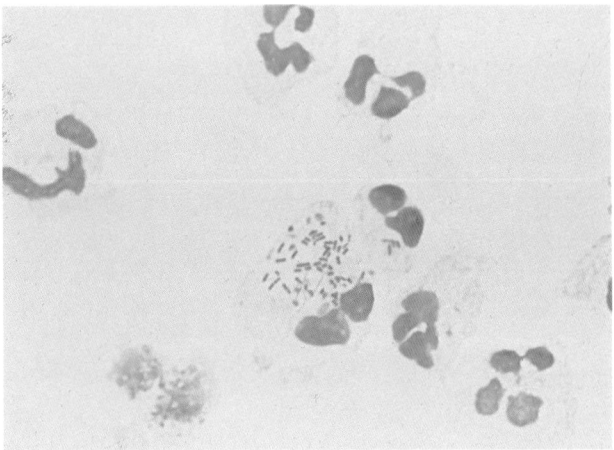

infections, convulsive disorders, and chronic granulocytic leukemia. Cases of basophilic meningitis associated with malignant lymphoma have been reported.[20]

Lupus erythematosus cells are rarely seen in the CSF.[21]

Malignant cells from a variety of neoplasms may be encountered in the CSF.[22,23] A CSF examination is particularly valuable in the diagnosis of metastatic carcinoma, leukemic and lymphomatous involvement of the meninges, and certain primary CNS tumors.[24] Of the primary CNS tumors, medulloblastoma is more likely to be associated with malignant cells in the CSF than are gliomas and meningiomas.[10,13] When cells from metastatic tumors are detected in the CNS, melanoma and carcinoma of the lung, breast, and gastrointestinal tract are the most common primary tumors.[10,13] Malignant cells in the CSF may occur singly or, more frequently, in clumps. Clumps of ependymal cells or choroid plexus cells, atypical lymphoid cells, and macrophages may be mistaken occasionally for tumor cells.

Immunoenzymatic studies using immunoalkaline phosphatase or immunoperoxidase techniques performed on cytocentrifuge preparations may be very helpful in the diagnosis. *Glial fibrillary acidic protein* (GFAP), which appears to be a building block of a type of intermediate filament, is found in normal and neoplastic astrocytes and ependymal cells. A positive reaction to GFAP is seen in tumor cells from patients with astrocytoma, glioblastoma, and ependymoma. Negative staining of tumor cells with anti-GFAP and positive staining with antikeratin or carcinoembryonic antigen suggests metastatic carcinoma to the brain.

CLINICAL CORRELATIONS

In *bacterial meningitis,* the leukocyte count may be higher than 50,000/µL; in the early stages of the disease, more than 90% of these leukocytes are neutrophils (Figure 40). In the very early stages of meningococcal meningitis, however, the PMN count may be as small as 10%. In addition to neutrophils, moderate numbers of lymphocytes, monocytes, and macrophages are seen. Successful treatment with antibiotics is usually associated with the rapid disappearance of neutrophils, while monocytes and macrophages become more prominent. Pathogenic organisms are often identified using a Gram stain (Figures 41 and 42). In some cases, intracellular organisms are also easily identified with the routine Wright's stain (Figure 43). Occasionally, leukocytosis of the CSF may persist despite successful antibiotic therapy. Such persistent pleocytosis is particularly associated with *Hemophilus influenzae* meningitis.[25]

Bacterial meningitis without CSF pleocytosis may be seen, particularly in patients with a defective host defense mechanism.[26] In addition to the absence of pleocytosis, the CSF glucose and protein may initially be normal in some cases of bacterial meningitis, and there may be delayed growth of the organism in cultures. It is recommended that the CSF be very carefully examined for gram-positive and gram-negative organisms, and, if clinically indicated, another lumbar puncture be performed.

Viral meningitis may be associated with mild or severe leukocytosis that is predominantly composed of lymphocytes. It is important to note, however, that neutrophils may predominate initially (Figure 44). This granulocytic phase may last from a few hours to several days. Many different types of medium-sized and large reactive lymphocytes are encountered (Figure 45). The reactive lymphocytes must be differentiated from lymphoblasts seen in acute lymphoblastic leukemia (ALL). In ALL, the lymphoblasts are generally uniform in size, shape, and appearance, while in reactive lymphocytosis, many different types of lymphocytes are present. Reactive lymphocytes have more cytoplasm and more clumped nuclear chromatin than do lymphoblasts in ALL. In the later stages of viral meningitis, lymphocytes decrease in number, while monocytes and macrophages become more evident.

Approximately 80% of the patients with untreated *acute lymphoblastic leukemia* (ALL) and approximately 60% of the patients with acute myeloblastic leukemia have leukemic cells in the CSF at some stage of the disease (Figures 46 and 47). With the increasing length of survival in patients receiving treatment, however, the incidence of relapse with CNS involvement has increased. High-risk factors associated with meningeal involvement include a high WBC count, youth, and splenomegaly. Therefore, CSF specimens should be examined in all patients with acute leuke-

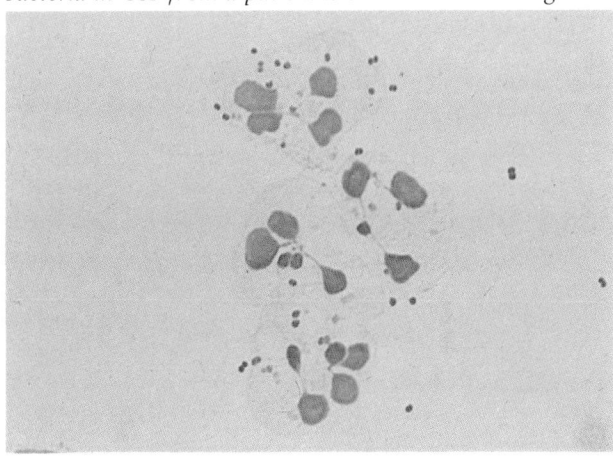

FIGURE 42. *Gram's stain showing numerous gram-negative bacteria in CSF from a patient with* Neisseria meningitidis.

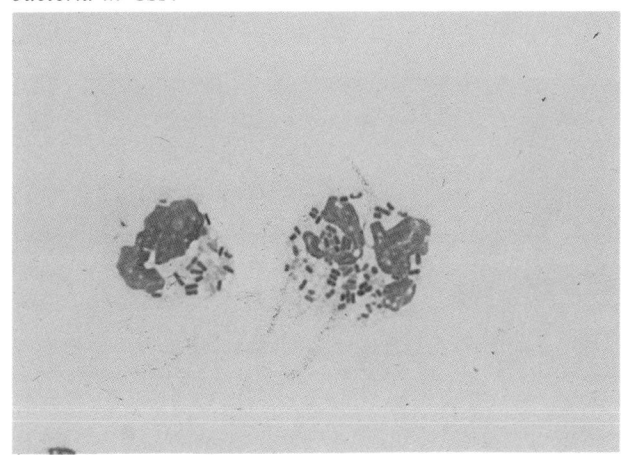

FIGURE 43. *Bacterial meningitis with multiple intracellular bacteria in CSF.*

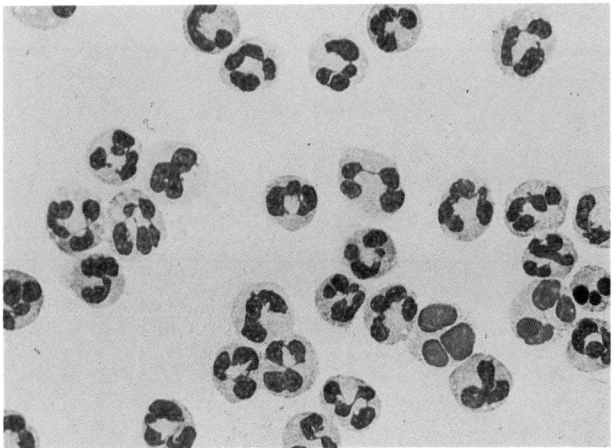

FIGURE 44. *A predominance of neutrophils in the CSF seen in the early phase in this patient with viral meningitis.*

FIGURE 45. *A spectrum of reactive (transformed) lymphocytes seen in the CSF in viral meningitis.*

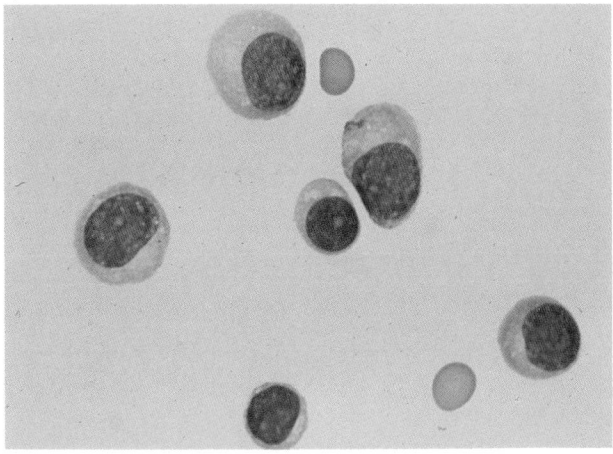

FIGURE 46. *Acute lymphoblastic leukemia in CSF. Note the uniformity of the blast cells.*

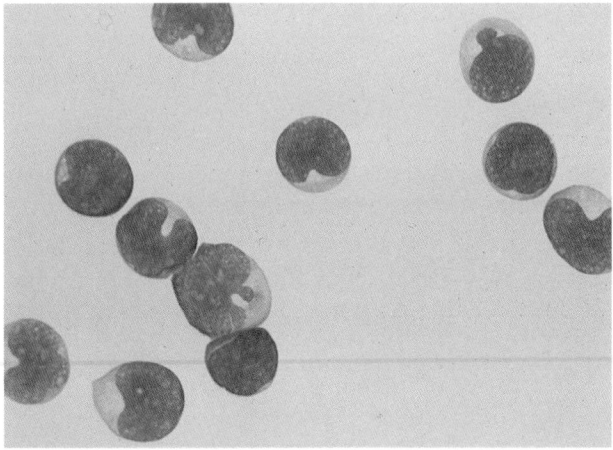

FIGURE 47. *Acute myeloblastic leukemia in CSF. Easily identifiable myeloblasts are seen.*

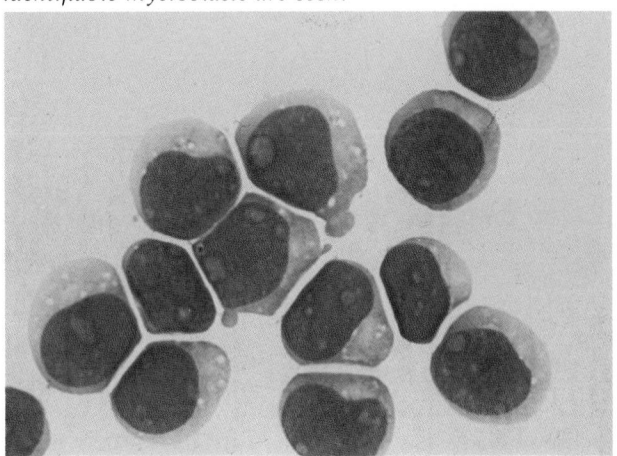

mia.[27–29] The treatment of ALL now includes skull irradiation combined with intrathecal chemotherapy or intrathecal drug therapy alone to eradicate any meningeal leukemia.

When many blasts are present in the smear, making a correct diagnosis is usually not difficult. The uniformity of the leukemic cells is the characteristic feature (Figures 46 and 47). However, when only a few cells are present, it may be extremely difficult to distinguish leukemic cells from atypical or activated lymphocytes or, sometimes, from atypical monocytes.[30] It should be emphasized that an elevated CSF leukocyte count does not necessarily mean that leukemia is present, nor does a normal cell count exclude leukemic infiltration.[27,28] An occasional lymphoblast is present in diseases other than leukemia; as mentioned, viral, bacterial, and fungal meningitis may be associated with lymphoblast-like cells in the CSF. Irradiation of the brain and intrathecal chemotherapy may also be associated with atypical mononuclear cells.

The CSF may be contaminated with peripheral blood during the puncture, and, occasionally, bone marrow may be aspirated from puncture of a vertebral body (Figure 22). The problem with contamination is especially great in specimens prepared by filtration. The filter method is extremely efficient in collecting a small number of lymphoblasts, and the telltale erythrocytes are lysed by alcohol. A false-positive diagnosis of leukemia may be avoided if the diagnosis of leukemia is made only in the presence of an increased total cell count, and only when immature or abnormal cells constitute at least 40% to 60% of the total cell population.[27] If leukemia is to be diagnosed correctly, it is essential that the specimen be adequate (greater than 2 mL) and the cells be well preserved.

Cytochemical studies using peroxidase and esterase stains may be helpful in the diagnosis (Figure 48). Terminal deoxynucleotidyl transferase (TdT), a DNA polymerase enzyme, is present in lymphoblasts from all patients with the non-B, non-T common ALL type and in most T-cell ALL but is rarely positive in lymphoblasts from the rare B-cell ALL[31] (Figure 49). It is very unusual for TdT to be present in blasts from patients with acute myeloblastic leukemia, and TdT is not present in reactive CSF mononuclear leukocytes. The identification of TdT may be very useful in identifying ALL cells in the CSF, even when cell counts are below 10/cu mm.[32] Terminal deoxynucleotidyl transferase is identified in cold absolute methanol–fixed smears, using an immunofluorescent or immunoperoxidase procedure. A careful correlation of clinical, cytologic, and immunologic findings is essential in each case.

In contrast to acute leukemias, involvement of CNS with chronic lymphocytic and myelogenous leukemia is distinctly unusual (Figure 50).

Tumor cells in CSF indicate that the leptomeninges have been seeded widely by tumor. This applies to metastatic and primary CNS tumors (Figures 51 through 57). Malignant cells are usually not seen in the CSF when the tumor is limited to the brain and the pial membrane has not been broken.[33]

Small-cell carcinoma of the lung (oat cell carcinoma) may be differentiated from acute leukemia by the former's tendency to form cell clusters and by the presence of more cytoplasm (Figure 58). Medulloblastoma and metastatic neuroblastoma cells resemble lymphoblasts, but clustering of cells with nuclear molding by adjacent cells and rosette formation are typical of these tumors.[27] The rosette formation, however, may not be apparent in smears of CSF.

Leptomeningeal involvement has been reported in 5% to 27% of the patients with diffuse *non-Hodgkin's lymphoma*.[34–36] It has been suggested that lymphoma cells spread directly from the medullary cavity along tissue planes through the dura and subarachnoid space.[34] The most common lymphomas with CNS involvement are lymphoblastic lymphoma (Figure 59), diffuse large-cell ("histiocytic") lymphoma, and small non-cleaved cell (undifferentiated Burkitt's) lymphoma. Involvement of the CNS in nodular lymphomas, small-lymphocytic (well-differentiated) lymphomas, and Hodgkin's disease is uncommon. Since lymphoblastic and small non-cleaved cell lymphomas are the most common types of malignant lymphoma in childhood, children have a relatively high incidence of CNS involvement.

Morphologically, the lymphoblastic lymphomas, when involving the CSF, have an appearance identical to ALL. The small non-cleaved lymphomas are characterized by intermediate-sized lymphocytes having moderately abundant, deep blue–staining cytoplasm (Wright's stain) containing vacuoles and a nucleus with slightly clumped chromatin pattern and one or several prominent nucleoli (Figure 60). A cytologic

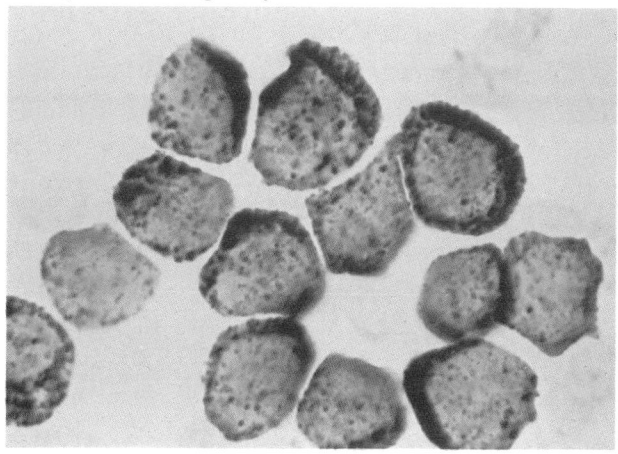

FIGURE 48. *Blast cells clearly identified as myeloblasts in CSF specimen using the peroxidase stain.*

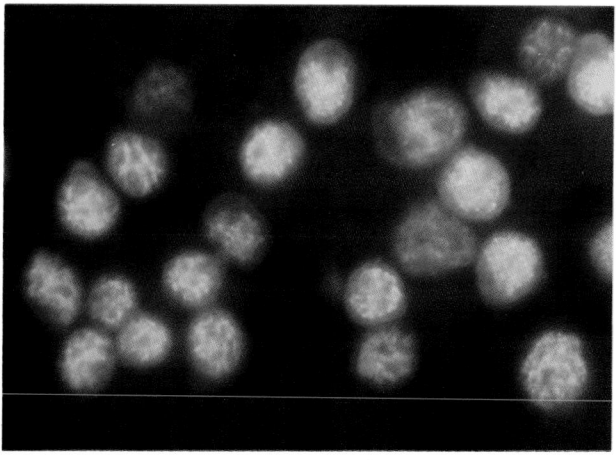

FIGURE 49. *Terminal deoxynucleotidyl transferase is seen on nuclei of blast cells from a patient with acute lymphoblastic leukemia (immunofluorescent method).*

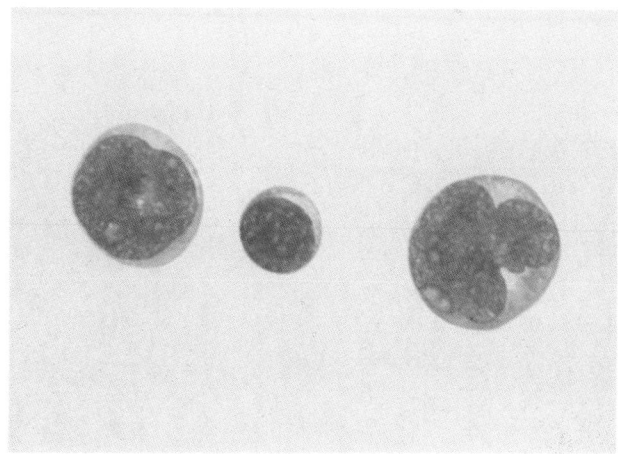

FIGURE 50. *Two blasts and one small lymphocyte in CSF sample from a patient with chronic myelocytic leukemia in blast crisis.*

FIGURE 51. *Glioblastoma cells in CSF.*

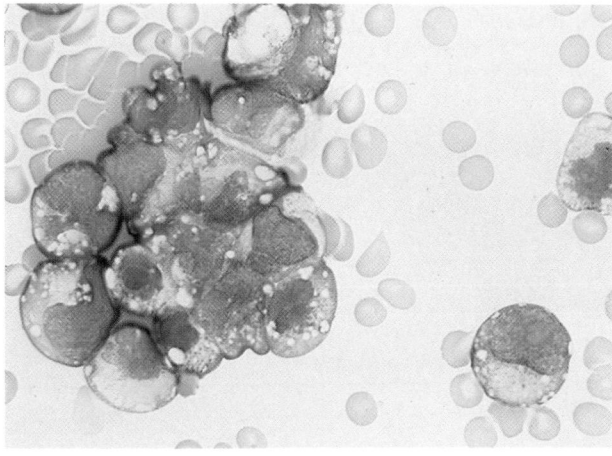

FIGURE 52. *Clustering of malignant cells in CSF in a patient with medulloblastoma.*

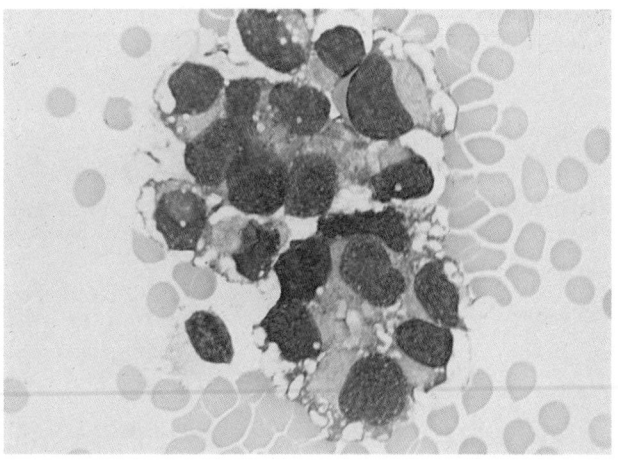

FIGURE 53. *Clump of cells in CSF specimen from a patient with metastatic neuroblastoma resembling metastatic oat cell carcinoma.*

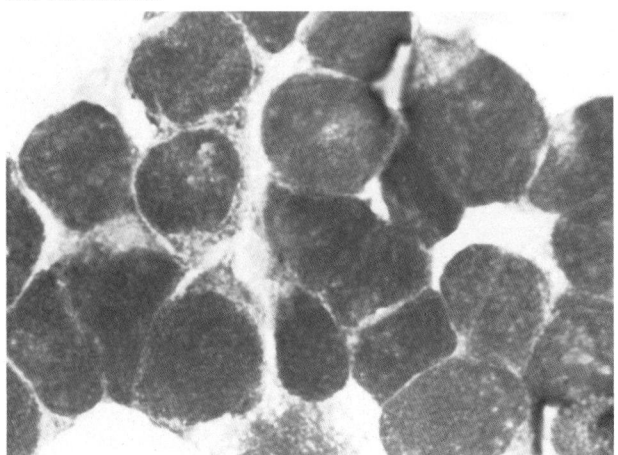

FIGURE 54. *Metastatic rhabdomyosarcoma cells in CSF sample from a patient with primary tumor in the eye.*

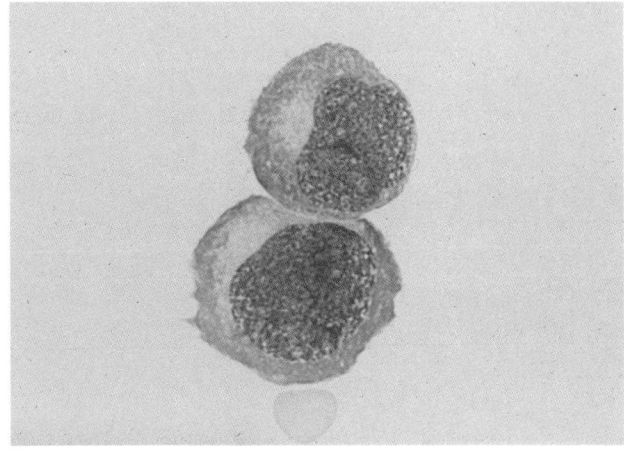

FIGURE 55. *Typical "cannonball" formation of metastatic breast carcinoma.*

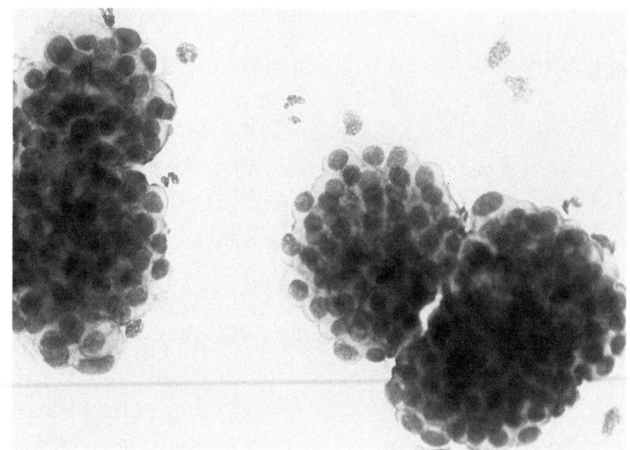

FIGURE 56. *Higher-power view of breast tumor cells seen in Figure 55.*

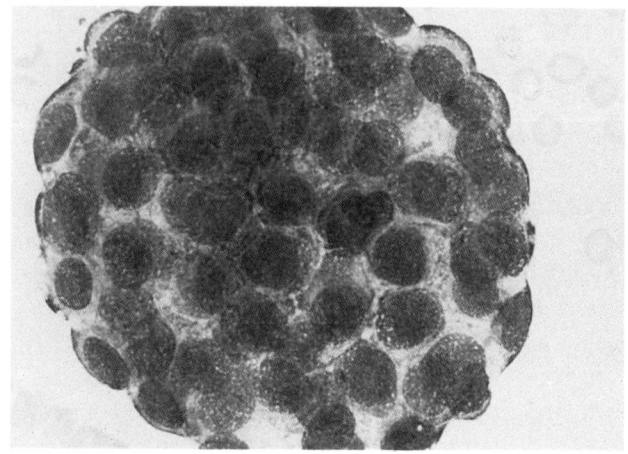

evaluation of the CSF is the most useful test for diagnosis and for monitoring response to therapy.

As with acute leukemias, in malignant lymphomas there is danger of a false-positive diagnosis, particularly when only a few cells are present. The presence of atypical, reactive, or activated lymphocytes may be mistaken for a large-cell lymphoma. Immunologic cell markers may be useful in the diagnosis of malignant lymphomas. Almost all small non-cleaved cell lymphomas and many large-cell lymphomas have monoclonal B-cell markers, and the TdT enzyme can be identified in all lymphoblastic lymphomas. The major problem in performing studies for immunologic markers on cells from CSF is that the number of cells obtained is frequently inadequate.

Iatrogenic conditions should also be considered when making diagnoses based on laboratory examination of the CSF. When a lumbar puncture has been repeated eight to 12 hours after the initial puncture, the CSF may contain increased numbers of neutrophils, monocytes, macrophages, and occasional macrophages showing erythrophagocytosis.[13]

Pneumoencephalography and myelography may lead to pleocytosis consisting of lymphocytes, neutrophils, monocytes, macrophages, and eosinophils in varying numbers. An increased number of monocytes and macrophages may be present for two to three weeks after the procedure is performed.[13]

Intracranial shunts for hydrocephalus may be associated with monocytosis and increased numbers of macrophages and eosinophils (see Figure 39).[13] The eosinophilic pleocytosis in particular may be striking and may represent an allergic reaction to the shunt.

Neonatal intracranial hemorrhage, which includes subdural, primary subarachnoid, intracerebellar, and periventricular (intraventricular and/or intracerebral) hemorrhage, has become an important neurologic disturbance, particularly in premature infants. Subdural hemorrhage, which is caused by trauma, is now uncommon due to advances in obstetrics technology. Primary subarachnoid hemorrhage is relatively common but is usually not clinically significant. Intracerebellar hemorrhage may be seen in 15% to 25% of premature infants at autopsy. More recently, periventricular hemorrhage has become recognized as a major clinical entity in the premature infant. In the great majority of patients, the periventricular hem-

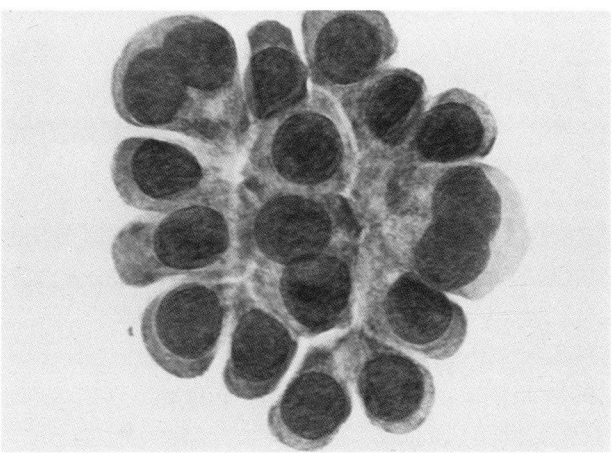

FIGURE 57. *Another cytologic appearance of metastatic breast carcinoma cells in the CSF.*

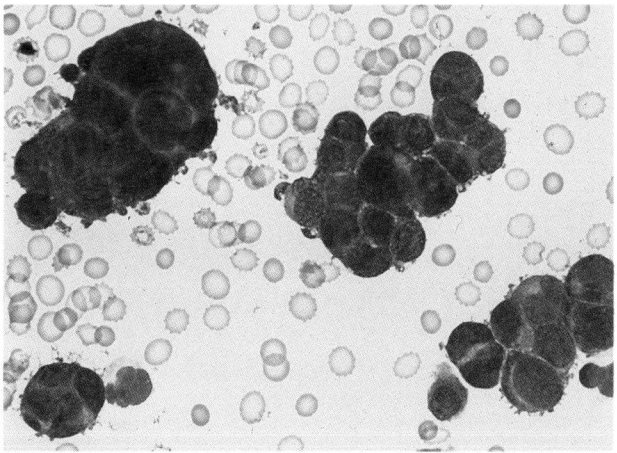

FIGURE 58. *Characteristic clumping of cells and molding of nuclei in metastatic oat cell carcinoma of the lung.*

FIGURE 59. *Lymphoblastic lymphoma involving the CSF. The cells are similar to those seen in acute lymphoblastic leukemia but, as illustrated here, usually have more nuclear convolutions.*

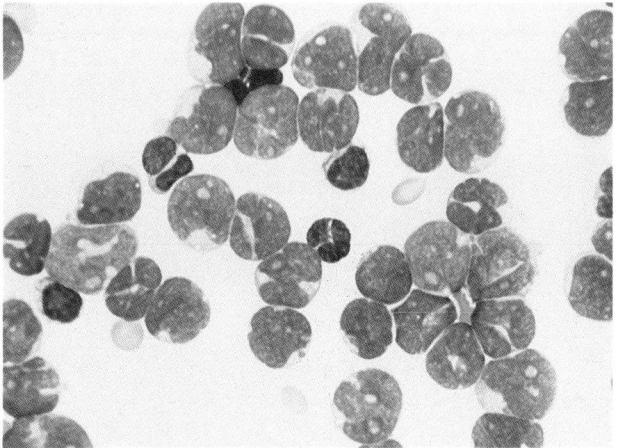

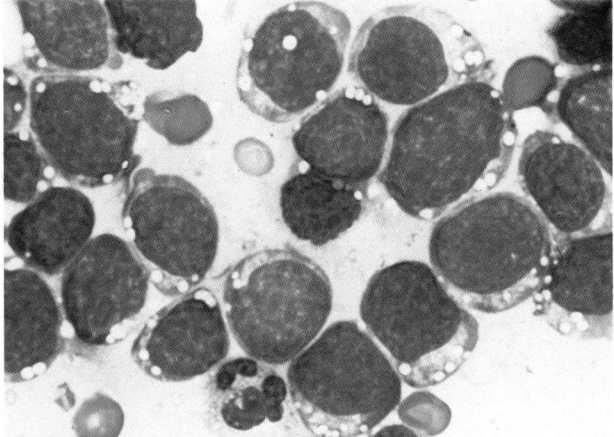

FIGURE 60. *Burkitt's lymphoma in the CSF. The cells are characterized by blue cytoplasm with vacuoles and slightly clumped chromatin pattern.*

orrhages occur in the ventricular system. Therapy for intraventricular hemorrhage may include daily lumbar punctures to lower the intracranial pressure, to remove blood and protein, and to reduce the incidence of obstruction in the flow of CSF.

CHEMICAL ANALYSIS

Protein

The CSF contains less than 1% of the amount of protein found in plasma. The normal concentration of lumbar CSF total protein is most often quoted as 15 to 45 mg/dL. However, these figures are not rigid, and reliable reference intervals vary considerably, depending on the method of analysis. As a result, an upper level of 60 mg/dL has been reported for the ultraviolet spectrophotometric method.[2] In addition, age is an important variable. Newborns have relatively high CSF protein values, which compare with adult levels only after about three to six months. A recent study, involving high-risk neonates without meningitis, showed mean levels of 90 mg/dL for term infants and 115 mg/dL for preterm infants, with an upper level of 170 mg/dL.[3] Although the reasons for these high levels are not fully known, altered permeability of the blood-CSF barrier is the favored explanation. The total protein level slowly increases after the age of 40 years to a normal range of 30 to 60 mg/dL at 60 years and older.[2,37] These figures refer only to spinal fluid removed through a lumbar puncture. Cisternal and ventricular fluids have lower levels of total protein.[2]

Elevation of the total protein level is the most frequent pathologic finding in CSF examination. This elevation is nonspecific but is indicative of meningeal or CNS disease. Hence, elevations are seen in inflammatory processes, tumors, degenerative disorders, subarachnoid hemorrhage, and traumatic taps.[2] Mild elevations have also been reported with long-term administration of certain drugs, particularly the phenothiazines.

Levels of CSF protein below 15 mg/dL have been reported in some normal children older than 6 months of age, in cases of water intoxication associated with increased intracranial pressure, and in some leukemic patients. Low CSF protein levels have also been associated with CSF leakage from a dural tear, CSF rhinorrhea or otorrhea, hyperthyroidism, and some instances in which large amounts of fluid have been removed for pneumoencephalography and the CSF is diluted from the cisterna magna.[2]

Accurate determination of CSF protein levels is hampered by several factors, including the low concentration of protein, the presence of different types of protein (mainly albumin and globulin), and the small amount of fluid usually available for analysis. Many different methods have been used for quantitative estimation. The most common methods in use are *turbidimetric procedures* involving such agents as sulfosalicylic acid. These procedures are popular since they are rapid and easily performed and use instruments that are readily available. They are reasonably accurate but are deficient in that albumin is about four times more turbid than a comparable amount of globulin.[38] Another problem with these methods is that there is a linear relationship between temperature and turbidity; hence, reasonably constant temperature control is essential. In methods that combine sulfosalicylic acid and sodium sulfate or use trichloroacetic acid, reactions with albumin and globulin are more similar. Albumin should not be used as a standard when using turbidimetric methods.[38]

Some of the same difficulties are encountered in most of the *colorimetric techniques,* along with another problem: the reagent used often reacts with nonprotein nitrogenous substances. Although the Lowry[39] method's reliability is least affected by varying albumin-globulin ratios, a serious drawback exists in the interference from nonprotein compounds. Nevertheless, this is the generally accepted method with which others are compared. Bradford[40] recently published a protein-dye binding technique using Coomassie Brilliant blue G-250 that is both rapid and highly sensitive. The reliability of this method for estimating CSF total protein was subsequently questioned on the basis of apparent variations in color yield seen with pure proteins, as well as wider standard deviations than those seen with the Lowry method.[41] However, several recent studies suggest that the Coomassie blue method is suitable as long as it is properly standardized and appropriate precautions are taken.[42–44]

Theoretically, *spectrophotometry* at 210 to 220 nm has several advantages, including high sensitivity, similar absorption for albumin and globulin (since it is

the peptide bond that absorbs at this wavelength), and a small sample requirement. The major problem with this direct measurement is the interference of other substances such as nucleosides, nucleotides, ascorbic acid, various carboxylic acids, and drugs that also absorb light in the 210- to 220-nm range. The use of prior gel filtration of the CSF, however, eliminates these interferences, thus making spectrophotometry a highly reliable and valuable technique.[45,46] Normal values are a little higher than with other methods (lying in the upper limits of the reference interval at about 60 mg/dL), but the precision is better. Hence the only real drawback to the spectrophotometry method appears to be the need for high-quality instrumentation that is reliable at 210 to 220 nm.

Other less commonly used methods include the modified biuret test, dye binding, and immunologic procedures. A relatively recent and unique colorimetric micromethod has been described[47] that consists of the coprecipitation by trichloroacetic acid of protein and ponceau S dye, dissolution of the precipitate in weak alkali, and readings of total protein made at 560 nm. In this method, temperature control is not required, reliability is relatively unaffected by the albumin-globulin ratio, and the reagent appears not to react with nonprotein substances. Although this colorimetric micromethod gives lower values than either the Lowry or trichloroacetic acid methods, it correlates well with the findings of the reference Kjeldahl technique.

Protein Fractionation

The fractionation of spinal fluid protein may be of considerable value in the study of certain disorders. Most of the proteins present in normal serum have also been demonstrated in CSF. These include prealbumin, albumin, transferrin, fibrinogen, ceruloplasmin, haptoglobulins, α_2-macroglobulin, IgG, IgA, and others. Most of these substances are derived from plasma. Their relative concentrations correlate well with the hydrodynamic radii and less well with the molecular weights of the protein components. Some proteins, mainly the γ-globulins, can be produced within the CNS.

Spinal fluid proteins can be separated by *electrophoresis* using paper, cellulose acetate, agarose, and

TABLE 2–11. Reference Values by Source for Electrophoresis of CSF Proteins*

| | SOURCE | | |
| | KAPLAN $\overline{x} \pm$ SD, % | WINDISCH AND BRACKEN $\overline{x} \pm$ SD, % | BREEBAART ET AL† (MG/DL $\pm$ 2 SDs) |
PROTEIN			
Prealbumin	4.9 ± 1.2	3.8 ± 1.18	0.4 to 2.5
Albumin	61.5 ± 5.3	65.5 ± 5.34	7.0 to 34.0
α_1-Globulin	4.5 ± 1.4	3.6 ± 1.32	0.7 to 3.6
α_2-Globulin	6.7 ± 1.8	6.8 ± 2.15	0.9 to 4.0
β-Globulin	13.7 ± 3.6	12.4 ± 2.62	1.9 to 7.5
γ-Globulin	8.8 ± 2.6	7.6 ± 2.36	0.7 to 4.3

Note: Data adapted from Kaplan,[48] Windisch and Bracken,[49] and Breebaart et al.[50]

*Figures in parentheses are SI-unit conversions.

†Study focused on subjects 20 to 40 years of age. The γ-globulin level was slightly higher in subjects older than age 40 years.

polyacrylamide gel. The major defined fractions include prealbumin, albumin, α_1-globulin, α_2-globulin, β-globulin including the τ-fraction, and γ-globulin. The τ-fraction, which represents a carbohydrate-deficient form of transferrin, is less conspicuous when the protein has not been denatured. Although fractionation studies have been conducted on unconcentrated fluid, it is recommended that the CSF be concentrated prior to electrophoresis. Many types of concentration techniques have been used[48–50] and have yielded reasonably similar reference values (Table 2–11).

Using paper electrophoresis, Ivers et al[51] found that the CSF of 72% of 144 patients with multiple sclerosis (MS) had increased γ-globulin levels. Many of these patients had a normal total protein level, a finding that has been repeatedly verified. However, the finding of an elevated γ-globulin level is not specific for this disease. Similar increases may be found in a variety of acute infections and in neurosyphilis, subacute panencephalitis, Guillain-Barré syndrome, meningeal carcinomatosis, and other neurologic conditions. Patients with cirrhosis, sarcoidosis, myxedema, collagen vascular disorders, multiple myeloma, and other conditions that are associated with increased levels of serum γ-globulin may also have increased levels of CSF γ-globulin. Hence a serum electrophoretic pattern may be imperative to interpret the CSF findings properly. Furthermore, it should be emphasized that it is the percentage of γ-globulin that is of major diagnostic significance and not its absolute value (normal γ-globulin level, less than 12% of total protein).

When polyacrylamide gel, isoelectric focusing, or electrophoresis on agarose or agar gel is used (in contrast to paper or cellulose acetate), the γ-globulins in spinal fluid from patients with MS migrate as discrete populations, forming so-called oligoclonal bands (Figure 61).[52–54] These abnormal patterns have been noted in 90% or more of patients with clinically active MS, making gel electrophoresis the single most sensitive and reliable method currently available for the diagnosis of this disorder.[54] However, the oligoclonal band finding is not specific for MS, since disorders that show increased CSF γ-globulin levels may also show oligoclonal bands in the CSF. In addition to the conditions already mentioned, the CSF in patients with Alzheimer's disease[55] and African Burkitt's lymphoma[56] involving the CNS has been shown to have characteristic banding. Moreover, oligoclonal bands in the CSF may not indicate MS if similar bands are present in the serum. It is recommended that high-resolution serum electrophoresis be performed in these instances, using agar gel or agarose gel. In addition, one should be aware that iophendylate, a radiocontrast dye used for myelography, interferes with CSF concentration and should be removed by centrifugation prior to electrophoretic analysis.[57]

Immunoglobulins

As indicated previously, proteins appear in the CSF either by diffusion across the blood-CSF barrier or by synthesis within the CNS. The normal plasma-to-CSF ratio for albumin is about 230.[2] The plasma-to-CSF IgG ratio is less well established, with values reported to be 370 to 800.[37,58] The plasma-to-CSF albumin ratio is decreased with traumatic tap, increased blood-CSF permeability, or impaired resorption. The plasma-to-CSF IgG ratio reflects both the synthesis of IgG in the CNS and blood-CNS barrier and blood-CSF permeability.

Kabat et al,[59] using the classic Tiselius technique for electrophoresis, were the first to note that the CSF γ-globulin level was increased in patients with neurosyphilis and MS. Approximately 65% of the patients with MS have increased CSF γ-globulin levels when these are expressed as a percentage of CSF total protein or CSF albumin.[2] Kabat et al and others[60] later developed an immunochemical method for CSF immunoglobulin quantitation that still serves as the reference technique. However, this method was too tedious for routine clinical work, and it was not until 1966 that the process of electroimmunodiffusion, suitable for use with small quantities of unconcentrated CSF, was described by Hartley et al.[61] This technique made it possible to study CSF immunoglobulins routinely and to establish reliable reference values for IgG and, possibly, IgA, in unconcentrated CSF. IgM, however, could not be detected in unconcentrated fluid. Hartley et al[61] also noted that the concentration of spinal fluid resulted in considerable destruction of the immunoglobulins, particularly IgG. A comparison of normal protein fractions in serum and CSF is given in Table 2–12.

In recent years, two additional techniques—*radial immunodiffusion* and *nephelometry*—have been introduced to measure IgG and albumin in the CSF. In radial immunodiffusion, the antigen being assayed diffuses radially through agar gel containing monospecific antiserum to that protein. A precipitin ring forms when the antigen-antibody complex approaches equivalence. The concentration of the antigen is proportionate to the square of the diameter of the precipitin ring.

Nephelometry is a quantitative determination of turbidity made by measuring light scattering. Immunoglobulins are quantitated by measuring either the rate of formation of the antigen-antibody complex or the total amount of complex. A report comparing radial immunodiffusion with nephelometry showed

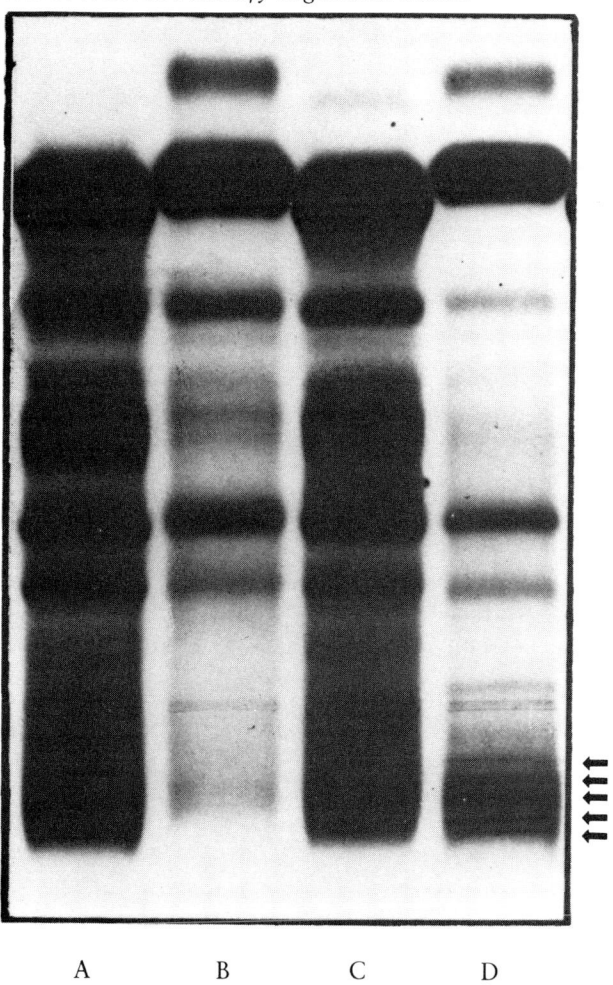

FIGURE 61. *Agarose gel electrophoresis of serum and CSF. Normal serum (A) and normal CSF (B) are compared with serum (C) and CSF (D) samples from patient with multiple sclerosis. Arrows identify oligoclonal bands.*

TABLE 2–12. Comparison of Normal Protein Ranges in CSF and Serum*

Protein	CSF, mg/dL (mg/L)	Serum, mg/dL (g/L)
Total protein	15–45 (150–450)	6,000–8,000 (60–80)
Albumin	10–30 (100–300)	3,500–5,000 (35–50)
IgG	0.7–4.0 (7–40)	800–1,500 (8–15)
IgA	0.0–0.4 (0–4)	90–450 (0.9–4.5)
IgM	0 (0)	6–250 (.06–2.5)

*Figures in parentheses are SI-unit conversions.

that the former had greater precision in measuring both IgG and albumin.[62] The nephelometric techniques, however, are much more rapid and convenient. Results are available within 1 to 60 minutes, depending on the system used.

Although the measurement of IgA and IgM is possible, it currently has no clinical usefulness. Total IgG measurement is also of little help. However, when an IgG measurement is expressed as a percentage of the CSF total protein or, more accurately, as a percentage of albumin, since albumin is more precisely measured, valuable information can be obtained. Approximately 75% of the patients with MS will have an elevated IgG ratio using CSF total protein or CSF albumin measurements. Unfortunately, reported normal ratios vary considerably, probably because of the use of different standards and antiserum samples. Reliable interpretation of these ratios is possible if one considers the upper limits to be 12% for IgG to total protein and 25% to 28% for IgG to albumin in normal CSF.[58] These ratios are more important than absolute IgG measurements because they "correct" for increased IgG in the CSF caused by increased permeability of the blood-CSF barrier and because they provide evidence that the increased IgG is produced locally, within the CNS.

A more sophisticated and recommended method of correction that allows for changes in the plasma proteins as well as for increased CSF-blood barrier permeability is the *IgG/albumin index*.[37]

$$\text{IgG/albumin index} = \frac{\text{CSF IgG/plasma IgG}}{\text{CSF albumin/plasma albumin}}$$

The normal range for this index is 0.34 to 0.58 (mean ± 2 SDs). About 85% of patients with MS have an increased IgG/albumin index.[37]

A recent study[63] has compared the CSF IgG/albumin index with the presence of oligoclonal bands in 149 patients; there were 23 with definite MS, 20 with possible MS, 20 with inflammatory neurologic disease, 65 with noninflammatory neurologic disease, and nine with no neurologic disease. The intensity of the oligoclonal banding was graded relative to the density of the prealbumin band. Both tests had a sensitivity of 88%; however, the specificity for the CSF IgG/albumin index was 95%, while that of oligoclonal bands was only 79%.[63] When cases with inflammatory neurologic disease were eliminated (which is generally done on the basis of other laboratory and clinical features), an elevated CSF IgG/albumin index together with the presence of oligoclonal banding had a specificity of 99% and a sensitivity of 79% for MS.

Link and Zetterwall[64] quantitated the CSF immunoglobulin κ and λ light chains. They pointed out that patients with MS may have IgG with an abnormal light chain distribution, most commonly an increase in the κ to λ ratio. Similar studies have been reported by Palmer et al.[65] These findings need further clinical evaluation, however, before their full significance is understood.

In MS, leukodystrophies, and other demyelinating syndromes, the myelin sheaths are selectively degraded. Demyelination can also occur as a secondary disorder in various intoxications, infections, vascular lesions, and other conditions. In these secondary disorders, not only myelin but other CNS components (eg, nerve cells and axons) are also degraded. In all of these conditions, *myelin basic protein* is released and appears in the CSF, where it can be accurately detected using radioimmunoassay.[66] The antiserum is produced by inoculating rabbits with guinea pig spinal cord that has been homogenized in complete Freund's adjuvant. Assays are performed on duplicate 0.5-mL samples of the CSF, and results are reported as negative (less than 4 ng/mL), weakly positive (4 to 8 ng/mL), or positive (greater than 8 ng/mL). Elevated levels have been found in patients with MS during exacerbations of the disease, while no myelin basic protein has been found during remission. It should be emphasized, however, that the assay for myelin basic protein is not specific for MS and should not be used as a definitive test for MS. The quantitation of myelin basic protein is indicated for the following purposes: (1) to follow the activity of the disease process; (2) to assist in the early diagnosis of MS prior to the appearance of oligoclonal bands; and (3) to assist in the diagnosis of MS in the 10% of patients in whom oligoclonal bands never develop.

Two recent studies compared several of the laboratory tests used in the diagnosis of multiple sclerosis. Bloomer and Bray[67] compared the search for oligoclonal bands, the calculation of the rate of CSF IgG synthesis, and the IgG/albumin ratio, while Gerson et al[68] compared the measurements of myelin basic protein, oligoclonal banding, and IgG as a percentage of total protein and albumin. Both groups reported that the search for oligoclonal bands was the single most useful test in helping to establish the diagnosis of multiple sclerosis and thus may be used in monitoring immunosuppressive therapy. It should be noted, however, that oligoclonal bands may occasionally be absent in multiple sclerosis.

The measurement of *C-reactive protein* by latex agglutination in the CSF of children with bacterial meningitis has been described.[69] The C-reactive protein was detected in 100% of patients (24/24) with culture-proven bacterial meningitis, as compared with 6% of patients (2/32) without bacterial meningitis.[69] C-reactive protein was considered to be more sensitive in differentiating between bacterial and nonbacterial meningitis than the CSF total leukocyte count, absolute number of neutrophils, CSF glucose or protein concentration, or Gram's staining of CSF.[69] More recently, Clarke and Cost,[70] using rate immunonephelometry, studied the use of serum C-reactive protein measurement in differentiating between septic and aseptic childhood meningitis. Their results indicated 100% sensitivity and specificity in differentiating between 17 cases of septic meningitis and 18 cases of aseptic meningitis. However, Philip and Baker,[71] using laser nephelometry, found that only two of 11 cases of neonatal meningitis (mainly group B streptococci) had CSF C-reactive protein levels greater than 1 mg/dL. On the basis of their data, they could not recommend the routine use of CSF C-reactive protein measurement in neonates with suspected sepsis and meningitis.

It appears that more information is needed before C-reactive protein can be recommended as a reliable early marker for bacterial meningitis or for differentiating between septic and aseptic meningitis.

Glucose

Glucose enters the CSF from plasma by two major mechanisms—diffusion and active transport. The former is influenced by the concentration and duration of the plasma glucose level. Hence changes in plasma glucose levels are not seen in the CSF until 30 to 90 minutes later. For this reason, it is preferable to analyze the plasma level at least 30 minutes before determining the CSF value. Otherwise an inaccurate interpretation may result.

After specimens are submitted, glucose analysis should be run without delay. Cerebrospinal fluid glucose levels have, historically, been interpreted in various ways. If a simultaneous plasma value is available, a normal CSF level should be about 60% to 70% of the plasma value. When the plasma level is not available, a commonly accepted reference range is 50 to 80 mg/dL,[2] with levels in the 40- to 50-mg/dL range considered equivocal. The use of this range assumes that the normal fasting plasma glucose levels are 65 to 100 mg/dL and is based on the use of highly specific methods for glucose analysis. A "bloody tap" will, of course, cause a false elevation. A more reliable reference interval for children is 45 to 100 mg/dL, a range recently arrived at[72] using meaningful nonfasting clinical specimens (obtained as patients entered the emergency room) and a significant population size (170 children).

An *elevated CSF glucose level,* either absolute or relative to the plasma glucose level, is evidence that hyperglycemia was present 0.5 to 2.0 hours before the specimen was obtained. It has no specific significance, however, unless the patient is diabetic and the

CSF glucose level is less than about 40% to 50% of the plasma value (possibly indicating meningitis).

Decreased glucose values, classically seen in patients with bacterial and tuberculous (or fungal) meningitis, may also be present in a variety of other conditions, such as hypoglycemia, primary or metastatic tumor involving the meninges, and subarachnoid hemorrhage caused by the release of glycolytic enzymes from RBCs. Occasionally, decreased levels are found in viral meningitis, but they are more frequently normal. Other conditions such as a brain abscess and neurosyphilis are usually associated with normal glucose levels.

There are several mechanisms used to explain low spinal fluid glucose levels in patients with bacterial meningitis. The initial mechanism proposed was glucose utilization by bacteria, a theory now known to be untenable in terms of the amount of glucose that can be metabolized by bacteria. A second proposal, the utilization of glucose by phagocytizing neutrophils, while tenable to some extent, has two major weaknesses. First, it fails to explain the low CSF glucose levels seen in tuberculous meningitis, where mononuclear cells predominate and few organisms are present. Second, the maximum amount of glucose used by leukocytes is small in comparison with the amount used by the brain. It has been argued that the major explanation for increased glucose utilization in bacterial meningitis is defective glucose transport and increased glycolytic activity in the brain.[73]

Although decreased CSF glucose levels in bacterial meningitis are commonly seen, it is not unusual to find normal values when cultures are positive. In their classic series of articles on bacterial meningitis involving 207 patients, Swartz and Dodge[74] reported low levels in only 55% of the cases of pneumococcal meningitis, in 53% of the meningitis cases caused by *Hemophilus influenzae,* and in 45% of the meningococcal meningitis cases. Other studies suggest that CSF glucose levels are decreased in a higher percentage of cases—especially in children, in whom low levels are reported in 60% to 80% of the cases.[72,75]

Elevated CSF lactate levels may be more frequently seen than a decreased glucose level in patients with bacterial meningitis.[76] In our study involving 73 consecutively seen cases of bacterial meningitis in children—83.6% of whom had *H influenzae*—64 (87%) had glucose levels below 40 mg/dL, but all 73 had CSF lactate levels higher than 30 mg/dL, and most (66, or 91%) had lactate levels higher than 40 mg/dL.[72]

The glucose oxidase test strips have long been considered useful in distinguishing between CSF and nasal secretions. Several studies have, however, shown that this test is of no clinical value.[77] Glucose can be demonstrated in most samples of nasal discharge, and the diagnosis of CSF rhinorrhea or otorrhea must be made by other methods such as the intrathecal administration of iodine 131–labeled serum albumin.[2] More information on this subject is given later in this chapter under "Detection of CSF Leakage."

Enzymes

Many studies have been conducted in an attempt to confirm an association between the levels of various enzymes and diseases involving the CNS. Yet despite frequent abnormalities in the enzyme levels of patients with such diseases, this field of study remains somewhat clouded regarding the value of these assays and their correlation with the diagnosis of various neurologic disorders.[78]

The clinical implications of *lactate dehydrogenase* (LD) assays of the CSF were first reported in the late 1950s.[79,80] It was demonstrated that the CSF levels of LD varied independently of plasma activity and that patients with CNS leukemia, lymphoma, metastatic carcinoma, and subarachnoid hemorrhage had consistently elevated LD values when compared with controls. In addition, marked increases occurred in patients with acute meningitis; these levels returned to normal after successful treatment. Subsequent studies not only confirmed these findings but showed that the LD assays were helpful in differentiating between acute bacterial and viral meningitis.[70,81,82] While the latter condition is usually associated with normal to mildly elevated LD activity,[75] increased levels usually can be seen in patients with bacterial meningitis who have received partial treatment.

One of the primary problems encountered in evaluating CSF specimens has been the lack of reliable reference values for many analytes, since large volumes of normal fluid are difficult to obtain. This problem is further complicated by enzyme analysis, since methodologies vary greatly and values change with substrate, buffer, and reaction conditions. As a result, reliable reference values for an adequate control sample have only recently become available.[72] In one study conducted by Knight et al,[72] the normal levels for LD were 1 to 25 units/L at 37° C, the 25 to 30 units/L range being equivocal. Bacterial meningitis is almost invariably accompanied by LD activities greater than 3.0 times the upper normal limit, while viral infections are associated with levels of less than 2.0 times this upper limit.[72,83] In addition to infection, total LD activity is increased in a variety of other conditions involving the CNS, including carcinomas, leukemia, lymphoma, and ischemic necrosis (stroke).[80,81,84]

It is important to remember that a "bloody tap" or fluid showing a recent or old hemorrhage will demonstrate significantly elevated LD levels. The RBCs contain 100 to 150 times the LD concentration of plasma, and plasma contains 15 to 20 times the LD activity of the CSF.

When the CSF is concentrated appropriately, *LD isoenzymes* can readily be studied. This technique has increased the specificity of enzyme analysis. Two reports[84,85] have shown that the normal CSF isoenzyme distribution is $LD_1 > LD_2 > LD_3 > LD_4 > LD_5$, with the last two isoenzymes making up no more than a small percentage of the total. Brain tissue, which is rich in LD, has a similar isoenzyme distribution but is more closely related to normal plasma, with a reversal in the distribution of isoenzymes LD_1 and LD_2—ie, $LD_2 > LD_1$. Consequently, the CSF of patients with various neurologic disorders (hydrocephalus, increased intracranial pressure, and chronic epilepsy) that are associated with mild elevations of total LD shows a "normal" distribution.

In bacterial meningitis, the CSF isoenzyme pattern is usually the exact opposite of that in normal CSF, with $LD_5 > LD_4 > LD_3 > LD_2 > LD_1$.[81,83] Although some cases vary slightly, LD_5 is invariably the dominant isoenzyme. Isoenzymes LD_4 and LD_5 predominate in granulocytes and are presumed to be the major enzyme source. In viral meningitis, the CSF isoenzyme pattern is usually a combination of that seen in the brain and lymphocytes; ie, $LD_2 > LD_1 > LD_3$ or $LD_2 > LD_3 > LD_1$[84,85]; lymphocytes contain predominantly LD_2 and LD_3. High levels of LD_1 and LD_2 in the CSF of patients with viral and bacterial meningitis are thought to be associated with severe CNS damage

and a poor prognosis.[2] In CNS childhood leukemia (acute lymphoblastic), the distribution of isoenzymes is essentially that of purified lymphoblasts, the major components being $LD_4 > LD_3 > LD_5$.

Like LD, *aspartate aminotransferase* (AST, formerly GOT) is normally present in the CSF, but in smaller quantities than in serum. Although reliable reference intervals have not been established, it is known that AST in CSF increases with age. As with LD, one must be careful in evaluating enzyme activities performed on "bloody taps" or xanthochromic fluid, since AST is about ten times more concentrated in RBCs than in plasma, and plasma has much more enzyme activity than spinal fluid.

The CSF and serum AST levels vary independently of each other. Increased AST levels in the CSF have been noted in some patients with brain tumors, cerebral infarction, and contusion (but not concussion); elevated values have also occurred within 48 hours of seizure activity in adults and after CNS radiation and/or chemotherapy.[78,86] Levels of AST and LD were measured in the CSF of dogs with experimentally produced infarcts.[87] Aspartate aminotransferase activities peaked at about 100 hours and gradually returned to normal by 15 days. The degree of elevation correlated well with the size of the tissue damage. Aspartate aminotransferase has been subsequently studied in great detail in patients with cerebral infarction and other conditions. However, the value of these reports is limited by the marked differences among methodologies and/or reference ranges used for measuring CSF AST.[78] Much the same can be said about LD with regard to many of the earlier studies using this enzyme. As a result, the measurement of AST in CSF has not heretofore been very helpful in the evaluation of CNS disorders.[78,81]

However, an interesting study[88] was recently published in which levels of the CSF enzymes LD, AST, creatine kinase (CK), and angiotensin-converting enzyme (ACE) were assessed as a group in differentiating between cortical and lacunar infarctions. Lacunar infarction syndromes are caused by small-vessel hypertensive disease, while cortical infarctions are thought to be caused by embolic phenomena. When the latter is suspected, carotid artery angiography may be warranted, while in the former cases, angiography is not helpful. In many cases, there may be confusion as to which type of stroke has occurred. Donnan et al[88] have shown that a marked elevation in level of at least one of the three CSF enzymes (LD, AST, or CK) occurs in 80% of cases of cortical stroke, while no elevation of CK, AST, or ACE levels is seen in the lacunar strokes. There was only a mild increase in LD levels noted in the patients with lacunar strokes. The same authors concluded that, in certain instances, the measurement of these enzymes may be of use in distinguishing between cortical and lacunar stroke, a precise diagnosis of which is important for clinical management, to enter the patient in stroke treatment trials, or to describe new syndrome types.

Creatine kinase is normally present in brain tissue, where it is thought to participate in maintaining adequate supplies of ATP, and in skeletal muscle and myocardium. It is not present in RBCs.

Elevated CSF CK levels have been reported, with a few exceptions, in patients with acute subarachnoid hemorrhage, hydrocephalus, cerebral infarction, muscular dystrophy, brain tumors, and various other conditions associated with increased intracranial pressure.[78] The degree of CK elevation may be of help in evaluating the prognosis in cases of head trauma. Florez et al[86] showed (1) significant elevations of CK in patients with mild concussions, as compared with CK levels of controls, (2) a significant elevation of CK in patients with moderate to severe concussions, as compared with levels in those having mild concussions, and (3) significantly higher CK levels in patients who died, as compared with levels in patients with moderate to severe concussions who survived. Serum CK levels were even more strikingly elevated and appeared to be primarily related to the degree of external trauma.[86] Nevertheless, these authors felt that total CK levels were probably not of prognostic significance and suggested further studies, including isoenzyme measurements. The only other CSF enzyme shown to be elevated in mild cases of head trauma was malate dehydrogenase, although more severe trauma also resulted in elevations of CSF LD and AST.[86]

In addition to total CK, the measurement of *CK isoenzymes* would appear to be more useful, since it is more specific. Several studies have shown that CSF CK isoenzymes have essentially the same distribution as that found in normal brain tissue and are composed primarily of CK-BB (97% to 98% BB, 0.9% MB, and 1.7% MM).[78] Sherwin et al[89] measured CSF CK in 185 patients with various neurologic disorders, including tumors, MS, intervertebral disk disease, and epilepsy. The total CK level was increased in 70 of these, and only CK-BB was detected.

Although CK-BB is relatively specific for brain tissue, an elevated value remains nonspecific, and, except for possible prognostic value in head injuries, neither the measurement of total CK nor that of CK-BB in CSF appears to be of any current value in evaluating CNS disorders.

Lysozyme (muramidase) is a low–molecular-weight protein (~15,000 daltons) that actively catalyzes the breakdown of mucopolysaccharides in bacterial cell walls. The lysozyme concentration is very high in neutrophils and monocytes. Lysozyme is also present in considerable quantities in the gastrointestinal tract and kidneys.

In normal persons, the lysozyme concentration in CSF is either absent or barely detectable (less than 0.5 μg/mL).[90] The highest values are seen in patients with acute bacterial meningitis. The levels appear to correlate both with the CSF protein concentration and the number of neutrophilic leukocytes.[90] As a result, CSF lysozyme concentration is usually normal in patients with viral meningitis.[91] Elevated levels have been reported in patients with cerebrovascular disease, MS, intracranial hemorrhage, epilepsy, cerebral atrophy, and various tumors.[78,90,91] Newman et al[92] reported prominent lysozyme elevations in patients with both primary and metastatic brain tumors, with the degree of elevation reflecting the nature and degree of tumor involvement. They also reported no activity in patients with Hodgkin's disease involving the CNS or Guillain-Barré syndrome (acute febrile polyneuritis). High concentrations, however, are to be expected in cases of acute myeloblastic and acute monocytic leukemia and in true histiocytic lymphoma when these disorders affect the CNS. Elevated levels have also been reported in cases of CNS sarcoidosis in which the enzyme was present in the epithelioid cells of the sarcoid granuloma.[93] One might also expect increased CSF lysozyme activities in patients with other granulomatous disorders.

Tumors of the CNS may have no direct association with the appearance of lysozyme in CSF as long as the CSF cytologic test and chemistry study findings are normal.[94,95] Rather, the enzyme's presence in CSF in these conditions is directly related to the protein concentration and/or the accompanying inflammatory cells that are present. Thus the presence of lysozyme in CSF may not be an accurate indicator of either CNS tumor or inflammation. It appears that lysozyme measurement currently has negligible value as a specific aid in the diagnosis of any CNS disease.

Several other enzymes have been measured in the CSF in an attempt to correlate their activities with various disease processes. These include ribonuclease, cholinesterase, arginine esterase, adenylate kinase, and dopamine-β-hydroxylase.[78] At this time, however, more research is needed to evaluate fully the potential usefulness of measuring these enzymes in the study of CNS disorders.

Ammonia, Amines, and Amino Acids

Increased levels of *ammonia* in the CSF are seen in patients with a variety of liver diseases that lead to hepatic encephalopathy, including Reye's syndrome in children. In addition, elevated values occur in hypercapnea.[96] In all of these conditions, elevated CSF levels appear to correlate with the degree of encephalopathy. Normal CSF values of ammonia are about half those found in blood.

Several investigators have shown that *glutamine* correlates well with the severity of hepatic encephalopathy. This compound is synthesized by the brain from ammonia and glutamic acid and provides the means whereby ammonia is removed from the CNS. However, as more ammonia and glutamic acid react, other intermediates in cerebral metabolism, such as α-ketoglutarate, are depleted. This loss of critical metabolic intermediates may be one of the contributing factors in the development of hepatic encephalopathy.

The CSF concentration of glutamine is increased in about 75% of patients with Reye's syndrome.[97] Normal values of CSF constituents (eg, ammonia) depend on the methodology used. When glutamine is deaminated with sulfuric acid and the liberated ammonia is measured by either Nessler's reagent or phenolhypochlorite,[98,99] the upper limit of the normal range is approximately 20 mg/dL. When ammonia is measured enzymatically, the upper level of the normal range is 15 mg/dL.[2]

Some researchers have suggested that the *biogenic*

amines (5-hydroxytryptamine, norepinephrine, and dopamine) act as synaptic transmitters in the CNS.[100] Each amine is thought to function in a distinct system of the brain: 5-hydroxytryptamine (serotonin) in the limbic structures, norepinephrine in the central autonomic system, and dopamine in the extrapyramidal system. These compounds are formed from precursor aromatic amino acids that enter the brain from the blood, become ring-hydroxylated, and then are decarboxylated to form the specific aromatic amine.

Although these substances are not readily measured in the CSF, some of their metabolites are, such as 5-hydroxyindoleacetic acid (5-HIAA) from 5-hydroxytryptamine and homovanillac acid (HVA) from dopamine. In contrast to what is seen in the peripheral nervous system, vanillylmandelic acid is apparently not the end-product of norepinephrine metabolism. The major end-product is now known to be *3-methoxy-4-hydroxyphenylethylene glycol* (MHPG), a compound currently being measured in urine as an aid in the differential diagnosis and treatment of the affective disorders (depression and mania). Earlier observations that certain pharmacologic agents produced alterations in affective states and also in the disposition and metabolism of CNS catecholamines served as the stimulus for research on the possible role of norepinephrine metabolism changes in producing affective disorders.[100] From these studies, the idea arose in the mid-1960s[101] that subgroups of patients with depressive states could be identified by differences in norepinephrine metabolism. Since then, numerous reports have provided data supporting this hypothesis, and from this body of evidence has emerged the practice of measuring urinary MHPG levels in depressed patients.[102–105] Unfortunately, CSF MHPG levels have not proven to be a reliable indicator in these cases.

Vanillic acid is also found in the CSF and is presumably derived through a related pathway.[102,106] Although the CSF concentration of vanillic acid exceeds that of MHPG,[106] its measurement has no known current clinical value.

The measurement of *HVA* and *5-HIAA* has been thought to provide an index of CNS disease. This appears to be true in part, as the concentrations of both 5-HIAA and HVA have been shown to be significantly decreased in the caudate nucleus and fluid from the lateral ventricle in patients with Parkinson's disease[100,107,108] and in patients with presenile or senile dementia.[93,100–102,107–109] Decreased CSF levels of HVA have also been reported in certain cases of chronic alcoholism (chronic alcoholic ataxia, "abstinence syndrome," and Wernicke-Korsakoff's syndrome).[110] Since these metabolites are actively transported out of the CSF, it is common to measure their concentration before and after probenecid administration. Probenecid competitively inhibits CSF-to-blood transport of HVA and 5-HIAA[111] so that their levels rise in normal individuals to a greater extent than in patients with parkinsonism. These findings may be more difficult to demonstrate in CSF samples taken from the lumbar sac, since the fluid there is less homogeneous.[112] As knowledge in this rapidly changing field has advanced, it has become clear that the lumbar CSF concentration of amine metabolites is influenced by age, sex, diet, drugs, state of physical activity, diurnal rhythms, volume of the CSF sample, and the way it is stored.[113,114]

Various other metabolites in the CSF have been reported recently. It appears that palmitic acid is present in normal CSF in greater concentration than any other organic acid.[115] Stearic acid is also prominently present. In one study, significant amounts of 3-methoxy-4-hydroxyphenylethanol were found in 28 of 37 samples of normal fluid.[115] The clinical value, if any, of measuring these compounds will have to await further investigations.

γ-*Aminobutyric acid* (GABA), a major inhibitory neurotransmitter in the mammalian CNS, has received the greatest attention of the amino acid transmitters.[116–118] It is well established that there is a marked decrease in GABA-containing neurons in the basal ganglia of patients with Huntington's disease. Studies have shown that CSF levels of GABA are also decreased in patients with this disorder and possibly in patients with Alzheimer's disease as well.[119,120] Using a sensitive radioreceptor assay, it has been shown that patients with Huntington's disease have a mean CSF GABA level of 119 picomole/mL, as compared with control patients, who have a mean level of 230 picomole/mL.[118] Although only three patients with Alzheimer's disease were studied, their mean value of CSF GABA was essentially the same as that of patients with Huntington's disease.

Another interesting compound is γ-*hydroxybutyric acid* (GHB), a metabolite of GABA.[121] This is a neuroactive substance that has several potent neuropharmacologic and neurophysiologic effects.[122,123] Snead[122] found a higher concentration of GHB in the CSF of young infants than in older children and a higher concentration in the latter than in adults. The highest concentrations of all were found in children who had seizures.[116] Whether the measurements of GABA or GHB in CSF will have any routine clinical application or not must await further developments.

Other amines and amino acids have been measured in the CSF. One finding of possible significance is the report of increased amounts of *ethanolamine* in the CSF of autistic children.[124] It appears possible that a subgroup of autistic children may have a brain disorder related to the abnormal metabolism of this compound. Elevated concentrations of *glycine* in plasma are also seen in a wide variety of metabolic disorders. Two of these disorders, albeit rare, are most easily detected by appropriate analysis of the CSF. The first of these is ketotic hyperglycinemia, in which plasma elevations of glycine appear to be caused by the accumulation of one or more organic acids that are products of the branched-chain amino acids. Examples of ketotic disorders include propionic acidemia, isovaleric acidemia, and methylmalonic acidemia.

However, most children with nonketotic hyperglycinemia, the second type of disorder, have no apparent organic acid abnormality. This is a heterogeneous group of disorders, but in some cases, a severe illness develops early in childhood that is usually fatal. In these cases, but not in the ketotic disorders, the CSF glycine levels are increased 15 to 30 times the normal level. The basic defect appears to be the absence of a glycine cleavage enzyme.[125]

Homocarnosinosis is a familial metabolic disorder, characterized by elevated levels of *homocarnosine* (a dipeptide composed of GABA and histidine). In patients with this disorder, the homocarnosine levels are 20 times that seen in normal controls.[126]

Although amines and amino acids are not measured routinely—and most of these measurements are currently of little practical value—they may prove to have considerable diagnostic value in the future.

Electrolytes

The measurement of CSF *sodium* is not considered to be clinically useful in the diagnosis of neurologic disorders. The levels of sodium found in the CSF parallel those found in serum but appear to fluctuate less in cases of hyponatremia and hypernatremia.

Reference intervals for CSF *potassium,* as determined by several groups of investigators, are consistently in the 2.6 to 3.1 mmole/L range,[127] a much lower and more narrow interval than for plasma (3.5 to 5.0 mmole/L). There is essentially no fluctuation of CSF potassium levels with systemic acid-base abnormalities; hence the routine measurement of CSF potassium has little clinical importance in these situations. On the other hand, significant changes in potassium levels have been reported in cisternal fluid following cardiac arrest and may give some indication of the degree of cerebral damage.[128] This increase is significantly greater in those patients who do not regain consciousness, as compared with those who do.

Unlike most other CSF constituents, CSF *chloride* is present in higher concentrations than in plasma, the normal range being approximately 115 to 130 mmole/L in CSF. Plasma levels are quite labile, and changes are rapidly reflected in the CSF. As a result, any condition characterized by hypochloremia or hyperchloremia will show comparable changes in the CSF. In the past, determination of CSF chloride concentrations was thought to be helpful in the diagnosis of meningitis, particularly the tuberculous type, in which decreased levels are consistently seen. This finding, however, merely reflects the hypochloremia usually seen in most patients with meningitis, regardless of the cause. Therefore, CSF chloride measurements are not considered to be of any current value in the diagnosis of meningitis or any other neurologic disorder.

Spinal fluid contains approximately half the concentration of the total *calcium* in plasma, and this concentration is essentially equal to that of the nonprotein-bound or diffusable calcium in plasma. Changes in concentration of ionized serum calcium are rapidly reflected in the CSF. Active transport is another operating mechanism. In contrast to calcium concentrations, the CSF concentrations of *magnesium* are normally maintained at levels averaging 30% greater than those in serum. Patients with infectious diseases and apparently some with ischemic brain disease lose their ability to maintain this high concentration in the CSF.[129]

There appears to be no known clinical use for the measurement of either calcium or magnesium in the CSF.

pH and Acid-Base

In 1917, Levinson[130] first demonstrated that patients with acute bacterial meningitis show a decrease in the CSF *pH.* More recently, this measurement, along with that of CSF lactate, has been shown to be helpful in the early diagnosis of bacterial meningitis, although the laboratory value of CSF lactate is probably a more reliable indicator (see section entitled "Lactate").[131]

In recent years, the measurements of pH, PCO_2, and *bicarbonate* in the CSF have received considerable attention.[132,133] However, from a clinical standpoint, these CSF measurements are still in the experimental phase, although they may soon prove to be clinically useful. For example, the consistent finding that acute cerebral edema following head trauma is frequently preceded by a persistent reduction in CSF bicarbonate levels may prove helpful information in these cases.[134] Other conditions, such as hypoxia and salicylate intoxication, may prove to be more easily managed when these measurements are routinely available.

Lactate

The measurement of CSF *lactate* is now widely considered to be an important adjunct in the early diagnosis of bacterial meningitis, as well as in the differential diagnosis of viral and bacterial meningitides.

Increased levels of CSF lactate in patients with tuberculous and meningococcal meningitis were first noted by Nishimura[135] in 1924, and four years later it was concluded that the changes in CSF lactic acid concentration were a better index of the progress of the infection than were the changes in glucose content.[136] However, primarily because of the technical difficulties in measuring lactic acid accurately, its use greatly declined and its potential value became generally unknown. The usefulness of CSF lactate measurement in the early diagnosis of bacterial meningitis and as an early indicator in separating bacterial from viral meningitis began with the introduction of better methodology.[137–140] Controni et al[139] studied 396 patients for the early detection of bacterial meningitis: CSF lactate levels were elevated in all 62 patients with proven bacterial or mycoplasma meningitis. All 334 patients without bacterial meningitis had normal lactate values, as did 15 patients with aseptic meningitis. In addition, antecedent antibiotic therapy did not compromise the reliability of the test. Several more recent studies have supported these results.[140–143] However, it is now known that a small number of patients with viral meningitis will have equivocal or even mild elevations of CSF lactate levels.[72,138,140] Hence, despite the value of CSF lactate measurement as indicated here, some have questioned its routine use.[144,145]

The mechanism for elevated CSF lactate levels appears to be tissue hypoxia caused by increased intracranial pressure with subsequent impairment of the central blood supply. Therefore, any condition associated with decreased blood flow or deficient oxygenation of the brain can cause increased lactate levels.[146,147] Such conditions include intracranial hemorrhage, brain abscess, cerebral arteriosclerosis, hypotension, low arterial P_{CO_2}, primary and metastatic malignant conditions, traumatic brain injuries, and idiopathic seizures.[2] Xanthochromic fluid specimens invariably show high lactate levels originating from RBCs and should probably not be analyzed for lactate, since the results are usually misleading.

Lactate in the CSF, as well as in other body fluids, is readily and accurately measured using either enzymatic or gas-liquid chromatographic techniques.[138–143] Both methods yield essentially identical results. Reliable reference intervals are in the 9.0 to 26.0 mg/dL range (1.13 to 3.23 mmole/L).[72,148] Values in the 26- to 30-mg/dL range are considered equivocal. Patients with very early cases of bacterial meningitis may occasionally have values in the equivocal range, although in most cases the levels will exceed 35 to 40 mg/dL. On the other hand, lactate levels associated with viral meningitis will usually fall below 25 mg/dL and almost invariably below 35 mg/dL. It is important that appropriate serologic tests be carried out to identify infections caused by mycoplasma. Cultures in these cases are negative, but lactate levels are usually elevated.[139] If the serologic studies are not carried out, mycoplasma infection may be mistaken for viral meningitis with high lactate values.

The aforementioned reference intervals refer to older children and adults. Neonates have higher lactate levels, which fall into the aforementioned ranges about 10 days after birth.[149] Newborns have a mean level of 24.7 mg/dL, with a range of 10 to 40 mg/

dL.[149] At 11 to 20 days of age, the mean lactate level is 12.9 mg/dL, with a range of 10.4 to 24.4 mg/dL.[149]

Tumor Markers

Many studies have been carried out on CSF in search of biochemical markers for CNS tumors. They include, in addition to several enzymes already discussed (LD, AST, lysozyme, and others), carcinoembryonic antigen, α-fetoprotein, human chorionic gonadotropin, β-glucuronidase, cyclic nucleotides, adenohypophyseal hormones (eg, corticotropin, growth hormone, and thyrotropin), somatostatin, desmosterol, polyamines (spermine, spermidine, and putrescine), astroprotein, and β$_2$-microglobulin.[150–155] Although most of these substances are of interest, and some have definite potential value, the routine measurement of biochemical tumor markers in CSF currently has limited clinical value.

Levels of α-*fetoprotein*, a glycoprotein produced by yolk sac elements, are elevated in the CSF of patients with embryonal carcinoma.[156] *Astroprotein,* a cerebroprotein (glial fibrillary acidic protein), is a specific marker for fibrillary astrocytes in the normal brain, as well as for reactive astrocytes and astrocytoma cells.[153] The measurement of this protein in CSF by an immunochemical method has been reported in patients with primary brain tumors.[154] Increased astroprotein levels were seen in 43.3% of patients with glial tumors and 66.7% of those with glioblastomas.[154] Further studies correlating CSF astroprotein levels with the clinical course of the disease and tumor size and location are needed before the full value of this measurement can be accurately assessed.

β-$_2$-Microglobulin (β$_2$M) is usually measured in the urine. It has also been measured in other body fluids, including CSF, where it has been evaluated as an indicator of inflammation and malignant conditions. Serial β$_2$M levels measured by a radioimmunoassay have been shown to correlate with the clinical appearance and disappearance of CNS involvement in patients with leukemia and lymphoma.[157] Serum and CSF β$_2$M determinations were useful in the early diagnosis of CNS involvement and in the monitoring of intrathecal therapy in these patients.[157] The measurement of CSF β$_2$M, in conjunction with lactoferrin and lysozyme measurement, may be of clinical value in discriminating between bacterial and viral infections and possibly between malignant and benign cerebral tumors.[158] However, since β_2M is a nonspecific marker, it should only be used as an ancillary tool, and CSF levels should be checked against serum levels.[157] The involvement of CSF by leukemia or lymphoma is likely when CSF levels exceed serum levels.[157]

β-Subunit of human chorionic gonadotropin is usually elevated in the CSF of patients in whom choriocarcinomas, gonadotropin-producing teratomas, or germinal cell testicular carcinomas have metastasized to the CNS.[159] The level of β-subunit of human chorionic gonadotropin appears to be related to the tumor activity during therapy, and the CSF changes may precede clinical or radiographic evidence of metastasis.[159]

β-Glucuronidase and carcinoembryonic antigen may be useful markers of early metastatic involvement of the leptomeninges, particularly with lung and breast carcinoma.[160] It should be noted that elevated β-glucuronidase levels are also seen in bacterial and fungal meningitis.[160]

Miscellaneous Biochemical Measurements

Urea, uric acid, zinc, phosphorus, ethanol, various hormones, peptides, and a wide variety of other substances have been measured in the spinal fluid and, in some cases, reference values have been established.[2] None of these measurements has current clinical value.

Detection of CSF Leakage

The diagnosis of rhinorrhea and otorrhea may be difficult, particularly when the fluid sample is small. The most common methods are roentgenography, radioactive cisternography, intrathecal staining, and chemical analysis of glucose, protein, and electrolyte content of the fluid obtained from the nose or ear.

A more recent method is based on the demonstration of an extra band of transferrin located in the β_2 fraction of protein electrophoresis of CSF.[161] The β_2-transferrin present in CSF is not present in serum, nasal secretions, saliva, tears, or perilymph and endolymph.

MICROBIOLOGIC EXAMINATION

Appropriate microbiologic examination is essential for every patient in whom the clinical findings suggest even the slightest possibility of meningitis. The major

reasons for this are as follows: (1) untreated bacterial meningitis is a lethal disease capable of rapid progression; (2) early treatment with appropriate antibiotic therapy is curative; and (3) the selection of adequate antimicrobials depends on the knowledge of a specific causative agent, which often requires in vitro susceptibility testing.

The CSF should be cultured and a gram stain performed. In addition, blood cultures should be obtained in cases where meningitis is suspected, as they will be positive in 40% to 60% of such cases. Blood cultures may provide the only definitive clue as to the causative agent. Cultures of CSF will be positive in about 90% of suspicious cases. Septicemia is less common in meningococcal meningitis (32% of blood cultures positive) than in *Hemophilus influenzae* and *Streptococcus pneumoniae* (60% to 90% of blood cultures positive).[162] Routine cultures of specimens from the pharynx or external ear are not usually helpful.

Bacterial Meningitis

Bacterial meningitis is most commonly caused by *Hemophilus influenzae* (Figure 41), *Neisseria meningitidis* (Figure 42), and *Streptococcus pneumoniae*. Although figures vary with the study and patient population, these three organisms accounted for 147 (71%) of 207 cases in one study that included all age groups.[163] *Streptococcus pneumoniae* was the most frequent organism isolated, accounting for 56 cases, as compared with 52 caused by *H influenzae*.[163] However, when studies are limited to children, *H influenzae* accounts for up to 80% of the cases.[72] The majority of the remaining cases are caused by *Staphylococcus aureus*, β-hemolytic and other streptococci, and various enteric microorganisms and are associated with epidural empyema, brain abscess, neurosurgical procedures, or head trauma. Pneumococcus is the most common cause of meningitis in patients with CNS rhinorrhea occurring after head trauma.

Rare cases of meningitis caused by *Listeria monocytogenes* (easily confused with diphtheroids on Gram's staining)[164] or *Mima-Herellea* (which morphologically may resemble *H influenzae* or *N meningitidis*)[164,165] may be seen. In addition to these and other unusual organisms, uncommon bacterial origins may include episodes of simultaneous mixed meningitis caused by two or more bacterial species.[166,167] Furthermore, one should be aware that unusual serotypes may be seen. For example, *H influenzae* type B is clearly the predominant serotype, but rare cases of other serotypes may be encountered.[168] In adults, such organisms are especially seen in immunosuppressed patients. When *N meningitidis* is the offending organism, groups B and C are most common. However, groups Y and W-135 are being seen with increasing frequency.[169,170]

Hemophilus influenzae meningitis, encountered almost exclusively in children between 2 months and 6 years of age, makes up well over 60% of the cases of postneonatal meningitis. The gram-negative enteric organisms (chiefly *Escherichia coli*) have been the predominant pathogens in systemic neonatal infections. This situation has now changed with the emergence of group B β-hemolytic streptococcus as a major pathogen.[171] Currently, group B streptococci *(Streptococcus agalactiae)* and *E coli* together account for approximately 70% of neonatal meningitis and septicemia.[171] These infections are acquired primarily during birth from organisms normally present in the maternal genital and intestinal tracts. It is of interest that of the 100 known *E coli* K antigens, 80% of the neonatal infections are associated with the K_1 strain. The most common streptococcal serotype seen in neonatal meningitis is the group B III, which contains a polysaccharide capsule similar in composition to the *E coli* K_1.[171] These two antigens may play an important role in the pathogenesis of neonatal meningitis caused by these two organisms. Neonatal meningitis due to group B β-hemolytic streptococci is associated with less morbidity and mortality than other organisms.[172]

The significance of the isolation of certain organisms from CSF is not always appreciated. In a recent study of 43 patients, eight different species of an α-hemolytic streptococci were recovered.[173] Only eight patients (19%) had significant infections based on bacteriologic, laboratory, and clinical findings. Thirty-five (81%) of the isolates were considered contaminants, *Streptococcus mitis* being the most frequent single organism identified (in 49% of cases).[173] The lumbar puncture skin site was considered the most likely source for these contaminants.[173]

A quality gram stain of the sedimented CSF, examined by an expert microbiologist, will yield an accurate presumptive diagnosis in the majority of cases (up to 80%), although its reliability is probably considerably lower in most institutions. The most common diagnostic errors include the misinterpretation of precipitated dye or stained debris for gram-positive organisms and the mistaking of stained nuclear fragments or precipitated protein for gram-negative bacteria, especially pleomorphic *H influenzae* (Figure 41), or dead bacteria in collection tubes. The major problem with the gram stain is its apparent lack of sensitivity (demonstrated in the high percentage of false-negative results). In an attempt to improve this problem, acridine orange, a fluorochrome stain, has been proposed as potentially superior to the gram stain in the direct microscopic examination of all clinical specimens, including CSF.[174] It has been recommended, however, that all positive smears using acridine orange be reexamined with the gram stain to confirm the results and determine the gram reaction of the microorganisms.[174] This last is important for appropriate early antibiotic therapy. We believe that Gram's stains performed on cytocentrifuge smears increase the sensitivity. With this preparatory method the cell morphologic structure is better preserved and the intracellular organism is easily identified. Organisms can often be easily identified with the Wright's stain alone.

Another critical step that may enhance the sensitivity of the staining technique is the appropriate initial handling of CSF. It has been recommended that the sediment of all spinal fluid specimens be examined after centrifugation at 1,500*g* for 15 minutes.[175] Higher bacterial recovery has been seen following centrifugation than after filtration, especially in patients who have received antibiotics.[175] In addition to problems with false-negative results using the gram stain, there is the time delay for culture results and the frequency of negative cultures. As a result, the measurement of CSF glucose, lactate, and other nonspecific chemical markers has become more important, along with the use of counterimmunoelectrophoresis and the *Limulus* lysate test, all of which help in accelerating the laboratory diagnosis of bacterial meningitis.

Most cases of bacterial meningitis are, fortunately, easily and rapidly diagnosed, and ancillary diagnostic aids are not needed. The value of the latter lies in the 20% to 30% of cases in which the gram stain is negative but meningitis is suspected because of the clinical picture and/or other laboratory abnormalities (eg, pleocytosis and an increased CSF protein level). Ancillary diagnostic aids may also be useful in cases of early meningitis where all initial laboratory measurements are normal.[162,176–179] It is with these two types of cases that measurement of CSF lactate and, possibly, LD may be of help, both in the differential diagnosis of viral and bacterial meningitis and in the differentiation of "developing" meningitis from no CNS disease. It may also be of benefit in preventing meningitis following additional lumbar punctures in a patient with bacteremia but not meningitis.[179]

The hematogenous dissemination of tubercle bacilli to the brain and meninges may result in chronic meningitis or simulate an intracranial neoplasm. Children who have miliary tuberculosis at the time of primary infection are at greater risk of contracting CNS tuberculosis than adults who have the disease in a disseminated form. In suspected cases, an acid-fast stain of the sedimented CSF and appropriate cultures are needed. The number of organisms is usually small, and patience is needed in examining the smears. The fluorescent rhodamine stain may be more sensitive than the Ziehl-Neelsen method.[2] Chemical determinations are frequently helpful, as the CSF lactate level will be elevated above 30 mg/dL, the glucose level decreased below 35 mg/dL, and the protein level increased in most cases. These findings, plus the presence of increased numbers of leukocytes, predominantly mononuclear, should arouse suspicion that the case might be one of tuberculous meningitis.

Aseptic (Viral) Meningitis

Aseptic (viral) meningitis is a relatively common disease, especially in children. Its early laboratory differentiation from bacterial meningitis is usually not difficult since the CSF, in the usual case, differs from the CSF in bacterial meningitis in total leukocyte count, differential cell count, and glucose, lactate, and protein levels. Occasionally, however, the distinction may be difficult since these laboratory markers lack specificity and may overlap in the two diseases. The final diagnosis may be one of exclusion with negative bacterial cultures. Viral cultures of CSF are rarely requested because most clinicians believe the results are too delayed to be helpful in managing the patient's condition. However, the results of a recent report involving 390 patients over a two-year period are not consistent with this philosophy.[180] Of 390 patients who had CSF viral cultures, 111 were discharged with a specific final diagnosis of aseptic meningitis, meningoencephalitis, or both. It was concluded that the specific diagnosis of meningitis of a viral origin saved a minimum of 70 hospital days of unnecessary antibiotic therapy.[180] In addition to cultures, viruses may be demonstrated in the CSF with immunofluorescent and immunoperoxidase techniques.[181]

Viral meningitis may be caused by a variety of infectious agents. The most common agents identified are the enteroviruses, which account for approximately 80% of the cases for which an origin can be determined. A specific agent was established in only 20% of all cases reported to the Centers for Disease Control in 1976.[182] The determination of origin through the isolation of a specific agent should now approach 50% and may be as high as 70% during an epidemic occurring over a short period and involving a single agent.[180,183] Other viruses that may occasionally be identified include mumps virus, arboviruses, herpes simplex virus, and the lymphocytic choriomeningitis virus. Adenoviruses and rhinoviruses are rarely implicated. Echoviruses have only rarely been isolated as the causative agent in aseptic meningitis. In a report of an epidemic of aseptic meningitis caused by echovirus type 7, the majority of patients were younger than 1 year of age.[184] Interestingly, CSF neutrophilic pleocytosis was identified in 66% of these cases.[184] It is important to emphasize that the earlier in the clinical course the specimen is collected, the more probable it is that the virus will be identified. Viruses should also be sought in the feces (enteroviruses and herpesvirus), urine (mumps), saliva (herpesvirus and mumps), and throat washings (enteroviruses, lymphocytic choriomeningitis viruses, and herpesvirus). Since viremia occurs prior to the onset of meningitis, blood examination is not a good method for identifying viruses.

Fungal Meningitis

The most frequent causes of fungal meningitis are *Cryptococcus neoformans*, *Candida* sp, and *Coccidioides immitis*.[185] Approximately 50% of these cases occur in the immunocompetent patient as chronic infections. The CSF usually shows neutrophilic pleo-

FIGURE 62. *India ink preparation demonstrating* Crypto-coccus neoformans. *Magnification, ×850.*

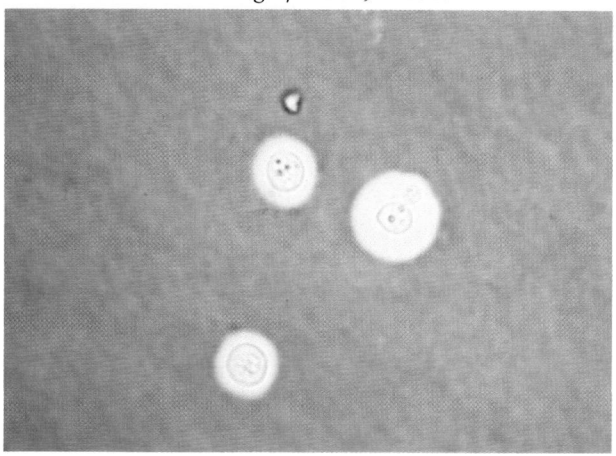

FIGURE 63. Cryptococcus neoformans *found in CSF sample from a patient receiving therapy for Hodgkin's disease.*

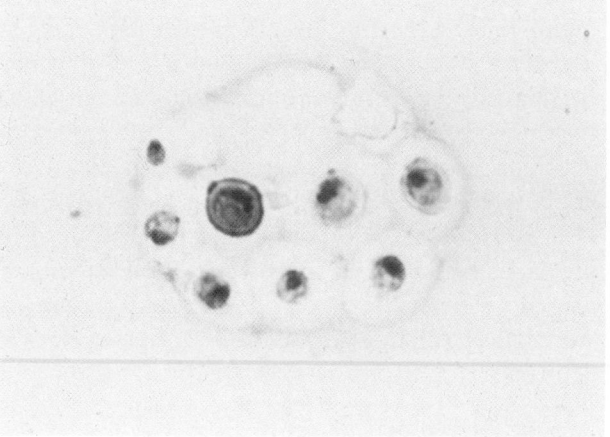

cytosis (40 to 400/cu mm, although mononuclear cells predominate), increased total protein, and decreased glucose levels.

The India ink preparation is useful for the detection of such fungal meningitides as *C neoformans* (Figure 62). This organism resembles mononuclear cells on Wright's staining (Figure 63) and stains positively with periodic acid–Schiff and methenamine silver stains. However, both India ink preparation and Gram's stain are relatively insensitive and require the staining of many organisms. Culture of a membrane filter using a biphasic medium is a much more sensitive test.[185]

Until recently, patients suffering from cryptococcosis were considered to be essentially nonresponsive immunologically. However, various serologic tests that are both diagnostically and prognostically helpful are now available. These methods include an indirect fluorescent antibody technique, tube agglutination and charcoal particle agglutination tests for cryptococcal antibodies, and a latex slide agglutination test for cryptococcal antigen. The last test is the current procedure of choice, since it is highly specific, has both diagnostic and prognostic value, and is widely used.[186,187] It can be used with both serum and CSF. False-positive reactions are rare, and the test results correlate well with those of cultural methods (92% correlation). A positive latex test result with CSF at any titer is usually indicative of active CNS disease. The titer is usually proportional to the extent of the infection. Increasing titers suggest spread of the infection and a poor prognosis, while declining titers indicate a good therapeutic response.

In primary *amebic meningoencephalitis*, organisms such as *Acanthamoeba* sp and *Nagleria* sp are difficult to identify on stained smears. Wet mount preparations, immunofluorescent methods, and electron microscopy may be helpful in the diagnosis.

DETECTION OF MICROBIAL ANTIGENS

Counterimmunoelectrophoresis

The technique of counterimmunoelectrophoresis (CIE) is essentially the familiar Ouchterlony gel-diffusion to which an electric current has been applied. At the pH used (usually 8.6), the water-soluble antigen is strongly negative and migrates toward the anode. The antibody is also negatively charged. Since the antibody charge is so weak, however, it is pulled in a counter direction by the endosmotic forces toward the cathode. The antigen and antibody therefore meet near the center, where they combine and precipitate to form a visible band.

The first clinical application of CIE was in 1970, when Gocke and Howe[187a] used the method for the identification of the hepatitis B antigen in serum. Shortly thereafter, it was shown to be useful in demonstrating the presence of the antigens of *Streptococcus pneumoniae* and *Neisseria meningitidis*. Improvements in the technique have now made it a reasonably simple, rapid, and reliable method for identifying a variety of bacterial antigens and a few antibodies.[188–191]

Although applicable to the measurement of all body fluids, including serum and urine, CIE is particularly valuable in cases of suspected bacterial meningitis. Specific bacterial identification can be made within less than an hour of receipt of the spinal fluid. Counterimmunoelectrophoresis is especially useful in cases of partially treated patients, who make up a significant percentage of cases admitted to a hospital. Unfortunately, not all microorganisms are detectable by this technique. Currently, the method is reliable for detecting most types of *S pneumoniae*, *H influenzae*, group B streptococci, *N meningitidis*, and *E coli*. These organisms, however, are by far the most common ones seen in childhood meningitis, so most infections can be diagnosed by this procedure.

Although the technique is highly specific, it lacks some degree of sensitivity. Occasional cases are seen in which the CIE measurement is negative but cultures are positive. The number of false-negative values from CIE can be substantially reduced if the CSF is concentrated prior to use. Even when this is done, however, a negative CIE value and positive culture can sometimes occur. In these situations, organisms are usually rare, and cultures usually show only one to three colonies and require a 36- to 48-hour incubation period before the organisms are recognized. Results of serum and urine analysis by CIE, although less often positive when compared with those of CSF analysis, are of assistance in many cases. When CSF, serum, and urine specimens are evaluated simultaneously, the diagnostic accuracy approaches 100%.[191]

Although CIE has heretofore been the immunologic method of choice for the rapid detection of microbial antigens, particularly in the diagnosis of meningitis, it has certain disadvantages in comparison with more recent techniques. These disadvantages include the need for specialized equipment and highly trained personnel and the method's comparative lack of sensitivity. The effectiveness of CIE is influenced not only by the system employed and the reagents used, but also by the concentrations of the bacterial antigens. Fung and Wicher[192] have shown that a minimum blood concentration of 10^3 colony-forming units per milliliter was needed for *S pneumoniae* and *H influenzae* before antigens could be detected in serum, while 10^6 colony-forming units per milliliter were needed for group B streptococcal detection.

Several other techniques are now available for microbial antigen detection, including *staphylococcal coagglutination*, *latex agglutination*, and *radioimmunoassay*. Staphylococcal coagglutination depends on protein A of staphylococci binding to the Fc fragment of some subclasses of IgG, leaving the antigen-specific Fab fragment exposed on the surface. Commercial test reagents are available for the streptococcal groups *H influenzae* and *S pneumoniae*. Latex particles sensitized with partially purified globulin fractions are available commercially for detecting antigens of *H influenzae*, *N meningitidis* groups A and C, and *S pneumoniae*.

The major advantages of the coagglutination and latex methods are that they are rapid (10 to 15 minutes) and easy to perform and require no special equipment. In addition, they appear to be more sensitive than CIE,[193–197] although not all investigators are in complete agreement on this point.[198,199] A recent comparative evaluation of these methods revealed an apparent 100-fold greater sensitivity for the latex method, as compared with that of CIE and coagglutination for detecting *H influenzae* type B. The major drawback to these methods appears to be the occurrence of nonspecific agglutinations with many body fluids. Nonspecific reactions may be reduced by heating the specimen for a short period (two to ten minutes). With the use of hybridoma techniques for production of monospecific antibodies, more sensitive and specific reagents will be developed. Radioimmunoassay is, as might be expected, the single most sensitive method.[193] Antigen detection still remains an adjunct to CSF culture.

Limulus Lysate Gelation Test

The horseshoe crab *Limulus polyphemus* is a creature of prehistoric origin found, mysteriously enough, only on the eastern coasts of continents. Circulating within it are cells known as amebocytes. These cells contain a copper complex that gives them a blue color. A lysate of the amebocytes was found to coagulate in the presence of extremely small quantities of endotoxin. This finding led Levin and Bang[200] to develop a relatively simple, rapid, and reliable test that detects endotoxin in various body fluids. It has now been shown to be particularly helpful in the early diagnosis of meningitis caused by gram-negative organisms.[201,202] Its use in the diagnosis of gram-negative sepsis has been less clear-cut and technically more difficult.

The *Limulus* test, using CSF, is an excellent adjunct to the measurement of lactate and to bacterial antigen methods in the rapid diagnosis of bacterial meningitis. Levels of lactate in the CSF are usually elevated in all types of bacterial meningitis. However, they may also be abnormal in a variety of noninfectious processes. When the test results are positive, CIE measurement is highly specific, yet it lacks sensitivity and its effectiveness is limited to a relatively small group of microorganisms. Results of the *Limulus* test are positive in essentially all gram-negative infections, including *H influenzae*, *E coli*, *N meningitidis*, *Proteus morganii*, *Citrobacter freundii*, and *Pseudomonas aeruginosa*. Since a wide variety of gram-negative organisms are known to cause sepsis and meningitis in neonates, the test is particularly helpful in the newborn, where rapid diagnosis and treatment are so important.

Since endotoxin is ubiquitous and contamination widespread, adequate precautions must be taken when this test is performed.[203]

Tests for Neurosyphilis

The lack of a completely reliable laboratory test for the diagnosis of neurosyphilis means that such a diagnosis can be quite difficult to establish and must be based primarily on clinical findings. This is further complicated by a rising incidence of atypical forms of syphilis, by the increasing subtlety of clinical findings, and by the fact that nontreponemal serologic tests are not sensitive enough to be of great help in this diagnosis.[204]

Tests for syphilis are basically of two types—those that measure nonspecific antibodies (reagins) and those that measure specific treponemal antibodies. The nonspecific reaginic tests (serologic tests for syphilis) include the VDRL, rapid plasma reagin, Mazzini, and Kolmer tests, among others. The specific tests use a variety of preparations of the treponemal antigen, including *Treponema pallidum* immobilization, fluorescent treponemal antibody (FTA), fluorescent treponemal antibody with absorption (FTA-ABS), and the microhemagglutination test for *T pallidum*, among others. The FTA-ABS test has generally replaced the *T pallidum* immobilization test and is considered to be the current standard treponemal test.

The reagin tests, while quite satisfactory for screening patients for syphilis by using serum samples, lack the sensitivity to evaluate the CSF adequately. As a result, CSF samples from at least 40% of patients with neurosyphilis will have a negative VDRL result.[205–207] On the other hand, a false-positive VDRL result in CSF is rare, so the test is still indicated for detecting a CSF syphilitic response. Escobar and associates[206] recommend the highly sensitive FTA test for screening spinal fluid for neurosyphilis. As this test lacks some specificity, however, producing a few false-positive results, the FTA-ABS and VDRL were recommended for all fluid specimens giving a positive FTA result. However, a more recent report questions the diagnostic value of using the FTA-ABS test with CSF.[208] One should be aware that a negative serum FTA-ABS test result essentially excludes the diagnosis of neurosyphilis and generally makes examination of the CSF unnecessary. In addition, the microhemagglutination test for *T pallidum* complements the FTA-ABS test and may replace it in the future because it is easier to perform.

More than 90% of mothers of neurosyphilitic infants will have positive serum VDRL and FTA results. Since the antibodies identified in these tests are primarily IgG, they cross the placenta. Hence, cord blood samples will also be positive for syphilis, regardless of whether the infant has congenital syphilis or not. If available, the specific FTA-ABS-IgM test for specific infant antibodies is also helpful. In any event, the infant's CSF should be examined, since asymptomatic neurosyphilis is common in infants with the congenital form of the disease.[207]

REFERENCES

1. Cutler RWP, Spertell RB: Cerebrospinal fluid: A selective review. *Ann Neurol* 11:1–10, 1982

2. Krieg AF: Cerebrospinal fluids and other body fluids, in Henry JB (ed): *Clinical Diagnosis and Management by Laboratory Methods,* ed 16. Philadelphia, WB Saunders Co, 1979, pp 635–657

3. Sarff LD, Platt LH, McCracken GH: Cerebrospinal fluid evaluation in neonates: Composition in high-risk infants with and without meningitis. *J Pediatr* 88: 473–477, 1976

4. McCracken GH: Neonatal septicemia and meningitis. *Hosp Pract* 11:89, 1976

5. Novak RW: Lack of validity of standard corrections for white blood cell counts of blood-contaminated cerebrospinal fluid in infants. *Am J Clin Pathol* 82: 95–97, 1984

6. Osborne JP, Pizer B: Effect on the white cell count of contaminating cerebrospinal fluid with blood. *Arch Dis Child* 56:400–401, 1981

7. Chow G, Schmidley JW: Lysis of erythrocytes and leukocytes in traumatic lumbar punctures. *Arch Neurol* 41:1084–1085, 1984

8. Sheth KV: Cerebrospinal and Body Fluids Cell Morphology through a Hematologist's Microscope, *American Society of Clinical Pathologists workshop manual.* Chicago: ASCP, 1978

9. Dyken PR: Cerebrospinal fluid cytology: Practical clinical usefulness. *Neurology* 25:210–217, 1975

10. Kolmel HW: Atlas of Cerebrospinal Fluid Cells, ed 2. New York: Springer-Verlag, 1977

11. Pappu LD, Purolit DM, Levkoff AH: CSF cytology in the neonate. *Am J Dis Child* 136:297–298, 1982

12. Oehmichen M, Domasch D, Wiethölter H: Origin, proliferation and fate of cerebrospinal fluid cells. *J Neurol* 227:145–150, 1982

13. Oehmichen M: Cerebrospinal Fluid Cytology. *An Introduction and Atlas.* Philadelphia: WB Saunders Co. 1976

14. Kruskall MS, Carter SR, Ritz LP: Contamination of cerebrospinal fluid by vertebral bone marrow cells during lumbar puncture. *N Engl J Med* 308:697–700, 1983

15. Moser RP, Robinson JA, Prostko ER: Lymphocyte subpopulations in human cerebrospinal fluid. *Neurology* 26:726–728, 1976

16. Oehmichen M, Huber H: Supplementary cytodiagnostic analysis of mononuclear cells of the cerebrospinal fluid using cytological markers. *J Neurol* 218: 187–196, 1978

17. Traugott U: T and B lymphocytes in the cerebrospinal fluid of various neurological diseases. *J Neurol* 219:185–197, 1978

18. Bosch I, Oehmichen M: Eosinophilic granulocytes in cerebrospinal fluid: Analysis of 94 cerebrospinal fluid specimens and review of the literature. *J Neurol* 219: 93–105, 1978

19. Kuberski T: Eosinophils in the cerebrospinal fluid. *Ann Intern Med* 91:70–75, 1979

20. Glasser L, Corrigan JJ, Payne C: Basophilic meningitis secondary to lymphoma. *Neurology* 26:899–902, 1976

21. Nosanchuk JS, Kim CW: Lupus erythematosus cells in CSF. *JAMA* 25:2883–2884, 1976

22. Balhuizen JC, Bots GTAM, Schaberg A, et al: Value of cerebrospinal fluid cytology for the diagnosis of malignancies in the central nervous system. *J Neurosurg* 48:747–753, 1978

23. Gondos B: Cytology of cerebrospinal fluid: Technical and diagnostic considerations. *Ann Clin Lab Sci* 6:152–157, 1976

24. Bigner SH, Johnston WW: The cytopathology of cerebrospinal fluid: I. Nonneoplastic conditions, lymphoma and leukemia. *Acta Cytol* 25:335–353, 1981

25. Chartrand SA, Cho CT: Persistent pleocytosis in bacterial meningitis. *J Pediatr* 88:424–426, 1976

26. Fishbein D, Palmer DL, Porter KM: Bacterial meningitis in the absence of CSF pleocytosis. *Arch Intern Med* 141:1369–1372, 1981

27. Aaronson AG, Hajdu SI, Melamed MR: Spinal fluid cytology during chemotherapy of leukemia of the central nervous system in children. *Am J Clin Pathol* 63:523–537, 1975

28. Ducos R, Donoso J, Weickhardt U, et al: Sedimentation versus cytocentrifugation in the cytologic study of craniospinal fluid. *Cancer* 43:479–482, 1979

29. Drewinko B, Sullivan MP, Martin T: Use of the cytocentrifuge in the diagnosis of meningeal leukemia. *Cancer* 31:1331–1336, 1973

30. Gondos B, King EG: Cerebrospinal fluid cytology: Diagnostic accuracy and comparison of different techniques. *Acta Cytol* 21:542–547, 1976

31. Bradstock KF, Papageorgiou ES, Janossy G: Diagnosis of meningeal involvement in patients with acute lymphoblastic leukemia. *Cancer* 47:2478–2481, 1981

32. Casper JT, Lauer SJ, Kirchner PA: Evaluation of cerebrospinal fluid mononuclear cells obtained from children with acute lymphocytic leukemia: Advantages

of combining cytomorphology and terminal deoxynu-cleotidyl transferase. *Am J Clin Pathol* 80:666–670, 1983

33. Glass JP, Melamed M, Chernik NL: Malignant cells in the cerebrospinal fluid (CSF): The meaning of a positive CSF cytology. *Neurology* 29:1369–1375, 1979

34. Bunn PA, Schein PS, Banks PM, et al: Central nervous system complications in patients with diffuse histiocytic and undifferentiated lymphoma: Leukemia revisited. *Blood* 47:3–10, 1976

35. Young RC, Howser DM, Anderson T, et al: Central nervous system complications of non-Hodgkin's lymphomas. *Am J Med* 66:435–443, 1979

36. Herman TS, Hammond N, Jones SE, et al: Involvement of the central nervous system by non-Hodgkin's lymphoma: The Southwest Oncology Group experience. *Cancer* 43:390–397, 1979

37. Tibbling G, Link H, Ohma S: Principles of albumin and IgG analysis in neurological disorders: I. Establishment of reference values. *Scand J Clin Lab Invest* 37:385–390, 1977

38. Schriever H, Gambino S: Protein turbidity produced by trichloroacetic acid and sulfosalicylic acid at varying temperatures and varying ratios of albumin and globulin. *Am J Clin Pathol* 44:667–672, 1975

39. Lowry OH, Rosebrough NJ, Farr A, et al: Protein measurement with the Folinphenol reagent. *J Biol Chem* 193:265–275, 1951

40. Bradford MM: A rapid and sensitive method for the quantitation of microgram quantities of protein utilizing the principle of protein-dye binding. *Anal Biochem* 72:248–254, 1976

41. Peterson GL: Review of the Folin phenol protein quantitation method of Lowry, Rosebrough, Farr and Randall. *Anal Biochem* 100:201–220, 1979

42. Johnson JA, Lott JA: Standardization of the Coomassie Blue method for cerebrospinal fluid proteins. *Clin Chem* 24:1931–1933, 1978

43. Gadd KG: Protein estimation in spinal fluid using Coomassie blue reagent. *Med Lab Sci* 38:61–63, 1981

44. Hische EAH, van der Helm HJ, van Meegen MT, et al: Protein estimation in cerebrospinal fluid with Coomassie Brilliant Blue. *Clin Chem* 28:1236–1237, 1982

45. Patrick RL, Thiers RE: The direct spectrophotometric determination of protein in cerebrospinal fluid. *Clin Chem* 9:283–295, 1963

46. Igou PC: An evaluation of a gel filtration-spectrophotometric method for spinal fluid protein. *Am J Med Technol* 33:354–360, 1967

47. Pesce MA, Strande CS: A new micromethod for determination of protein in cerebrospinal fluid and urine. *Clin Chem* 19:1265–1267, 1973

48. Kaplan A: Electrophoresis of cerebrospinal fluid proteins. *Am J Med Sci* 253:549–555, 1967

49. Windisch RM, Bracken MM: Cerebrospinal fluid proteins: Concentration by membrane ultrafiltration and fractionation by electrophoresis on cellulose acetate. *Clin Chem* 16:416–419, 1970

50. Breebaart L, Becker H, Jongebloed FA: Investigation of reference values of components of cerebrospinal fluid. *J Clin Chem Clin Biochem* 16:561–565, 1978

51. Ivers RR, McKenzie BF, McGuckin WF, et al: Spinal-fluid gamma globulin in multiple sclerosis and other neurologic diseases. *JAMA* 176:515–519, 1961

52. Laterre EC, Callewaert A, Heremans JF, et al: Electrophoretic morphology of gamma globulins in cerebrospinal fluid of multiple sclerosis and other disease of the nervous system. *Neurology* 20:982–990, 1970

53. Link H, Muller R: Immunoglobulins in multiple sclerosis and infections of the nervous system. *Arch Neurol* 25:326–344, 1971

54. Johnson KP, et al: Agarose electrophoresis of cerebrospinal fluid in multiple sclerosis. *Neurology* 27:273–277, 1977

55. Williams A, Papadopoulos N, Chase TN: Demonstration of CSF gamma-globulin banding in presenile dementia. *Neurology* 30:882–884, 1980

56. Wallen WC, Biggar RJ, Levine PH, et al: Oligoclonal IgG in CSF of patients with African Burkitt's lymphoma. *Arch Neurol* 40:11–13, 1983

57. Wecksler WR, El-Shatory MD, Harris NS: Effects of two radiocontrast dyes on the detection of oligoclonal gamma globulins by high resolution agarose gel electrophoresis. *Am J Clin Pathol* 79:607–608, 1983

58. Tourtellotte WW, Tavolato B, Parker JA, et al: Cerebrospinal fluid electroimmunodiffusion. *Arch Neurol* 25:345–350, 1971

59. Kabat EA, Moore DH, Landow H: An electrophoretic study of the protein component in cerebrospinal fluid and their relationship to the serum proteins. *J Clin Invest* 21:571–577, 1942

60. Kabat EA, Glusman M, Knaub V: Quantitative estimation of the albumin and gamma globulin in normal and pathologic cerebrospinal fluid by immunochemical methods. *Am J Med* 4:653–662, 1948

61. Hartley TF, Merrill DA, Claman HN: Quantitation of immunoglobulins in cerebrospinal fluid. *Arch Neurol* 15:472–479, 1966

62. Joseph JC, Bermes EW: Comparison of protein values in cerebrospinal fluid by nephelometry and radial

immunodiffusion. *Ann Clin Lab Sci* 9:408–415, 1979

63. Pearl GS, Check IJ, Hunter RL: Agarose electrophoresis and immunonephelometric quantitation of cerebrospinal fluid immunoglobulins: Criteria for application in the diagnosis of neurologic disease. *Am J Clin Pathol* 81:575–579, 1984

64. Link H, Zetterwall O: Multiple sclerosis: Disturbed kappa: lambda light chain ratio of immunoglobulin G in cerebrospinal fluid. *Clin Exp Immunol* 6: 435–438, 1970

65. Palmer DL, Minard BJ, Witt NJ: IgG subgroups of multiple sclerosis dysproteins. *Am J Clin Pathol* 59:140, 1973

66. Cohen SR, Herndon RM, McKhann GM: Radioimmunoassay of myelin basic protein in spinal fluid. *N Engl J Med* 295:1455–1457, 1976

67. Bloomer LC, Bray PF: Relative value of three laboratory methods in the diagnosis of multiple sclerosis. *Clin Chem* 27:2011–2013, 1981

68. Gerson B, Cohen SR, Gerson IM, et al: Myelin basic protein, oligoclonal bands, and IgG in cerebrospinal fluid as indicators of multiple sclerosis. *Clin Chem* 27:1974–1977, 1981

69. Corrall CJ, Pepple JM, Moxon ER, et al: C-reactive protein in spinal fluid of children with meningitis. *J Pediatr* 99:365–369, 1981

70. Clarke D, Cost K: Use of C-reactive protein in differentiating septic from aseptic meningitis in children. *J Pediatr* 102:718–720, 1983

71. Philip AGS, Baker CJ: Cerebrospinal fluid C-reactive protein in neonatal meningitis. *J Pediatr* 102: 715–717, 1983

72. Knight JA, Dudek SM, Haymond RE: Early (chemical) diagnosis of bacterial meningitis-cerebrospinal fluid glucose, lactate, and lactate dehydrogenase compared. *Clin Chem* 27:1431–1434, 1981

73. Menkes JH: The causes for low spinal fluid sugar in bacterial meningitis: Another look. *Pediatrics* 44: 1–3, 1969

74. Swartz MN, Dodge PR: Bacterial meningitis: A review of selected aspects. *N Engl J Med* 272:779–787, 1965

75. Feldman WE: Cerebrospinal fluid lactic acid dehydrogenase activity: Levels in untreated and partially antibiotic-treated meningitis. *AJDC* 129:77–80, 1975

76. Controni G, Rodriquez WJ, Hicks JM, et al: Cerebrospinal fluid lactic acid levels in meningitis. *J Pediatr* 92:379–384, 1977

77. Hull HF, Morrow G: Glucorrhea revisited: Prolonged promulgation of another plastic pearl. *JAMA* 234:1052–1053, 1975

78. Savory J, Brody JP: Measurement and diagnostic value of cerebrospinal fluid enzymes. *Ann Clin Lab Sci* 9:68–79, 1979

79. Wroblewski F, Decker B, Wroblewski R: Activity of lactate dehydrogenase in spinal fluid. *Am J Clin Pathol* 28:269–271, 1957

80. Wroblewski F, Decker B, Wroblewski R: The clinical implications of spinal-fluid lactic dehydrogenase activity. *N Engl J Med* 258:635–639, 1958

81. Lending M, Slobody LB, Mestern J: Cerebrospinal fluid glutamic oxalacetic transaminase and lactic dehydrogenase activities in children with neurologic disorders. *J Pediatr* 65:415–421, 1964

82. Neches W, Platt M: Cerebrospinal fluid LDH in 287 children, including 53 cases of meningitis of bacterial and non-bacterial etiology. *Pediatrics* 41: 1097–1103, 1968

83. Feldman WE: Cerebrospinal fluid lactic acid dehydrogenase activity. Levels in untreated and partially antibiotic-treated meningitis. *AJDC* 129:77–80, 1975

84. Nelson PV, Carney WF, Pollard AC: Diagnostic significance and source of lactate dehydrogenase and its isoenzymes in cerebrospinal fluid of children with a variety of neurological disorders. *J Clin Pathol* 28: 828–833, 1975

85. Beaty HN, Oppenheimer S: Cerebrospinal-fluid lactic dehydrogenase and its isoenzymes in infections of the central nervous system. *N Engl J Med* 279: 1197–1202, 1968

86. Florez G, Cabeza A, Gonzalez JM, et al: Changes in serum and cerebrospinal fluid enzyme activity after head injury. *Acta Neurochir* 35:3–13, 1976

87. Wakim KG, Fleisher GA: Effect of experimental cerebral infarction on transaminase activity in serum, cerebrospinal fluid and infarcted tissue. *Proc Staff Meet Mayo Clin* 31:391–399, 1956

88. Donnan GA, Zapf P, Doyle AE, et al: CSF enzymes in lacunar and cortical stroke. *Stroke* 14:266–269, 1983

89. Sherwin AL, Norris JW, Bulcke JA: Spinal fluid creatine kinase in neurologic disease. *Neurology* 19: 993–999, 1969

90. Constantopoulos A, Antonakakis K, Matsaniotis N, et al: Spinal fluid lysozyme in the diagnosis of central nervous system tumors. *Neurochirurgia* 19:169–171, 1976

91. Rabe EF, Curnen EC: The occurrence of lysozyme in the cerebrospinal fluid and serum of infants and children. *Pediatrics* 38:147–153, 1951

92. Newman J, Cacatian A, Josephson AS, et al: Spina fluid lysozyme in the diagnosis of central-nervous tumors. *Lancet* 1:756–759, 1974

93. Mason DY, Robert-Thomson P: Spinal-fluid lysozyme in diagnosis of central-nervous-system tumours. *Lancet* 2:952–953, 1974

94. DiLorenzo N, Palma L: Spinal-fluid lysozyme in diagnosis of central-nervous-system tumours. *Lancet* 1:1077, 1976

95. DiLorenzo N, Palma L, Ferrante L: Cerebrospinal fluid lysozyme activity in patients with central nervous system tumors. *Neurochirurgia* 20:19–22, 1977

96. Jaikin A, Agrust A: Cerebrospinal fluid glutamine concentration in patients with chronic hypercapnea. *Clin Sci* 36:11–14, 1969

97. Glasgow AM, Dhiensiri K: Improved assay for spinal fluid glutamine, and values for children with Reye's syndrome. *Clin Chem* 29:642–644, 1974

98. Whitehead TP, Whittaker SRF: A method for the determination of glutamine in cerebrospinal fluid and the results in hepatic coma. *J Clin Pathol* 8:81–84, 1955

99. Hourani BT, Hamlin EM, Reynolds TB: Cerebrospinal fluid glutamine as a measure of hepatic encephalopathy. *Arch Intern Med* 127:1033–1036, 1971

100. Moir ATB, Ashcroft GW, Crawford TBB, et al: Cerebral metabolites in cerebrospinal fluid as a biochemical approach to the brain. *Brain* 93:357–368, 1970

101. Schildkraut JJ: The catecholamine hypothesis of affective disorders: A review of supporting evidence. *Am J Psychiatr* 122:509–522, 1965

102. Maas JW, Landis DH: In vivo studies of the metabolism of norepinephrine in the central nervous system. *J Pharm Exp Ther* 163:147–162, 1968

103. Maas JW: Biogenic amines and depression: Biochemical and pharmacological separation of two types of depression. *Arch Gen Psychiatry* 32:1357–1361, 1975

104. Schildkraut JJ, Orsulak PJ, Schatzberg AF, et al: Toward a biochemical classification of depressive disorders. *Arch Gen Psychiatry* 35:1427–1433, 1978

105. Moyer TP, Maruta T, Richelson E, et al: The implications for antidepressant therapy for measurement of urinary MHPG. *Mayo Clin Proc* 57:665–667, 1982

106. Ebinger G, Verheyden R: On the occurrence of vanillic acid in human brain and cerebrospinal fluid. *J Neurol* 212:133–138, 1976

107. Johansson B, Roos BE: *Proceedings of the Eighth International Congress of Neurology,* Vienna, Verlag der Wiener Medizinischen Akademic, 1965, vol 4, p 141

108. Bernheimer H, Birkmayer W, Hornykiewicz O: Homovanillic acid in the cerebrospinal fluid in Parkinson's syndrome and other diseases of the CNS. *Wien Klin Wochenschr* 23:417–419, 1966

109. Gottfries CG, Gottfries I, Roos BE: Homovanillic acid and 5-hydroxyindoleacetic acid in the cerebrospinal fluid of patients with senile dementia, presenile dementia and parkinsonism. *J Neurochem* 16:1341–1345, 1969

110. Roos BE, Silfverskiold BP: Homovanillic acid in cerebrospinal fluid of alcoholics. *N Engl J Med* 288:1358–1359, 1973

111. Kartzinel R, Ebert MH, Chase TN: Intravenous probenecid loading effects on plasma and cerebrospinal fluid probenecid levels on monoamine metabolites in cerebrospinal fluid. *Neurology* 26:992–996, 1976

112. Jakupcevic M, Lackovic Z, Stefoski D, et al: Nonhomogeneous distribution of 5-hydroxyindoleacetic acid and homovanillic acid in the lumbar cerebrospinal fluid of man. *J Neurol Sci* 31:165–171, 1977

113. Wood JH: Neurochemical analysis of cerebrospinal fluid. *Neurology* 30:645–651, 1980

114. Cutler RWP, Spertell RB: Cerebrospinal fluid: A selective review. *Ann Neurol* 11:1–10, 1981

115. Waterbury LD, Pearce LA: Separation and identification of neutral and acidic metabolites in cerebrospinal fluid. *Clin Chem* 18:258–262, 1972

116. Glaeser BS, Hare TA: Measurement of GABA in human cerebrospinal fluid. *Biochem Med* 12:274–282, 1975

117. Enna SJ, Snyder S: A simple, sensitive and specific radioreceptor assay for endogenous GABA in brain tissue. *J Neurochem* 26:221–224, 1976

118. Bóhlen P, Schechter PJ, van Damme W, et al: Automated assay of γ-aminobutyric acid in human cerebrospinal fluid. *Clin Chem* 24:256–260, 1978.

119. Enna SJ, Stern LZ, Wastek GJ, et al: Cerebrospinal fluid γ-aminobutyric acid variations in neurological disorders. *Arch Neurol* 34:683–685, 1977

120. Manyam NVB, Hare TA, Katz L, et al: Huntington's disease cerebrospinal fluid GABA levels in at-risk individuals. *Arch Neurol* 34:728–730, 1978

121. Roth RH, Giarman NJ: Conversion in vivo of γ-aminobutyric acid to γ-hydroxybutyric acid in the rat. *Biochem Pharmacol* 18:247–250, 1969

122. Snead OC III: Gamma hydroxybutyrate. *Life Sci* 20:1935–1944, 1977

123. Snead OC III, Brown GB, Morawetz RB: Concentration of gamma-hydroxybutyric acid in ventricular and lumbar cerebrospinal fluid. *N Engl J Med* 304:93–95, 1981

124. Perry TL, Hansen S, Christie RG: Amino compounds and organic acids in CSF, plasma, and urine of autistic children. *Biol Psychiatry* 13:575–586, 1978

125. Perry TL, Urquhart N, MacLean J, et al: Nonketotic hyperglycinemia: Glycine accumulation due to

absence of glycine cleavage in brain. *N Engl J Med* 292:1269–1273, 1975

126. Sjaastad O, Berstad J, Gjesdahl P, et al: Homocarnosinosis: II. A familial metabolic disorder associated with spastic paraplegia, progressive mental deficiency and retinal pigmentation. *Acta Neurol Scand* 53:275–290, 1976

127. Sambrook MA: The concentration of cerebrospinal fluid potassium during systemic disturbances of acid-base metabolism. *J Clin Pathol* 28:418–420, 1975

128. Siemkowicz E, Christiansen I, Sorensen S: Changes in cisternal fluid potassium concentration following cardiac arrest. *Acta Neurol Scand* 55:137–144, 1977

129. Woodbury J, Lyons K, Carretta R, et al: Cerebrospinal fluid and serum levels of magnesium, zinc, and calcium in man. *Neurology* 18:700–705, 1965

130. Levinson A: The hydrogen-ion concentration of cerebrospinal fluid: Studies in meningitis. *J Infect Dis* 21:556–570, 1917

131. Bland RD, Lister RC, Ries JP: Cerebrospinal fluid lactic acid level and pH in meningitis. *AJDC* 128:151–156, 1974

132. Wichser J, Kazemi H: CSF bicarbonate regulation in respiratory acidosis and alkalosis. *J Appl Physiol* 38:504–512, 1975

133. Plum F, Siesjo BK: Recent advances in CSF physiology. *Anesthesiology* 42:708–730, 1975

134. Katsurada K, Minami T, Ogawa M, et al: Cerebrospinal fluid acidosis and its possible relation to acute brain swelling. *Jpn J Surg* 2:131–140, 1972

135. Nishimura K: The lactic acid content of blood and spinal fluid. *Proc Soc Exp Biol Med* 22:322–324, 1924

136. Garcia T, Killian JA, De Sanctis A: The lactic acid and sugar content of the spinal fluid in meningitis. *Arch Pathol* 6:530, 1928

137. Pryce JD, Grant PW, Saul KJ: Normal concentrations of lactate, glucose and protein in cerebrospinal fluid, and the diagnostic implications of abnormal concentrations. *Clin Chem* 16:562–565, 1970

138. Bland RD, Lister RC, Ries JP: CSF lactic acid levels and pH in meningitis. *AJDC* 128:151–156, 1974

139. Controni G, Rodriquez WJ, Hicks JM, et al: Cerebrospinal fluid lactic acid levels in meningitis. *J Pediatr* 92:379–384, 1977

140. Brook I, Bricknell KS, Overturf GD, et al: Measurement of lactic acid in cerebrospinal fluid of patients with infections of central nervous system. *J Infect Dis* 137:384–390, 1978

141. Gastrin B, Briem H, Rombo L: Rapid diagnosis of meningitis with use of selected clinical data and gas-liquid chromatographic determination of lactate concentration in cerebrospinal fluid. *J Infect Dis* 139:529–533, 1979

142. Herold DA, Savory J, Bruns DE: Lactic acid in cerebrospinal fluid: Evaluation and application of an automated enzymatic assay. *Ann Clin Lab Sci* 11:416–421, 1981

143. Berg B, Gardsell P, Skansberg P: Cerebrospinal fluid lactate in the diagnosis of meningitis. *Scand J Infect Dis* 14:111–115, 1982

144. Rutledge J, Benjamin D, Hood L, et al: Is the CSF lactate measurement useful in the management of children with suspected bacterial meningitis? *J Pediatr* 98:20–24, 1981

145. Jordan GW, Statland B, Halsted C: CSF lactate in diseases of the CNS. *Arch Intern Med* 143:85–87, 1983

146. Kopetsky SJ, Fishberg EH: Changes in distribution ratio of constituents of blood and spinal fluid in meningitis. *J Lab Clin Med* 18:796–801, 1933

147. Paulson OB, Hansen EL, Christensen HS, et al: Cerebral blood flow, cerebral metabolic rate of oxygen and CSF acid-base parameters in patients with acute pyogenic meningitis and with acute encephalitis. *Acta Neurol Scand* 48(suppl 51):407–408, 1972

148. Knight JA, Dudek SM, Haymond RE: Increased cerebrospinal fluid lactate and early diagnosis of bacterial meningitis. *Clin Chem* 25:809–810, 1979

149. McGuinness GA, Weisz SC, Bell WE: CSF lactate levels in neonates. *AJDC* 137:48–50, 1983

150. Wasserstrom WR, Schwartz MK, Fleisher M, et al: Cerebrospinal fluid biochemical markers in central nervous system tumors: A review. *Ann Clin Lab Sci* 11:239–251, 1981

151. Heikkinen ER, Myllyla VV, Vapaatalo H, et al: Urinary and cerebrospinal fluid concentration of cyclic adenosine-3′, 5′-monophosphate in various neurological diseases. *Eur Neurol* 11:270–280, 1974

152. Cramer H, Ng LKY, Chase TN: Adenosine 3′, 5′-monophosphate in cerebrospinal fluid. *Arch Neurol* 29:197–199, 1973

153. Mori T, Mogami H, Benda P, et al: An astrocyte-specific cerebroprotein in normal brain and in human glioma. *Neurol Med Chir* 10:103–104, 1968

154. Hayakawa T, Morimoto K, Ushio Y, et al: Levels of astroprotein (an astrocyte-specific cerebroprotein) in cerebrospinal fluid of patients with brain tumors. *J Neurosurg* 52:229–233, 1980

155. Seidenfeld J, Marton LJ: Biochemical markers of central nervous system tumors measured in cerebrospi-

nal fluid and their potential use in diagnosis and patient management: A review. *JNCI* 63:919–931, 1979

156. Allen JC, Nisselbaum J, Epstein C, et al: Alpha-fetoprotein and human chorionic gonadotrophin determination in cerebrospinal fluid: An aid to the diagnosis and management of intracranial germ-cell tumors. *J Neurosurg* 57:368–374, 1979

157. Mavligit GM, Stuckey SE, Cabanillas FF, et al: Diagnosis of leukemia or lymphoma in the central nervous system by β₂-microglobulin determination. *N Engl J Med* 303:718–722, 1980

158. Hallgren R, Terent A, Venge P: Lactoferrin, lysozyme, and β₂-microglobulin levels in cerebrospinal fluid. *Inflammation* 6:291–304, 1982

159. Bagshawe KD, Harland S: Immunodiagnosis and monitoring of gonadotrophin-producing metastases in the central nervous system. *Cancer* 38:112–118, 1976

160. Schold SC, Wasserstrom WR, Fleisher M, et al: Cerebrospinal fluid biochemical markers of central nervous system metastases. *Ann Neurol* 8:597–604, 1980

161. Meurman OH, Irjala K, Suonpää J: A new method for identification of cerebrospinal fluid leakage. *Acta Otolaryngol* 87:366–369, 1979

162. Smales OR, Rutter N: Difficulties in diagnosing meningococcal meningitis in children. *Br Med J* 1:588, 1979

163. Swartz MN, Dodge PR: Bacterial meningitis: A review of selected aspects. *N Engl J Med* 272:725–731, 1965

164. Lavetter A, Leedom JM, Mathies AW, et al: Meningitis due to *Listeria monocytogenes*. *N Engl J Med* 285:598–603, 1971

165. Peyla TL, Burke EC: Mima polymorpha meningitis: Report of two cases of children. *Mayo Clin Proc* 40:236–239, 1965

166. Herweg JC, Middelcamp JM, Hartmann AF: Simultaneous mixed bacterial meningitis in children. *J Pediatr* 63:76–83, 1963

167. Keys TF, Wellman WE, Needham GM, et al: Bacterial meningitis: IV. Infections caused by multiple organisms. *Mayo Clin Proc* 41:179–185, 1966

168. Drayna CJ: Haemophilus influenzae type C meningitis. *JAMA* 244:146, 1980

169. Galaid EI, Cherubin CE, Marr JS, et al: Meningococcal disease in New York City, 1973 to 1978. *JAMA* 244:2167–2171, 1980

170. Brandstetter RD, Blair RH, Roberts RB: Neisseria meningitidis serogroup W-135 disease in adults. *JAMA* 246:2060–2061, 1981

171. McCracken GH: Neonatal septicemia and meningitis. *Hosp Pract* 11:89–97, 1976

172. Haslam RH, Allen JR, Dorsen MM, et al: The sequelae of group B beta-hemolytic streptococcal meningitis in early infancy. *AJDC* 131:845–849, 1977

173. Nachamkin I, Dalton HP: The clinical significance of streptococcal species isolated from cerebrospinal fluid. *Am J Clin Pathol* 79:195–199, 1983

174. Lauer BA, Reller LB, Mirrett S: Comparison of acridine orange and Gram stains for detection of microorganisms in cerebrospinal fluid and other clinical specimens. *J Clin Microbiol* 14:201–205, 1981

175. Murray PR, Hampton CM: Recovery of pathogenic bacteria from cerebrospinal fluid. *J Clin Microbiol* 12:554–557, 1980

176. Moore CM, Ross M: Acute bacterial meningitis with absent or minimal cerebrospinal fluid abnormalities. *Clin Pediatr* 12:117–118, 1973

177. Milne A, Hamilton W: Developing of normocellular bacterial meningitis. *NZ Med J* 84:6–8, 1976

178. Onorato IM, Wormser GP, Nicholas P: 'Normal' CSF in bacterial meningitis. *JAMA* 244:1469–1471, 1980

179. Teele DW, Dashefsky B, Rakusan T, et al: Meningitis after lumbar puncture in children with bacteremia. *N Engl J Med* 305:1079–1081, 1981

180. Chonmaitree T, Menegus MA, Power KR: The clinical relevance of 'CSF viral culture.' *JAMA* 247:1843–1847, 1982

181. Peters ACB, Versteeg G, Bots M: Nervous system complications of herpes zoster: Immunofluorescent demonstration of varicella-zoster antigen in CSF cells. *J Neurol Neurosurg Psych* 42:452–457, 1979

182. Meningitis associated with enteroviral infection—Texas, Canada, 1979. *MMWR* 29:341–343, 1980

183. Jarvis WR, Tucker G: Echovirus type 7 meningitis in young children. *AJDC* 135:1009–1012, 1981

184. Garza, DY, Conley FE: Culture-negative meningitis. *Lab Med* 13:439–441, 1982

185. Severence PJ, Kaufman CA: Diagnosis of cryptococcosis: comparison of various methods to detect cryptococcus neoformans. *Mykosen* 26:29–33, 1983

186. Kaufman L: Serodiagnosis of fungal disease, in Rose NR, Friedman H (eds): *Manual of Clinical Immunology*. Washington, DC, American Society for Microbiology, 1976, pp 371–372

187. Salom IL: Cryptococcal meningitis significance of positive antigen test on undiluted spinal fluid. *NY State J Med* 81:1369–1370, 1981

187a. Gocke DJ, Howe C: Rapid detection of Australia antigen by counterimmunoelectrophoresis. *J Immunol* 104:1031–1032, 1970.

188. Dorff GJ, Coonrod JD, Rytel MW: Detection by immunoelectrophoresis of antigen in sera of patients with pneumococcal bacteremia. *Lancet* 1:578–579, 1971

189. Edwards EA: Muehl PM, Peckinpaugh RO: Diagnosis of bacterial meningitis by counterimmunoelectrophoresis. *J Lab Clin Med* 80:449–454, 1972

190. Rytel MW: Counterimmunoelectrophoresis in diagnosis of infectious disease. *Hosp Pract* 10:75–82, 1975

191. Feigin RD, Wong M, Shackelford PG, et al: Countercurrent immunoelectrophoresis of urine as well as of CSF and blood for diagnosis of bacterial meningitis. *J Pediatr* 89:773–775, 1976

192. Fung JC, Wicher K: Minimum number of bacteria needed for antigen detection by counterimmunoelectrophoresis in vivo and in vitro studies. *J Clin Microbiol* 13:681–687, 1981

193. Leinonen M, Kayhty H: Comparison of countercurrent immunoelectrophoresis, latex agglutination, and radioimmunoassay in detection of soluble capsular polysaccharide antigens of *Hemophilus influenzae* type b and *Neisseria meningitidis* of groups A or C. *J Clin Pathol* 31:1172–1176, 1978

194. Ward JI, Siber GR, Scheifele DW, et al: Rapid diagnosis of *Hemophilus influenzae* type B infections by latex particle agglutination and counterimmunoelectrophoresis. *J Pediatr* 93:37–42, 1978

195. Thirumoorthi MC, Dajani AS: Comparison of Staphylococcal coagglutination, latex agglutination, and counterimmunoelectrophoresis for bacterial antigen detection. *J Clin Microbiol* 9:28–32, 1979

196. Wasilauskas BL, Hampton KD: Determination of bacterial meningitis: A retrospective study of 80 cerebrospinal fluid specimens evaluated by four in vitro methods. *J Clin Microbiol* 16:531–535, 1982

197. Marcon MJ, Hamoudi AC, Cannon HJ: Comparative evaluation of three antigen detection methods for diagnosis of *Hemophilus influenzae* type b disease. *J Clin Microbiol* 19:333–337, 1984

198. Dirks-Go SIS, Zanen HC: Latex agglutination, counterimmunoelectrophoresis, and protein A coagglutination in diagnosis of bacterial meningitis. *J Clin Pathol* 31:1167–1171, 1978

199. Webb BJ, Edwards MS, Baker CJ: Comparison of slide coagglutination test and counter-current immunoelectrophoresis for detection of group B streptococcal antigen in cerebrospinal fluid from infants with meningitis. *J Clin Microbiol* 11:263–265, 1980

200. Levin J, Bang FB: Clotable protein in limulus: Its localization and kinetics of its coagulation by endotoxin. *Thromb Diath Haemorrh* 19:186–197, 1968

201. Nachum R, Lipsfy A, Siegel SE: Rapid detection of gram-negative bacterial meningitis by the limulus lysate test. *N Engl J Med* 289:931–934, 1973

202. Dyson D, Cassaday G: Use of limulus lysate for detecting gram-negative neonatal meningitis. *Pediatrics* 58:105–109, 1976

203. Riegle L, Cooperstock MS: Limulus gelation test: Laboratory considerations. *Lab Med* 8:28–30, 1977

204. Hooshmand H, Escobar MR, Kopf SW: Neurosyphilis. *JAMA* 219:726–729, 1972

205. Harner RE, Smith JL, Israel CW: The FTA-ABS test in late syphilis: A serological study in 1985 cases. *JAMA* 293:545–548, 1968

206. Escobar MR, Dalton HP, Allison MJ: Fluorescent antibody tests for syphilis using cerebrospinal fluid: Clinical correlation in 150 cases. *Am J Clin Pathol* 53:886–890, 1970

207. McCracken GH, Kaplan JM: Penicillin treatment for congenital syphilis: A critical reappraisal. *JAMA* 228:855–858, 1974

208. Lee TJ, Sparling PF: Syphilis: An algorithm. *JAMA* 242:1187–1189, 1979

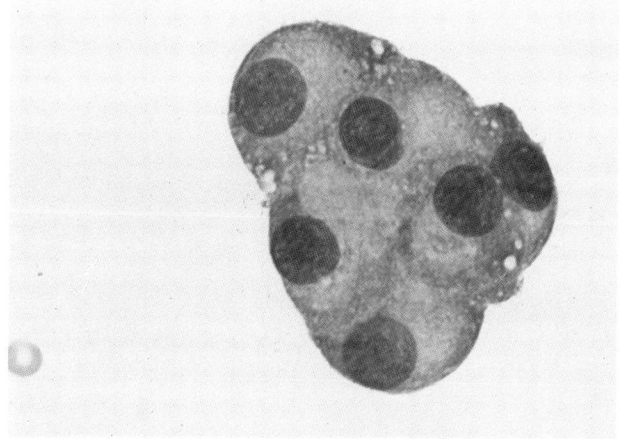

CHAPTER 3

Pleural &
Pericardial
Fluids

ANATOMY AND PATHOPHYSIOLOGY

The pleura encloses the lungs and consists of a thin membrane that forms a double layer. The two layers are contiguous, and the space between them forms the pleural cavity, which is lined by a single layer of mesothelial cells (the mesothelium). Normally, the contiguous layers of mesothelium are separated only by small amounts of fluid that facilitate movement of the two membranes against each other. The pleural cavity, therefore, is not a true cavity but only becomes so in the presence of disease causing the accumulation of fluid therein.

Similarly, the pericardial cavity is only a potential cavity formed by two serous membranes that are closely apposed to each other and separated by small amounts of serous fluid. This fluid allows the heart to move easily during contraction and relaxation. Fol-

lowing injury or the onset of disease, more fluid may accumulate within the cavity, causing a separation between the visceral and parietal pericardia.

The accumulation of fluid within the pleural or pericardial cavities is called an effusion. The aspiration of pleural fluid is called thoracentesis. In addition to its diagnostic uses, thoracentesis may have therapeutic benefit in the relief of pressure.

Pleural fluid is normally produced by the parietal pleura and absorbed by the visceral pleura. This is a continuous process. The fluid is formed by the filtration of plasma through the capillary endothelium; and its presence is dependent on the hydrostatic pressure in capillaries, plasma osmotic pressure, lymphatic resorption, and permeability of capillaries. Fluid is reabsorbed by lymphatic vessels and venules in the pleura.[1,2] Protein enters the pleural space from both

TABLE 3–1. Causes of Pleural Effusions

Transudates
  Acute atelectasis
  Congestive heart failure
  Cirrhosis with ascites
  Hypoproteinemia with nephrotic syndrome
  Postoperative abdominal surgery
  Postpartum effusion
  Peritoneal dialysis
  Superior vena cava obstruction

Exudates
  Infectious diseases
    Bacterial pneumonia (parapneumonic effusion)
    Tuberculosis
    Viral infection
    Fungal infection
    Parasitic infection
    Lung abscess
  Neoplastic disease
    Metastatic carcinoma
    Lung carcinoma
    Mesothelioma
    Lymphoma and leukemia
  Pulmonary embolization or infarction
  Collagen vascular disease
    Rheumatoid arthritis
    Systemic lupus erythematosis
  Gastrointestinal disease
    Pancreatitis
    Esophageal rupture
    Subphrenic abscess
    Hepatic abscess
  Postmyocardial infarction
  Trauma
    Hemothorax
    Chylothorax
  Chylous effusion
    Trauma
    Lymphoma
    Carcinoma
    Tuberculosis

pleural surfaces and leaves via the lymphatic vessels.[3]

Accumulation of pleural fluid (pleural effusion) may result from increased hydrostatic pressure in the circulatory system (congestive heart failure), decreased plasma osmotic pressure (hypoproteinemia), increased permeability of the capillaries in the pleura (bacterial pneumonia), and decreased lymphatic resorption. Approximately 300 mL of pleural fluid must be present before it can be detected by chest roentgenogram.

Causes of pleural effusions are listed in Table 3–1. The cause of pleural transudates, which are frequently bilateral and result from hydrodynamic imbalance, is usually diagnosed easily as congestive heart failure, nephrotic syndrome, cirrhosis, or malnutrition. The pathogenesis of exudative effusions is usually more difficult to diagnose. Pleural effusions often develop during the course of bacterial pneumonia and usually resolve spontaneously.

Unilateral pleural effusion, particularly on the right side, may occur when disease develops below the diaphragm, as in cirrhosis with ascites, subdiaphragmatic abscess, hepatic abscess, acute pancreatitis, and tumors. Pleural effusions are common in systemic lupus erythematosus but may also be associated with congestive heart failure or nephrotic syndrome. Rheumatoid arthritis may be associated with an inflammatory pleural reaction. Pleural effusions are common during the first few days after abdominal surgery but usually resolve spontaneously in such cases.[4] In the majority of the postoperative cases, they are associated with atelectasis, the presence of peritoneal fluid, or irritation of the diaphragm. Pleural effusion (transudate) is a common occurrence during the first 24 hours after birth. However, in the absence of any signs of cardiopulmonary disorders, no therapy is indicated.[5]

Accumulation of fluid in the pericardial cavity (pericardial effusion) is most frequently caused by damage to the lining of the cavity, together with an increase in capillary permeability.[6] In acute pericarditis, fibrinous exudate interferes with pericardial venous and lymphatic drainage and predisposes the patient to effusion.

Echocardiography provides a reliable method of diagnosing the causes of pericardial effusions; disorders associated with pericardial effusions are listed in Table 3–2. The major infectious agents responsible for pericarditis and pericardial effusion are viruses, especially the coxsackie group. Purulent bacterial and tuberculous effusions are less common than they used to be, but renal failure with uremia is commonly associated with pericardial effusion. Significant effusion is associated with the postinfarction syndrome (Dressler's), and cardiac rupture or acute aortic dissection rapidly produces a bloody effusion and cardiac tamponade. Metastatic tumors and, rarely, primary tumor of the pericardium (mesothelioma) are often associated with large effusions. Lung and breast carcinomas, together with lymphoma and leukemia, are the most common causes of secondary malignant effusions. Traumatic pericardial effusions caused by stab wounds or crush injuries may frequently result in cardiac tamponade.

TRANSUDATES AND EXUDATES

Effusions of pleural, pericardial, or peritoneal cavities may be divided into transudates and exudates. In general, transudates indicate that fluid has accumulated because of a systemic disease. A common disorder associated with transudates is congestive heart failure. Exudates are usually associated with disorders involving the pleural surfaces such as inflammation, malignant conditions, or infection (Table 3–1).

The first question that must be answered when a pleural effusion is discovered is whether the effusion is a transudate or an exudate. Although transudates and exudates frequently differ in such characteristics as color, appearance (clear vs cloudy or bloody), and cell count (Table 3–3), these assessments are unreliable in establishing which type of effusion is present. Classically, transudates have been differentiated from exudates by measuring their specific gravity and total protein content. According to these measurements, a transudate is an effusion in which the specific gravity is 1.015 or less and the total protein level is 3.0 g/dL or lower. It follows that exudates have a specific gravity greater than 1.015 and a total protein level greater than 3.0 g/dL. It is now recognized, however, that these simple criteria are unreliable. Melsom[7] demonstrated that, although the means of the total protein levels of transudates and exudates differed signifi-

TABLE 3–2. Causes of Pericardial Effusions
Infections
Viral
Bacterial
Tubercular
Fungal
Cardiovascular disease
Myocardial infarction
Postinfarction syndrome
Cardiac rupture
Congestive heart failure
Aortic dissection
Renal failure and uremia
Neoplastic disease
Mesothelioma
Metastatic carcinoma
Leukemia and lymphoma
Trauma
Coagulation disorders and anticoagulant therapy
Collagen vascular disease

cantly (2.5 g/dL vs 3.8 g/dL), their overlap was considerable, resulting in misclassification of the fluid specimen in about 30% of the cases (range for transudates, 1.0 to 4.7 g/dL; for exudates, 1.0 to 6.3 g/dL).

The most reliable tests for differentiating between a transudate and an exudate is the simultaneous analysis of the pleural fluid and serum for total protein and lactate dehydrogenase (LD) levels.[8,9] A transudate is an effusion in which the ratio of serous fluid total protein to serum total protein is less than 0.5, while the corresponding LD ratio is less than 0.6. Exudates have corresponding ratios higher than 0.5 and 0.6 (Table 3–3). It has also been suggested that transudates have LD levels lower than 200 units/L, while exudates have values higher than 200 units/L.[8] The problem with the use of the total LD activity value in this fashion is that it is affected, as are all enzyme assay results, by a wide variety of technical variables (eg, temperature of assay, concentration of substrate, and the "forward" or "backward" direction of the measured reaction). As a result, "200 units/L" does not have the same meaning in all laboratories.

TABLE 3–3. Findings Used to Distinguish Transudates from Exudates

Test	Transudate	Exudate
Gross examination	Clear Pale yellow	Usually cloudy Variably turbid, purulent, or bloody
WBC count	<1,000/µL	Variable, but usually >1,000/µL
Differential WBC findings	Mononuclear cells	Neutrophils early, mononuclear cells later
Glucose level	Same as in serum	Usually same as in serum
Total protein level	<50% of serum level	>50% of serum level
Lactate dehydrogenase (LD) activity	<60% of serum activity	>60% of serum activity
Fluid total protein to serum total protein ratio*	<0.5	>0.5
Fluid LD to serum LD ratio*	<0.6	>0.6

*These are currently the most reliable tests used to distinguish transudates from exudates.

It is of great clinical importance to classify the pleural fluid specimen accurately as an exudate or a transudate. Using results of the simultaneous testing of serum and pleural fluid protein and LD levels, together with those of a good clinical history and physical examination, an accurate assessment should be possible in more than 90% of patients with effusions. Once the fluid specimen is classified as a transudate, no further tests need be carried out. However, when the specimen is classified as an exudate, other studies are necessary to define the disease process further (Figure 64). Gram's staining, cultures, and counterimmunoelectrophoresis may be indicated if an infection is suspected. Cytologic tests and biopsy may be diagnostic in a case of a suspected malignant condition.

GROSS EXAMINATION

The first step in the investigation of pleural and pericardial effusions is the gross examination, which can play an important role in determining the pathogenesis of the effusion.[6,10] Massive pleural effusions that occupy the entire hemithorax are usually associated with a malignant disorder,[11] most commonly carcinoma of the lung (adenocarcinoma), followed by breast carcinoma. Cirrhosis of the liver and congestive heart failure may also be associated with massive effusions.

Transudates are usually clear and pale yellow and do not clot. Exudates are cloudy to purulent and often clot while standing because of the presence of fibrinogen. The latter fluid is usually associated with large numbers of leukocytes and an elevated protein content. A yellow, turbid fluid is associated with an infectious process; a greenish, turbid fluid is seen with rheumatoid arthritis; a milky-white fluid is found in chylothorax; a bloody fluid is associated with malignant disorders; and a viscous fluid is observed with mesothelioma. The presence of clearly visible pus is diagnostic of empyema. Anaerobic bacterial infection of the pleurae may produce fluid with a foul odor.

Hemorrhagic fluid may be present because of a traumatic tap, malignant disorder, pulmonary infarction, trauma, pancreatitis, or tuberculosis. It should be noted that only 2 mL or so of peripheral blood in 1,000 mL of pleural fluid will produce a blood-tinged appearance.[12] A traumatic tap must be distinguished from other sources of blood in the pleural fluid. In a traumatic tap, the blood is usually not distributed consistently and gradually clears as aspiration proceeds. The most common cause of a hemorrhagic effusion is a malignant disorder (usually lung cancer). True hemothorax, as may be seen in chest injuries, is associated with pure blood in the pleural cavity. A hematocrit reading is very helpful in differentiating between true hemothorax and hemorrhagic effusions. In a true hemothorax, the hematocrit of the fluid will be similar to that of the peripheral blood.

Chylous or so-called pseudochylous effusions are typified by milky-white pleural fluid (Figure 65). It should be emphasized, however, that the classic

FIGURE 64. *Summary of approach to laboratory investigation of pleural fluids. LD, lactic dehydrogenase.*

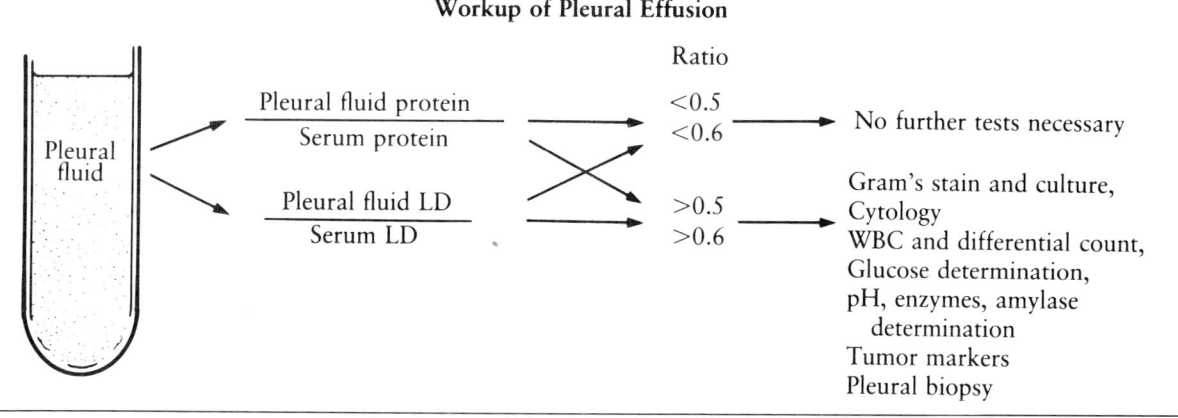

Workup of Pleural Effusion

milky-white appearance may be present in less than 50% of cases of chylous effusions. It may be yellow or green and turbid or even bloody. A true chylothorax is rare and results from leakage of the thoracic duct, which is usually caused by trauma or a malignant condition (lymphoma or carcinoma).[13] In rare cases, it may be the presenting sign of a lymphoma. Pseudochylous fluid, which may initially appear as chronic effusions in such conditions as rheumatoid arthritis or tuberculosis, has a milky or greenish appearance and sometimes a silky sheen. This appearance is the result of cellular debris and cholesterol crystals. Analysis of such fluids is further described under heading, "Chemical Analysis," subhead, "Lipids and Lipoproteins."

CELL COUNTS

Total leukocyte counts are of limited value in the differential diagnosis of pleural and pericardial effusions.[14] In general, leukocyte counts of less than 1,000/μL are associated with transudates, while leukocyte counts of more than 1,000/μL are seen with exudates. These values should not, however, be relied on to separate exudates from transudates, since there is considerable overlap.

The usefulness of the RBC count is also limited, which may be because it takes so little peripheral blood to turn the serous fluid red. However, RBC counts higher than 10,000/μL are highly suggestive of a malignant neoplasm, trauma, or pulmonary infarction.

MICROSCOPIC EXAMINATION

An examination of the cells present and a differential cell count should be performed on a stained smear made by using cytocentrifugation, a filter preparation (Millipore), or sedimentation methods. The cell types encountered in pleural, pericardial, and peritoneal fluids are neutrophils (polymorphonuclear leukocytes, eosinophils, and basophils), lymphocytes, plasma cells, mononuclear phagocytes (monocytes, histiocytes, and macrophages), mesothelial cells, and malignant cells. The following descriptions refer to the cells as seen in pleural, pericardial, and peritoneal fluids using a Romanovsky stain.

Mesothelial cells, which form the lining of pleural, pericardial, and peritoneal cavities, usually cause the most difficulty during the evaluation of the cell types present because they may be mistaken for malignant cells. During inflammatory processes, mesothelial cells undergo proliferation and often desquamate into the serous fluid (Figure 66). They may appear singly or in clusters (Figures 67 through 70). The cells are large and measure 12 to 30 μm in diameter. The cytoplasm is abundant, is light grey to deep blue, and may have a perinuclear zone of pallor, giving it a "fried egg" appearance (Figure 68). Cytoplasmic vacuoles of variable size are often seen. The nucleus is round to oval and occupies about one third to one half of the cell's diameter. The nuclear contour is usually smooth and regular. The chromatin is stippled and dark purple (Figure 71). One to three nucleoli may be seen. Some mesothelial cells resemble large plasma cells (Figure 72).

FIGURE 65. *Chylous pleural effusion typified by milky-white fluid.*

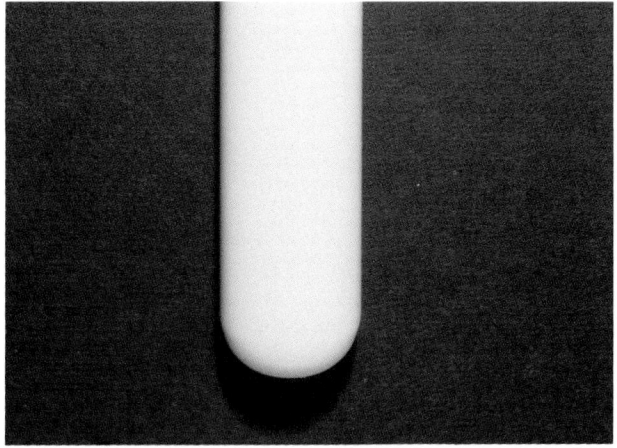

FIGURE 68. *Mesothelial cells with "fried egg" appearance.*

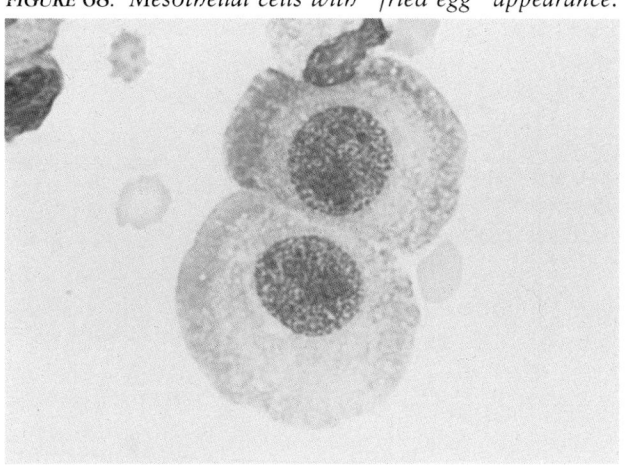

FIGURE 66. *Histologic section of pleura showing proliferation of mesothelial lining cells (hematoxylin-eosin stain).*

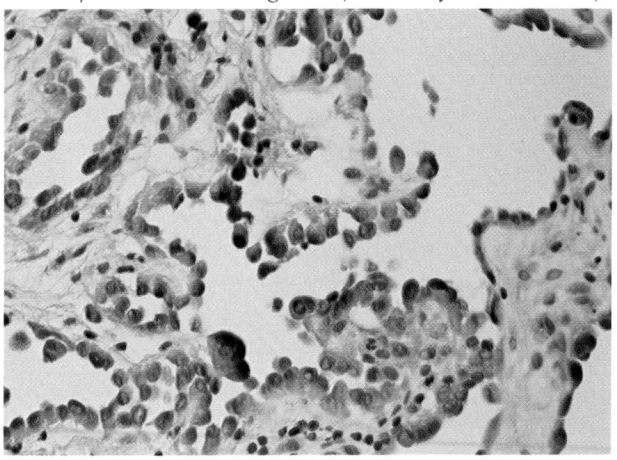

FIGURE 69. *Several mesothelial cells with more basophilic cytoplasm and several binucleated forms.*

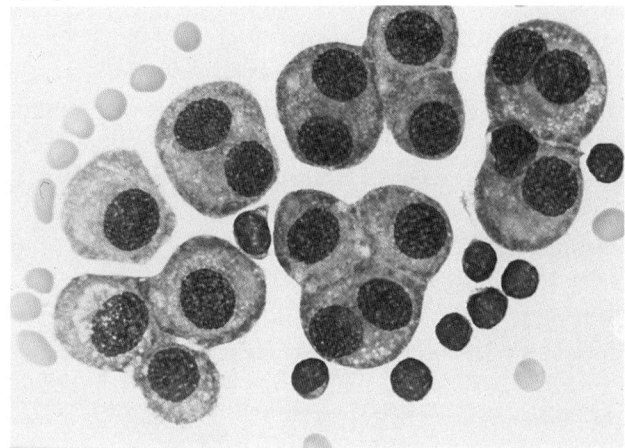

FIGURE 67. *Two mesothelial cells in pleural fluid.*

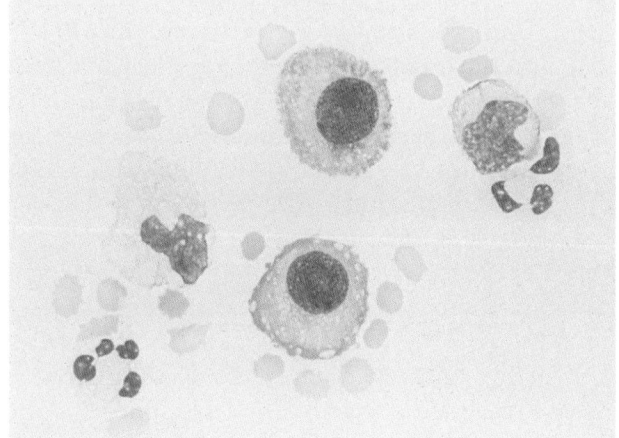

FIGURE 70. *Clump of mesothelial cells.*

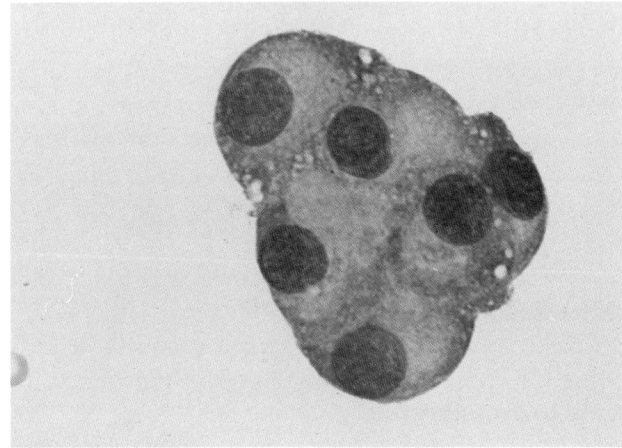

The mesothelial cells vary in appearance and often show atypical or so-called reactive changes. They are commonly mistaken for malignant cells. Mesothelial cells may be multinucleated, occasionally containing 20 or more nuclei; sometimes clusters or sheets of cells are seen (Figures 69, 73, and 74). Clustering may be caused by centrifugation and, in cases of long-standing effusion, may closely resemble malignant cells (Figures 75 and 76). Clumps of mesothelial cells may be distinguished from malignant cells by comparing their appearance within a clump with other, more readily identified mesothelial cells in the same smear and thereby recognizing the "family similarity." The uniform, regular arrangement of the cells usually indicates their benign origin. When the cell concentration is heavy, the specimen should be diluted to obtain optimal morphology.

Degenerative mesothelial cells may show pyknosis and karyorrhexis. Mesothelial cells may exhibit phagocytosis and transform into macrophages.[15] It may, therefore, be extremely difficult to differentiate between mononuclear phagocytes and intermediate forms of mesothelial cells. The nonspecific esterase stain is not useful in differentiating between mesothelial cells, mononuclear phagocytes, and malignant cells, since strong enzyme activity may be present in all of these cells.[15,16]

Mesothelial cells are seen in variable numbers in most effusions and are increased in sterile inflammations caused by such conditions as pneumonia, pulmonary infarction, and malignant disorders. In tuberculous pleurisy or when heavy concentrations of pyogenic organisms are present within the serous cavities, mesothelial cells are characteristically scarce.[17] This is probably due to a fibrinous exudate covering the mesothelial lining of the cavity.

Neutrophils (PMNs) differ in appearance in serous fluids. They may appear more or less identical to those seen in the blood (Figure 77) or may be difficult to recognize as PMNs.[17] In long-standing effusions, the granules may be decreased in number or lost. The nuclei may appear as densely stained spherical fragments and may be mistaken for nucleated RBCs (Figure 78). Occasionally, the cytoplasm may have a bluish color so that the PMN resembles a lymphocyte. In infected effusions, PMNs may show evidence of

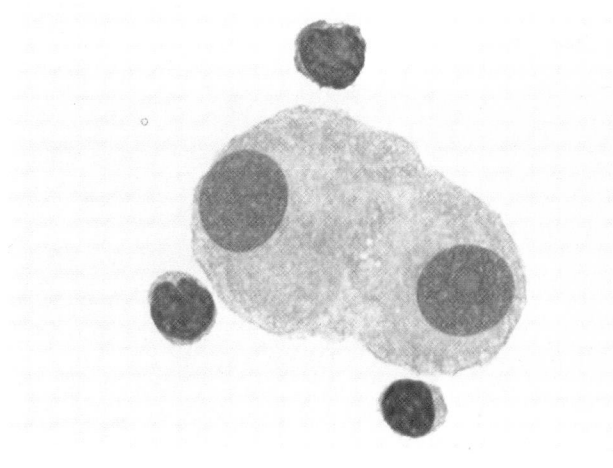

FIGURE 71. *Two mesothelial cells surrounded by three small lymphocytes.*

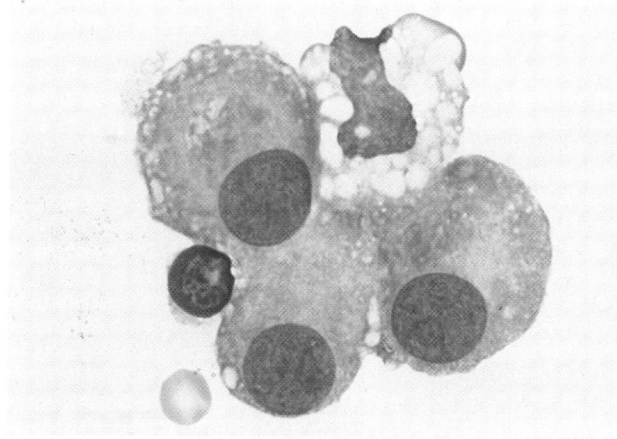

FIGURE 72. *Mesothelial cells resembling large plasma cells.*

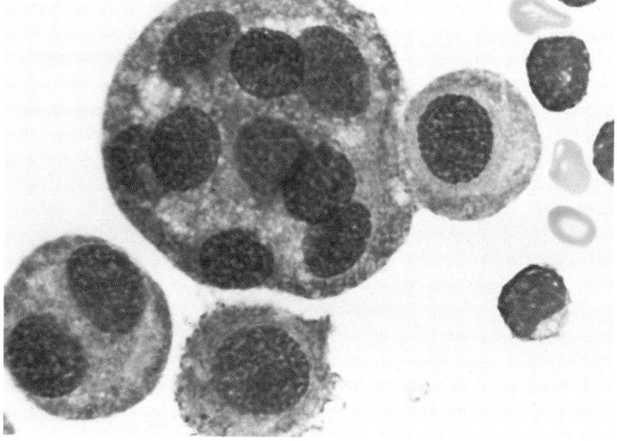

FIGURE 73. *Single and multinucleated mesothelial cells.*

FIGURE 74. *Very large mesothelial cell with multiple nuclei.*

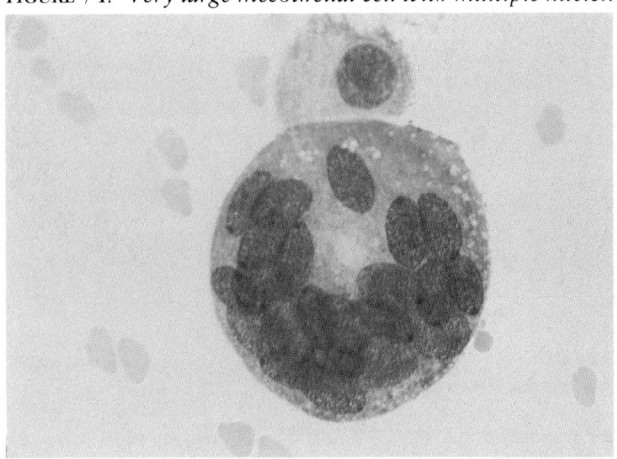

FIGURE 75. *Clump of mesothelial cells resembling tumor cells.*

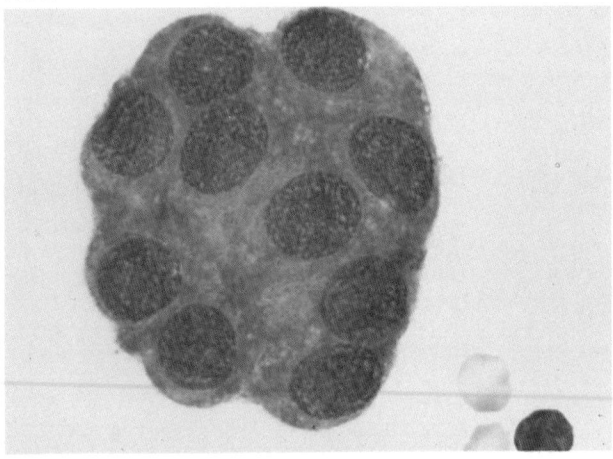

FIGURE 76. *Clump of hyperchromatic mesothelial cells that could be mistaken for malignant cells.*

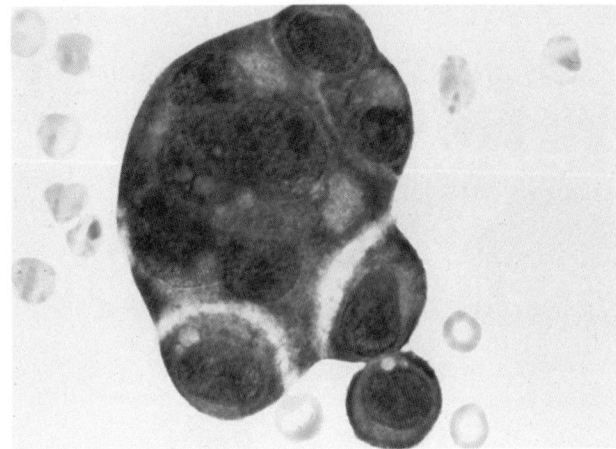

FIGURE 77. *Numerous neutrophils in patient with bronchopneumonia.*

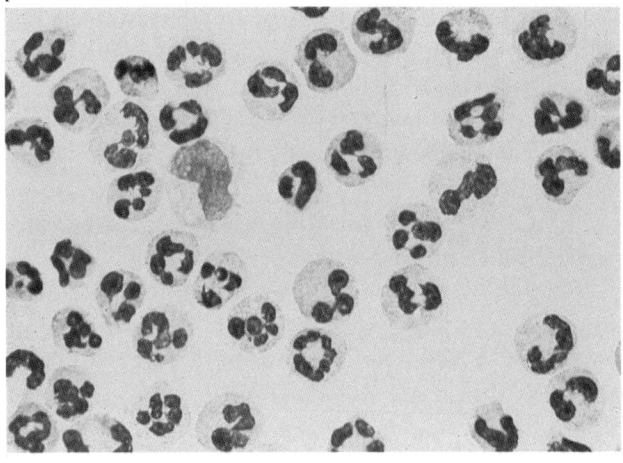

FIGURE 78. *Two degenerating neutrophils with nuclei appearing as dark, spherical fragments. When only one fragment is present, the neutrophil resembles a nucleated RBC.*

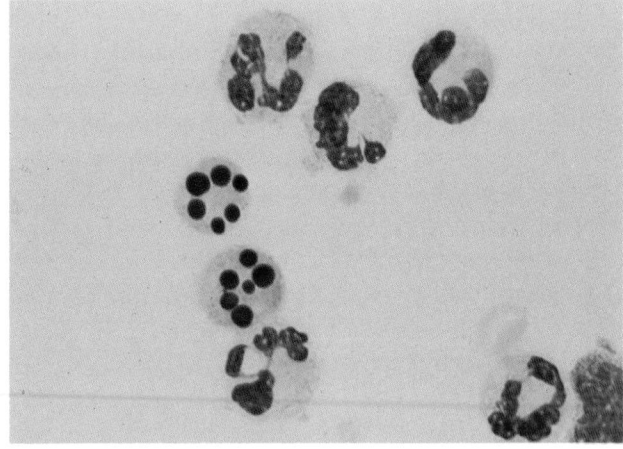

FIGURE 79. *Lymphocytes and neutrophils in pleural fluid sample from a patient with congestive heart failure.*

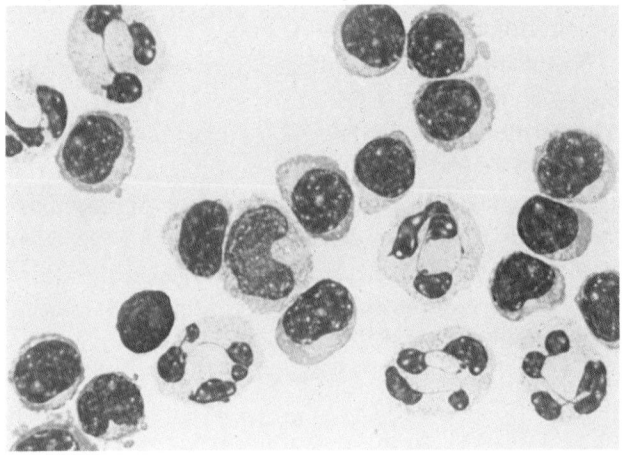

degeneration in the form of vacuolation, loss of granules, and blurred nuclei.

It is debatable how valuable a differential leukocyte count will be in the differential diagnosis. The number of PMNs present in different effusions may vary, but a predominance of PMNs suggests bacterial pneumonia, pulmonary infarction, or pancreatitis. Serous fluid neutrophilia is usually the initial cellular reaction to these conditions. Later there may be a predominance of mononuclear cells and mesothelial cells.

Lymphocytes are seen in variable numbers in most serous effusions (Figure 79). They may be small, medium-sized, or large, and they may exhibit reactive changes. The lymphocytes may have an immature appearance, suggesting lymphocytic leukemia or lymphoma if they represent the predominant cell type. Lymphocytic nucleoli are often more prominent in effusions than in the peripheral blood, and the nuclei may be cleaved (Figure 80). Some of the irregularity of the nuclear contours may be caused by centrifugation during the concentration process. Transformed or reactive lymphocytes (immunoblasts) may be present (Figures 81 and 82). These are large lymphocytes with abundant, deep-blue cytoplasm and often several prominent nucleoli. Tuberculous and malignant effusions frequently show a predominance of lymphocytes (Figures 83 and 84). In tuberculosis, the fluid characteristically shows lymphocytosis and only a few mesothelial cells. It should be emphasized, however, that the absence of lymphocytosis does not rule out either tuberculosis or malignant effusions. In non-Hodgkin's lymphoma, the malignant lymphocytes are generally uniform (monotonous) in size, shape, and staining characteristics. This is in contrast to benign conditions, in which there is usually a mixture of different types of lymphocytes. Lymphocytic pleural effusions may also be associated with leakage of the thoracic duct. A lesser degree of lymphocytosis may be seen in congestive heart failure and cirrhosis.

The detection of T- and B-lymphocytes in pleural effusions may aid in the differential diagnosis. In pulmonary tuberculosis, the number of T-lymphocytes in pleural fluid has been reported to be considerably higher than that in the peripheral blood.[18] The number of B-lymphocytes in pleural fluid is usually significantly lower than that in the peripheral blood of patients with pulmonary tuberculosis, pulmonary malignant disorders, or nonspecific pleuritis.[18] Similar

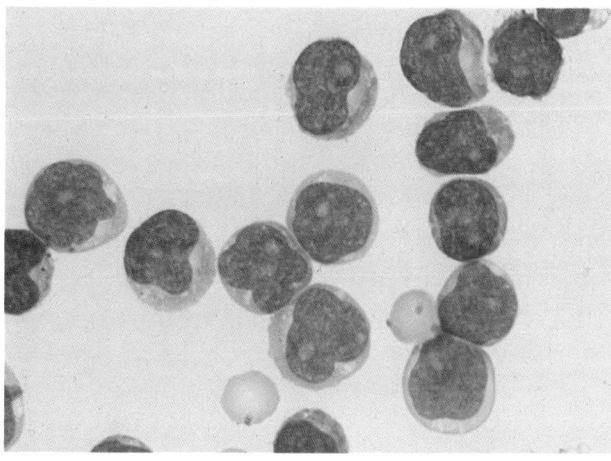

FIGURE 80. *Lymphocytes with irregular nuclear contours and moderately prominent nucleoli in a patient with viral pneumonia. The nuclear irregularities in this case are artifacts of the cytocentrifuge.*

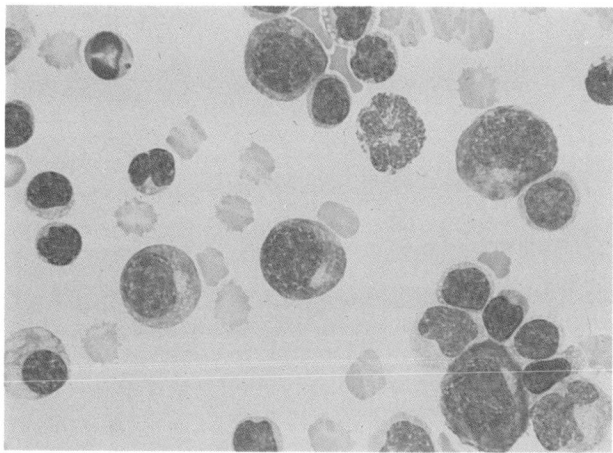

FIGURE 81. *Several reactive, transformed lymphocytes in pleural fluid sample from patient with pulmonary infarction.*

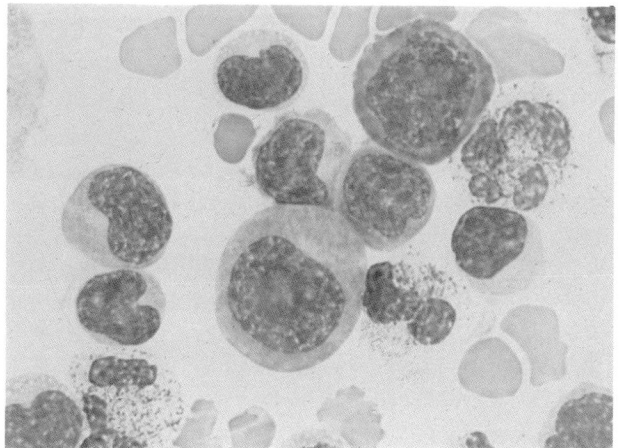

FIGURE 82. *Two transformed lymphocytes (immunoblasts) in pleural fluid sample from patient with pancreatitis.*

FIGURE 83. *Lymphocytosis in pleural fluid sample from patient with tuberculosis. Note absence of mesothelial cells.*

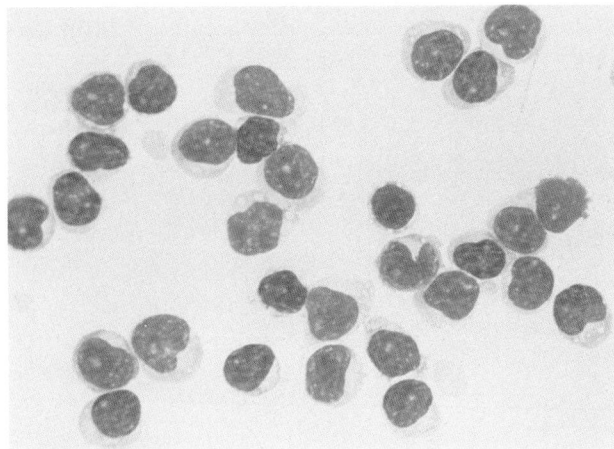

FIGURE 84. *Numerous lymphocytes and one malignant cell seen in pleural effusion in patient with metastatic colon adenocarcinoma.*

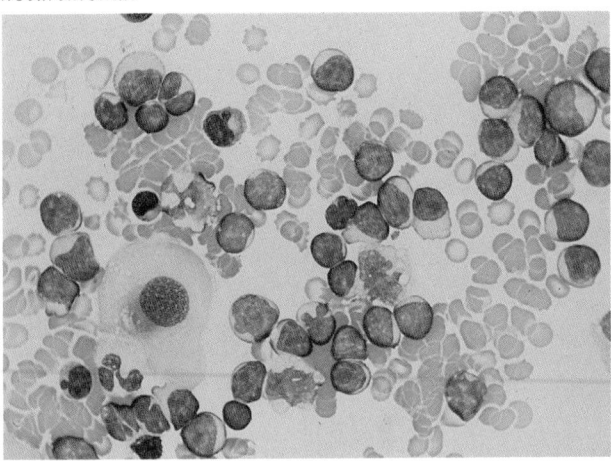

FIGURE 85. *Pleural effusion in patient with non-Hodgkin's lymphoma, small-lymphocytic type.*

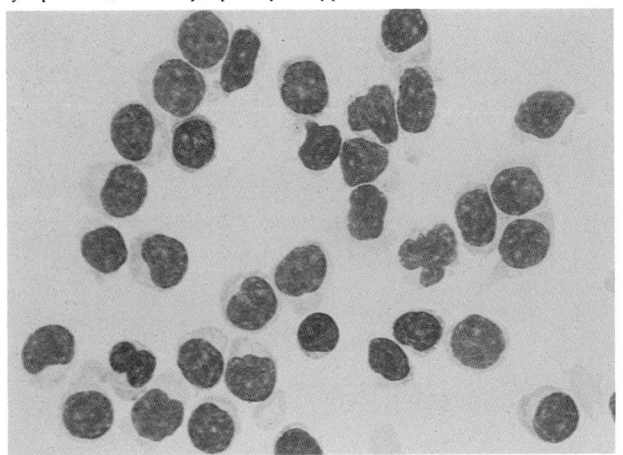

FIGURE 86. *Immunoenzymatic study using antibodies to heavy and light chains revealing a monoclonal B cell population and confirming that the lymphocytes in Figure 85 were malignant. Immuno–alkaline phosphatase stain with antibody to κ light chain shows strong activity (red staining).*

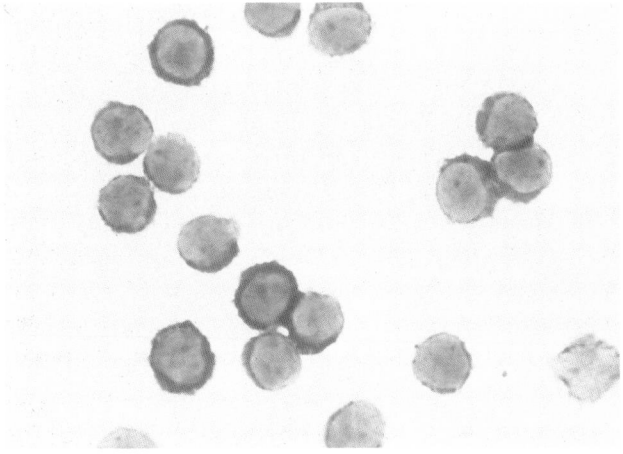

FIGURE 87. *Lymphocytes and plasma cell in pleural effusion from patient with rheumatoid arthritis.*

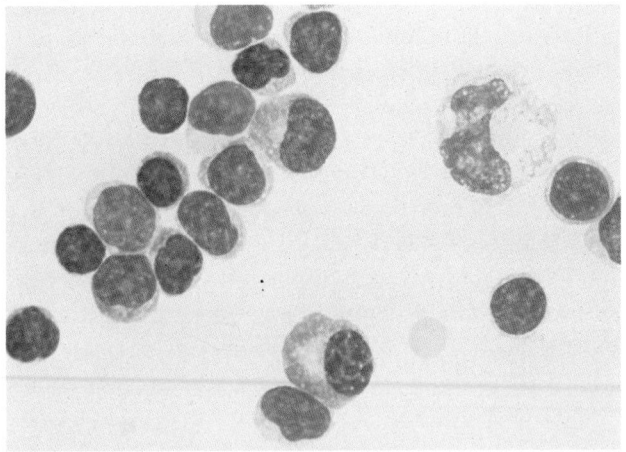

FIGURE 88. *Pleural fluid eosinophilia in patient with chronic renal failure. Two basophils are also seen. A small number of basophils commonly accompany eosinophils in a variety of conditions.*

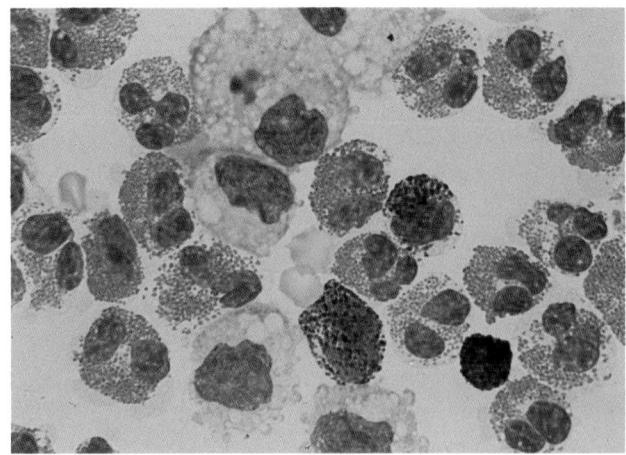

observations have been made in cases of malignant pleural effusion. The mean percentage of T-lymphocytes detected in pleural effusions of ten patients with nonmalignant disease (congestive heart failure, pulmonary emboli, tuberculosis, or hepatorenal syndrome) was 80.2%, and the mean percentage of B-lymphocytes was 7.4%.[19] The presence of a monoclonal B-cell population is usually associated with a malignant lymphoma (Figures 85 and 86).

Plasma cells may be seen in fluid specimens of patients with rheumatoid arthritis, malignant disorders, tuberculosis, and other conditions associated with lymphocytosis (Figure 87).

Pleural fluid *eosinophilia*, like blood eosinophilia, is nonspecific. It has been described in a number of disorders, including idiopathic effusions, infections, pneumothorax, neoplasms, infarction, chest trauma, subdiaphragmatic inflammation, congestive heart failure, collagen diseases, and hypersensitivity states (Figure 88).[20] The pleural fluid eosinophilia may or may not be accompanied by blood eosinophilia. When blood eosinophilia is also present, one should consider the possibility of hydatid disease, Löffler's syndrome, periarteritis nodosa, trauma, or Hodgkin's disease. Mast cells may accompany eosinophils, and 5% to 10% may be seen in pleural eosinophilia.[17] Eosinophilic pleural effusions are usually unilateral and frequently blood-tinged. Eosinophils are, however, seen very rarely in tuberculosis and malignant disorders.[21]

Mononuclear phagocytes (monocytes, histiocytes, and macrophages) are usually seen in variable numbers in pleural, pericardial, and peritoneal effusions.[17] Since both monocytes and mesothelial cells may be transformed into macrophages, the distinction between them is not always obvious (Figure 89). The terms "macrophage" and "histiocyte" are used synonymously in this book, although some authors distinguish between the two by defining the macrophages as those that show evidence of phagocytosis. Macrophages vary in size and have a diameter of 15 to 25 μm. The cytoplasm is pale grey, cloudy, and frequently vacuolated (Figure 90). Sometimes, very large (up to 50 μm) macrophages may be seen. So-called signet-ring cells are formed when the small vacuoles fuse, forming one or two large vacuoles that flatten the nucleus against the side of the cell membrane (Figure 91). The "signet-ring" cell is a descriptive term

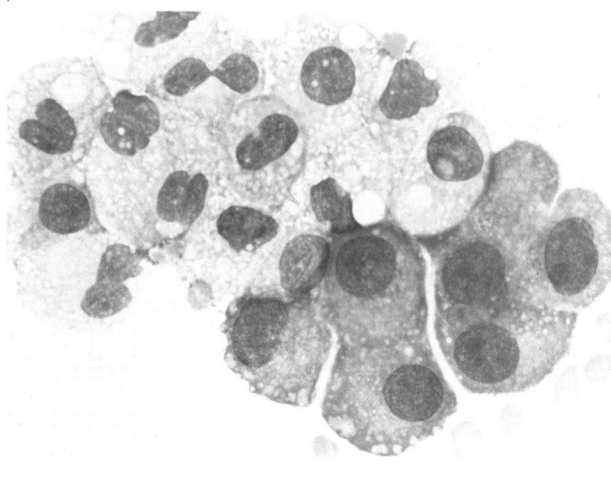

FIGURE 89. Mixture of macrophages (pale, vacuolated cytoplasm) and mesothelial cells (blue cytoplasm) in pleural fluid.

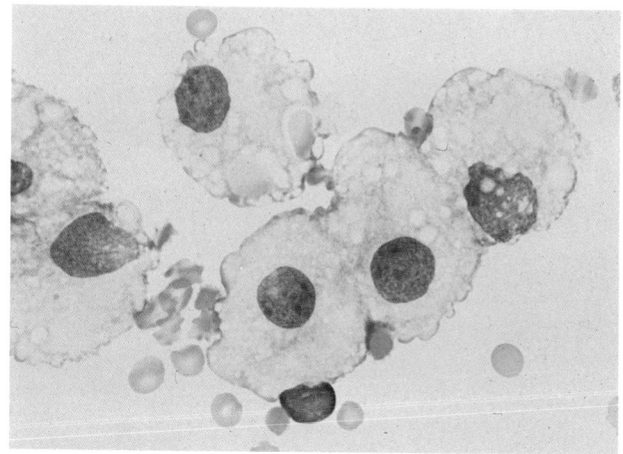

FIGURE 90. Macrophages, one showing erythrophagocytosis, in pleural effusion.

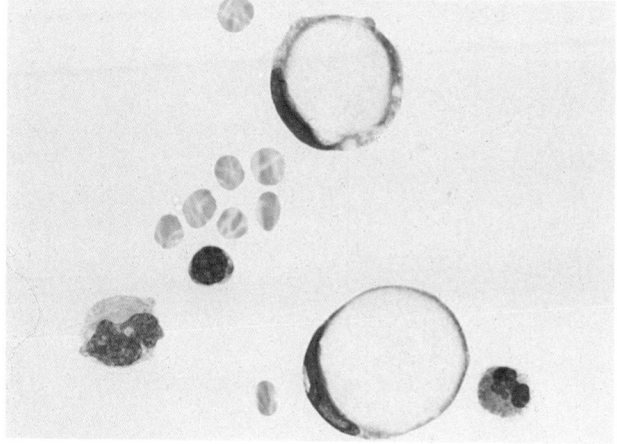

FIGURE 91. "Signet-ring" macrophages in pleural fluid.

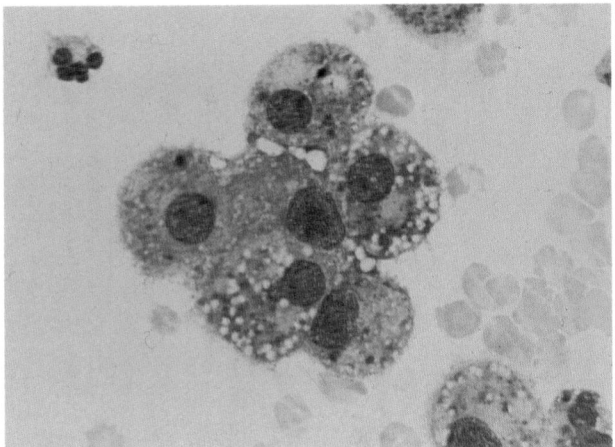

FIGURE 92. *Macrophages containing a variety of pigments.*

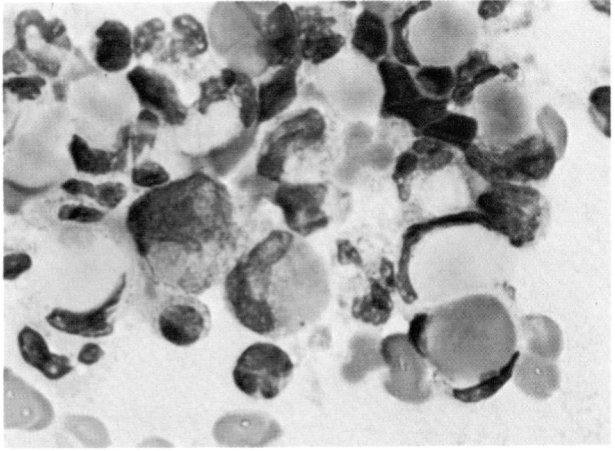

FIGURE 93. *Lupus erythematosus cells in pleural fluid.*

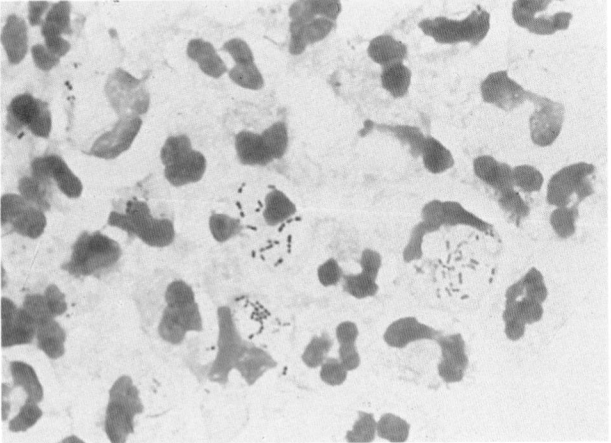

FIGURE 94. *Gram's stain of pleural effusion in patient with perforated esophagus. A mixed infection of gram-negative and gram-positive bacteria.*

and may be seen equally often in benign and malignant cells. Macrophages may contain phagocytosed RBCs, hemosiderin (brown or blue particles), portions of PMNs, carbon particles, or yellow bile pigment (Figure 92). Their numbers vary in both benign and malignant fluids and usually increase as the process becomes chronic.

In vivo *lupus erythematosus cell formation* has been reported in pleural, pericardial, and peritoneal fluids (Figure 93).[22]

CLINICAL CORRELATIONS

A *parapneumonic effusion* is a pleural effusion associated with bacterial pneumonia or lung abscess (Figures 94 and 95). Exudative effusions are seen in about 50% of all patients with bacterial pneumonia.[23] The leukocyte count in such cases ranges from 5,000 to 25,000/μL, with a predominance of neutrophils. Small pleural effusions are seen in patients with viral pneumonia and *Mycoplasma pneumoniae,* and an empyema is present when purulent fluid is aspirated. The leukocyte count is usually higher than 50,000/μL in these patients.

Effusions associated with tuberculosis are usually straw colored or occasionally serosanguineous. The leukocyte count is usually less than 10,000/μL and consists predominantly of small lymphocytes. The presence of a substantial number of mesothelial cells would not support a diagnosis of tuberculosis.

Pleural effusions are found in approximately 50% of the patients with *pulmonary embolism.*[24] When associated with *pulmonary infarction,* the effusions are usually small, serosanguineous exudates. Unfortunately, the fluid usually reveals no specific diagnostic features, and the results of both the gross and microscopic examinations are variable. In more than half of the effusions, the fluid is bloody and initially shows a predominance of PMNs. Later, lymphocytes and macrophages predominate. However, less than two thirds of the fluid samples tested in one study were exudates.[24] Thus, the presence of clear pleural fluid does not exclude the possibility of pulmonary embolism.

Rheumatoid pleural effusions are usually unilateral and have a yellow or yellowish green color. These effusions are usually associated with active arthritis and may be present for months or years.[25] The leukocyte count in such cases is usually less than 20,000/μL, and the majority of the cells are lymphocytes. The pleural fluid glucose concentration may be markedly decreased, and the pH is approximately 7.00.[26]

A pleural effusion is seen in approximately 10% of patients with *acute pancreatitis.*[27] It is usually found in the left pleural cavity but may be bilateral. The fluid is usually a serosanguineous exudate made up predominantly of PMNs. The fluid amylase level is at least twice as high as the serum level.

Bacterial pericarditis is characterized by leukocytosis (>1,000/μL) with a predominance of PMNs. Similar findings may be observed in patients with viral pericarditis and postmyocardial infarction syndrome.

Pleural and pericardial effusions may be seen in uremia and in patients undergoing *long-term dialysis.*[28,29] The pleural effusion is usually unilateral, serosanguineous, or hemorrhagic and contains a predominance of lymphocytes. The fluid is usually an exudate. Creatinine levels are similar to those found in the blood.

Neoplastic disease is one of the most common causes of pleural and pericardial effusions.[30,31] Therefore, the most important part of the laboratory investigation is the cytologic examination of the effusion for malignant cells. Pleural effusions develop in nearly half of the patients who have disseminated lung and breast cancer. Effusions are also common in patients with lymphoma,[32] mesothelioma, various sarcomas, and ovarian and gastrointestinal neoplasms. A true chylous effusion is often associated with lymphoma.[33] In determining the site of the primary tumor, it is helpful to consider the side of the pleural effusion (right or left pleural cavity) and the patient's sex. Ninety percent of malignant effusions originating from lung, breast, or ovarian tumors are ipsilateral to the primary tumor, and pleural metastases from primary sites other than the lung usually indicate tertiary spread from liver metastases.[34,35] Carcinoma or lymphoma is the most likely cause of bilateral effusions in the absence of congestive heart failure.

Malignant neoplasms produce pleural effusions through a number of different mechanisms.[30,36] The neoplasm may cause lymphatic and capillary obstruction, resulting in reduced absorption of fluid and protein. In addition, malignant cells may produce chem-

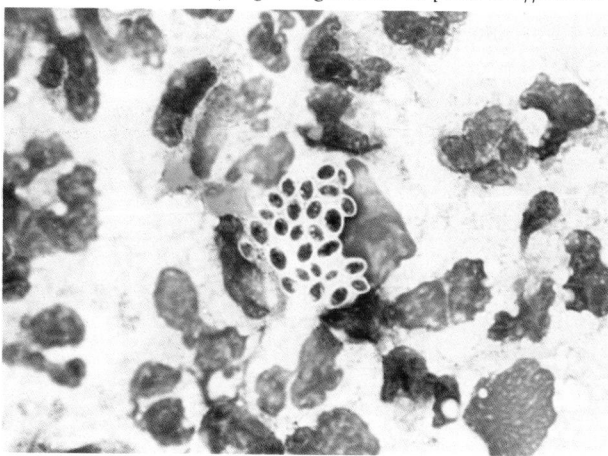

FIGURE 95. Candida *fungal organisms in pleural effusion.*

FIGURE 96.   *Characteristic clumping of tumor cells in pleural effusion.*

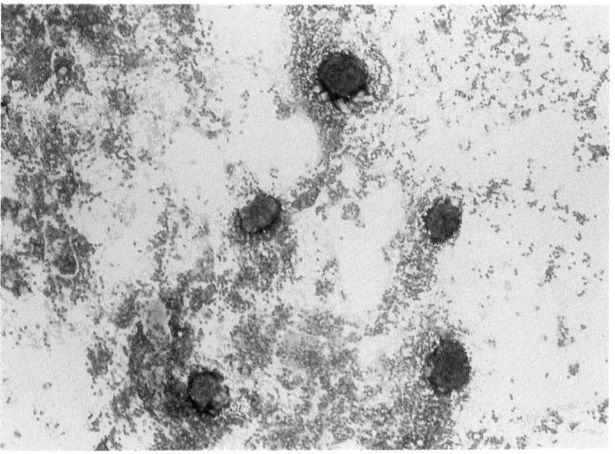

FIGURE 96.   *Characteristic clumping of tumor cells in pleural effusion.*

FIGURE 97.   *Clump of bizarre, vacuolated tumor cells from patient with metastatic adenocarcinoma.*

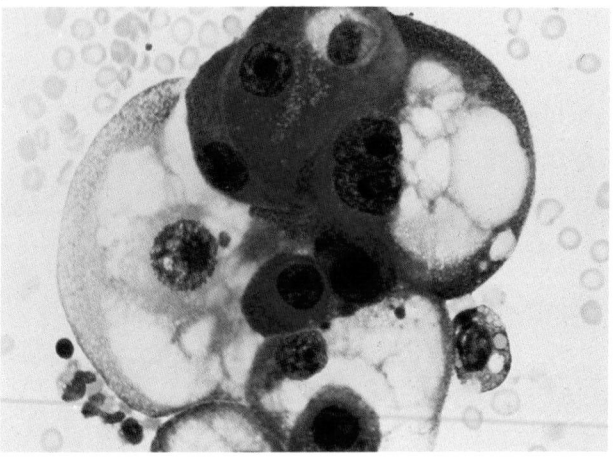

FIGURE 98.   *Typical molding of nuclei in oat cell carcinoma of the lung.*

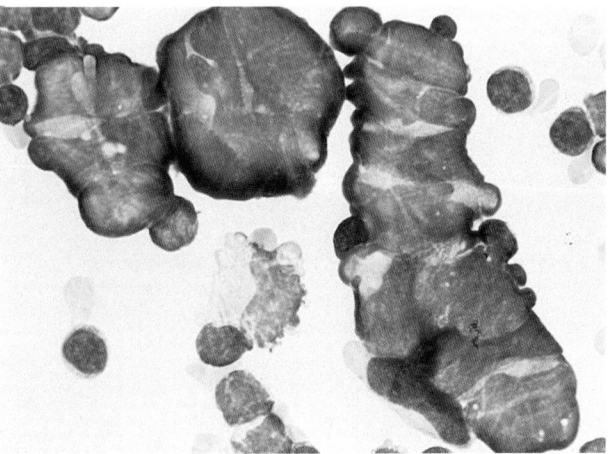

ical mediators that increase capillary permeability. Neoplastic lesions may also cause endobronchial obstruction with pneumonia or atelectasis. Occasionally, the tumor erodes a blood vessel, causing hemothorax. A massive bloody effusion in the absence of trauma is almost always caused by a malignant disorder.

Malignant effusions are usually exudates. The leukocyte count is variable and may show a predominance of lymphocytes, although serous fluid neutrophilia may also be present. The number of malignant cells found in effusions that are associated with malignant neoplasms varies.[30] Bilateral effusions are often associated with obstruction of the lymphatic vessels. When this occurs, a cytologic study of the effusion often reveals no malignant cells. In contrast, many malignant cells may be seen where there are free-growing tumor cells within the fluid and in the adjacent pleura. Exfoliation of solid tumor implants into the pleura is associated with a moderate number of tumor cells.

When a malignant effusion is suspected, a fluid specimen should be sent to the cytology laboratory. The smear, prepared as part of the routine examination of the pleural fluid in the clinical laboratory, should also be carefully examined for malignant cells. In general, the greater the number of methods that are employed to detect malignant cells, the better the physician's chances for arriving at a correct diagnosis. No single microscopic feature is absolutely diagnostic of malignant cells, but several points are helpful. Tumor cells frequently aggregate in clumps or cell balls and sometimes show gland-like formation (Figure 96). These clumps of cells are frequently best seen when the smear is scanned under low power. Malignant cells usually look distinctly different from cells encountered in benign fluids (Figure 97). They often have large nuclei with prominent, abnormally shaped nucleoli. The nuclear-to-cytoplasmic ratio is usually higher than that in normal cells. The malignant cells may be monomorphic (similar) or pleomorphic (variable in size and shape). The cytoplasm may be basophilic or vacuolated or may contain mucus.

Most malignant effusions are caused by *metastatic adenocarcinoma*. Tumors of this type may be associated with multiple round cell aggregates with or without giant vacuoles. In addition, the tumor cells may be isolated and bizarre, and monstrous forms may be seen (Figure 98). Atypical mesothelial cells may be difficult to distinguish from malignant cells, as mentioned, particularly when the former cells occur in clumps. Transmission-microscopic and scanning electron-microscopic techniques are occasionally helpful in distinguishing between atypical mesothelial cells and malignant cells.[37,38]

Oat cell carcinoma of the lung has a characteristic cell structure.[39] Cells of this type resemble large lymphocytes but are larger (about 20 μm). The nuclear chromatin is somewhat less fine than that found in lymphoblasts, and the nucleoli are usually indistinct. The cytoplasmic borders are indistinct and the cells are often seen in small groups, with the nuclei showing "molding" or a mosaic pattern (Figure 98). When occurring as single or separated cells, they may, however, be difficult to distinguish from lymphoma or lymphoblastic leukemia cells. Of primary lung carcinomas, adenocarcinoma, because of its peripheral location, is the most common cell type to involve the pleurae.

Pleural effusions are ultimately seen in approximately 50% of patients with *breast carcinoma*, with 50% to 80% of the effusions being ipsilateral to the primary tumor and about 10% bilateral.[40,41] The tumor cells characteristically are seen as tight, round clumps—so-called cannonballs (Figures 99 and 100). At times it may be difficult to differentiate between clumps of mesothelial cells and breast carcinoma cells (Figures 75, 76, 100, and 101). Immunoperoxidase studies performed on cytocentrifuge specimens may be very helpful in distinguishing between malignant and mesothelial cells (see "Tumor Markers").

Pleural effusions associated with malignant *lymphomas* may be chylous in nature. When an adequate number of malignant cells is present and when the observer is familiar with the variable appearance of reactive or benign transformed lymphocytes, it is usually not difficult to make a diagnosis of lymphoma.[42] Problems arise, however, in differentiating between a small lymphocytic lymphoma (well-differentiated lymphocytic lymphoma) and a reactive lymphocyte-rich effusion. Immunologic marker studies are very useful in such instances.[43] The identification of a monoclonal B-lymphocyte population is usually diagnostic of a non-Hodgkin's lymphoma (Figure 86). Similarly, the identification of T-cell markers and terminal deoxynucleotidyl transferase (TdT) (Figure 49)

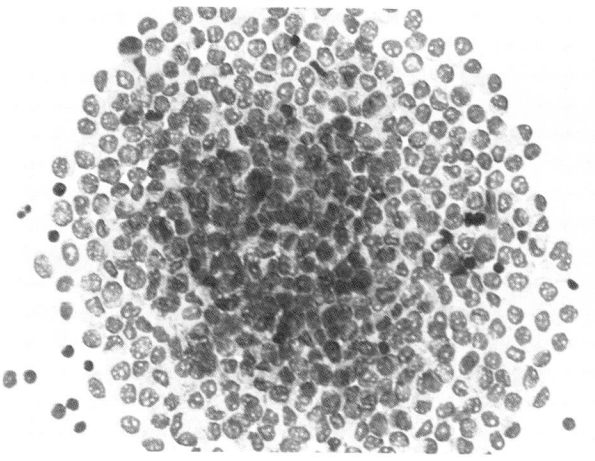

FIGURE 99. *Characteristic appearance of metastatic breast carcinoma in a pleural effusion.*

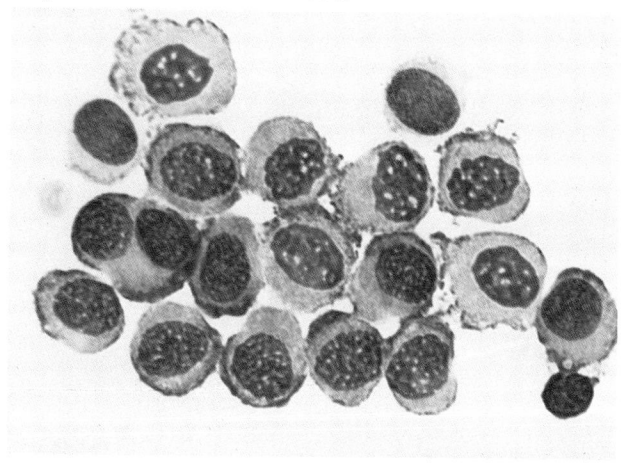

FIGURE 100. *Higher-power view of cells in Figure 99. When they occur singly outside the clump, these tumor cells look very similar to mesothelial cells.*

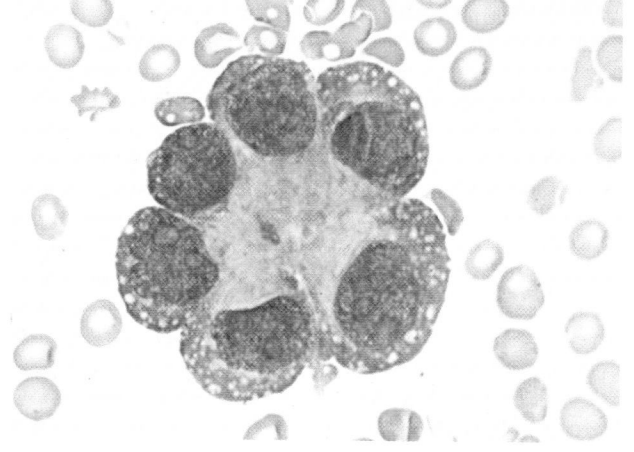

FIGURE 101. *Another morphologic appearance of metastatic breast carcinoma in a pleural effusion.*

is useful in the diagnosis of lymphoblastic lymphoma (Figures 102 through 104). The latter tumor is commonly located in the mediastinum, particularly in children. Considerable changes in the morphologic features of tumor cells, however, may occur when they are suspended in serous fluids. Thus we have seen cells, in patients with lymphoblastic lymphoma, with morphologic features closely resembling Burkitt's lymphoma (Figure 105). As lymphoblastic lymphoma cells are usually T cells and TdT-positive, while Burkitt's lymphoma cells are B cells and TdT-negative, immunologic markers can be of value in making a diagnosis. Effusions in *Hodgkin's disease* are usually associated with a mixed cell population consisting of benign-appearing small and transformed lymphocytes, eosinophils, and neutrophils. Recognizable neoplastic cells may not be seen.[42]

In *mesothelioma,* a pleural effusion is almost always present.[44] The fluid is characteristically viscous or gelatinous, resembling synovial fluid. Clumps of atypical mesothelial cells are seen, but it may be very difficult to differentiate between reactive and malignant mesothelial cells. One feature indicative of mesothelioma is morulae formation (cell grouping in clumps) with the cells showing considerable vacuolization (Figure 106).[45] The vacuoles are small and regular in size and usually centrally placed around the nucleus.[46] In contrast, the vacuoles (when present) in metastatic carcinoma are irregular in size and randomly located. The chromatin pattern is more irregular and coarsely reticular than that of benign mesothelial cells. While malignant mesotheliomas do not react to diastase para-aminosalicylic acid, pleural metastatic carcinomas usually do.[47] Elevated levels of acid mucopolysaccharides such as hyaluronic acid support the diagnosis of mesothelioma, as will be described later.

Other Studies

In addition to the examination of the pleural fluid, a needle biopsy of the pleura may significantly enhance the diagnostic yield.[48,49] This can be readily performed at the time of the initial thoracentesis or later, depending on the clinical situation and the laboratory results. A closed pleural biopsy should be performed on all undiagnosed exudates. An open thoracotomy or fiberoptic pleuroscopy may be useful for a definitive diagnosis. A pleural biopsy is particularly useful for the diagnosis of malignant disorders and tuberculosis. When biopsy is combined with cytologic examination, the diagnostic yield in malignant disorders is close to 90%.[50-51] If tuberculosis is suspected, a portion of the biopsy specimen should be submitted for culture.

Metastatic tumors of the pericardium and the heart are common in patients with advanced malignant disease. The most common tumors are carcinoma of the lung and breast (Figure 107), leukemia, and lymphoma. With a cytologic examination of the pericardial fluid, the type of malignant disorder can usually be defined.[52]

Chromosome examination of serous fluid may be helpful in the diagnosis of malignant effusion and adds another dimension to standard cytologic techniques. In one study, an effusion was considered malignant when at least 10% of cells in metaphase were hyperdiploid or contained a marker chromosome.[53] Using similar criteria, another study of 33 patients with malignant effusions yielded positive diagnoses in 91% (30 patients) using chromosome analysis, while cytologic examination in the same group yielded only 21 (64%).[53]

CHEMICAL ANALYSIS

Protein

The value of total protein measurement and the ratio of serous fluid total protein to serum total protein in classifying an effusion as an exudate or transudate was discussed previously. Electrophoretic techniques have been applied to the analysis of pleural fluid proteins, but patterns associated with specific causes have not been demonstrated.[55] On the other hand, the knowledge that inflammatory cells synthesize immunoglobulins locally suggests that their measurement in pleural fluid could be diagnostically useful. However, no correlation between the presence of specific immunoglobulins and clinical diagnosis has been demonstrated.[55]

Orosomucoid (α_1-acid glycoprotein; molecular weight, 45,000) is a small protein produced in the liver and is considered to be one of the principal serum components of the acute-phase reactant proteins. An early report suggested that its measurement in pleural and peritoneal fluids was helpful in distinguishing between neoplastic and non-neoplastic inflammatory ef-

FIGURE 102. *Numerous lymphoblasts and two mesothelial cells in a case of lymphoblastic lymphoma.*

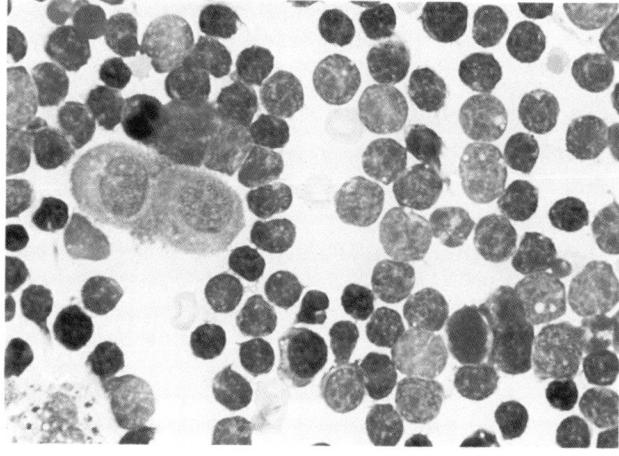

FIGURE 103. *Focal acid phosphatase activity in lymphoblastic lymphoma.*

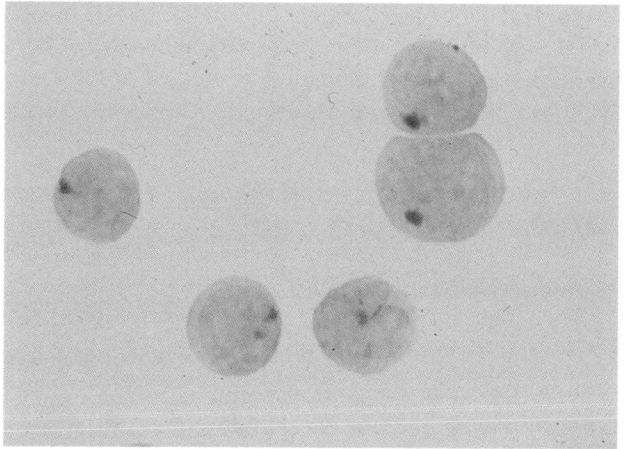

FIGURE 104. *T-lymphoblast with E-rosette. T cells characteristically form rosettes with sheep RBCs.*

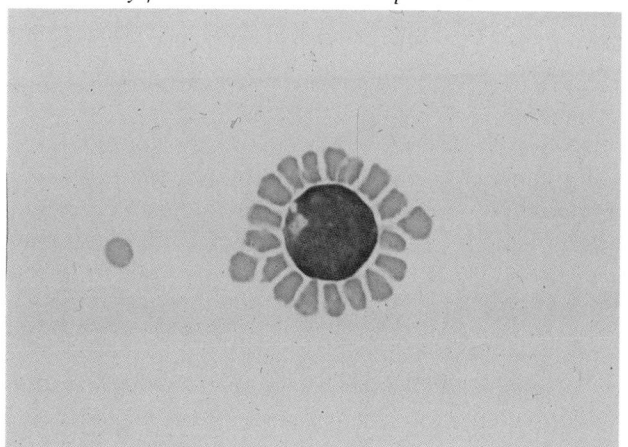

FIGURE 105. *Lymphoblasts in the pleural fluid from a patient with lymphoblastic lymphoma in the mediastinum. The cells, in this case, resemble those seen in Burkitt's lymphoma.*

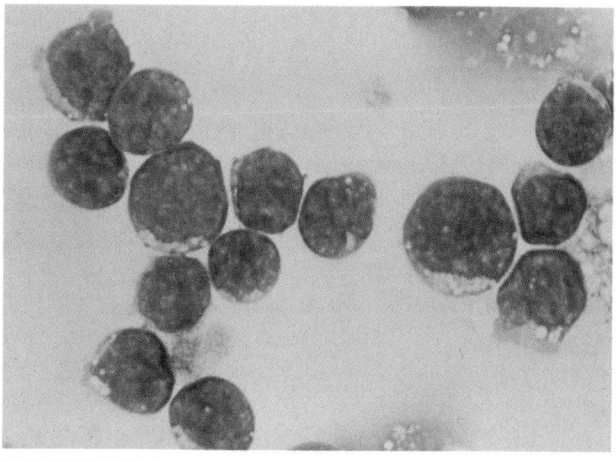

FIGURE 106. *Malignant mesothelial cells from pleural fluid in a patient with mesothelioma.*

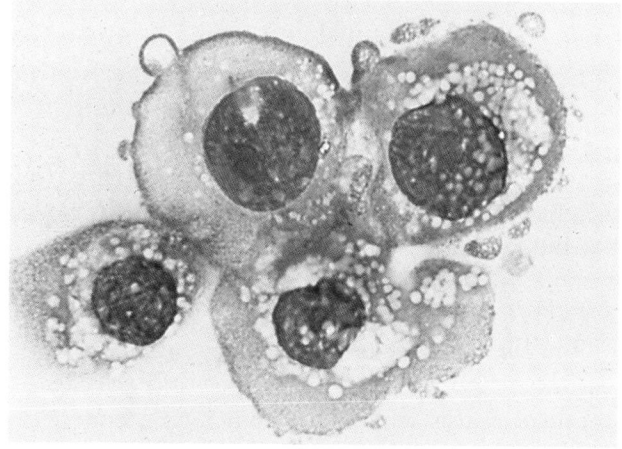

FIGURE 107. *Clumps of tumor cells in pericardial fluid sample from a patient with metastatic breast carcinoma.*

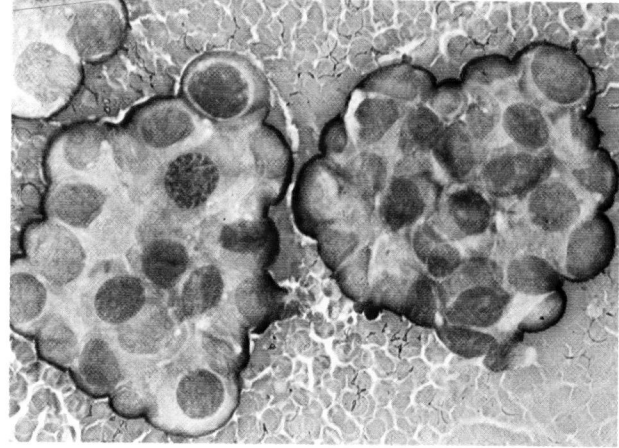

fusions.[56] Since then, several published reports have concluded that its measurement in serous fluids was not helpful in making this distinction.[57–59] Several other proteins, including β_2-microglobulin (β_2m) and ceruloplasmin, have been measured in serous effusions but have likewise shown no diagnostic usefulness.[57–59]

The measurement of β_2m in pleural effusions, however, has been reported to be useful in distinguishing among several disease processes.[60,61] This small protein is synthesized by most nucleated cells and especially lymphocytes. Its normal concentration in serum is 1.1 to 2.4 μg/mL, with a slight increase with advancing age.[60] Pleural fluid β_2m concentrations have been shown to be consistently higher than serum levels in effusions caused by malignant conditions (especially lymphomas), collagen disorders, and tuberculosis.[58,61]

Fibrinogen degradation products have been recently measured in pleural fluids.[62] Elevated levels were more consistently seen in effusions caused by malignant disorders, pulmonary embolism, and infection than those seen in transudates resulting from congestive heart disease.[63] It was suggested that concentrations higher than 40 μg/mL in patients with heart failure should lead one to suspect another reason for the effusion.[63]

Lipids and Lipoproteins

The clinical diagnosis of chylothorax (and chylous ascites) has been based on the appearance of the pleural fluid; that is, milky or creamy fluid is commonly considered synonymous with chyle. It is now recognized that the pseudochylous effusion (cholesterol-rich with low triglyceride levels) may also be indistinguishable in appearance from chyle. Pseudochylous effusion results from chronic pleural infection or inflammation caused by a variety of disorders.

Seriff et al[63] demonstrated the presence of chylomicrons in the effusion from a patient with chylothorax—and their absence in the patient's serum. Hence the authors suggested that the confirmatory test for chylothorax should be lipoprotein electrophoresis of the pleural fluid. Chylous effusions are associated with much higher triglyceride levels (mean, 249 mg/dL) than are the pseudochylous fluids (mean, 33 mg/dL), but there is no significant difference between the two groups in the cholesterol concentration.[64] Staats et al[64] suggested that lipoprotein electrophoresis is not necessary to confirm the presence of chylous fluid if the triglyceride level exceeds 110 mg/dL. However, lipoprotein analysis is recommended in the equivocal triglyceride range of 50 to 110 mg/dL.[64]

Glucose

The determination of glucose levels may be useful in pleural fluid analysis when one is dealing with an exudate. Glucose levels in pleural fluid below 60 mg/dL—or 40 mg/dL less than the simultaneous serum glucose level—are considered "decreased."[65] For the most reliable interpretation of glucose values, it is best to perform the thoracocentesis when the subject is fasting and measure both serum and pleural fluid glucose levels simultaneously. If the fluid specimen cannot be analyzed immediately, it should be frozen or collected in an appropriate container to prevent glycolysis. Although normal or elevated glucose concentrations are of no significance, decreased values may be seen in exudates resulting from (1) bacterial infections, especially when the exudate is purulent; (2) rheumatoid arthritis; (3) malignant pleuritis; and (4) tuberculous pleuritis.

The lowest levels of glucose are consistently seen in rheumatoid arthritis, in which values are below 20 to 30 mg/dL in 70% to 80% of cases and are frequently less than 10 mg/dL.[66,67] On the other hand, pleural fluid glucose levels are usually higher than 60 mg/dL in systemic lupus erythematosus (SLE).[68] Although glucose levels in effusions caused by malignant disorders, tuberculosis, or infections may be decreased, they are more often normal. In one study, the pleural fluid glucose level was below 60 mg/dL in only 13 (15%) of 88 patients with malignant pleuritis (primarily cases of metastatic carcinoma of the lung, breast, and ovary).[69]

Pericardial fluid glucose levels are frequently decreased in comparison with serum glucose levels in bacterial endocarditis and malignant effusions.

Enzymes

Pleural fluid *amylase* activity may be increased in a variety of conditions, including acute and chronic pancreatitis, pancreatic pseudocyst, esophageal rupture, and, rarely, primary or metastatic carcinoma of the lung. Amylase levels are considered "elevated" when they either exceed the upper limit of normal for serum or are significantly higher (usually 1.5 to 2.0 times or more) than those of a simultaneously analyzed serum specimen. Pleural effusions, especially those found in the left pleural cavity, occur in about 10% to 15% of patients with either acute or chronic pancreatitis, and amylase determinations may therefore be of considerable assistance in the differential diagnosis of an exudate.[65] In cases of acute pancreatitis, elevations in amylase levels probably are caused by lymphatic transport of pancreatic enzymes,[49] while in patients with chronic pancreatitis, elevations in levels are caused by internal pancreatic fistulas decompressing into the chest.[80] Since a pleural effusion may be the first sign of pancreatic disease, amylase activity should be measured in all unexplained effusions.[65]

Amylase activity may also be increased in pleural effusions occurring after esophageal rupture.[81] It is thought that the elevated amylase levels in these cases are of salivary gland origin. Verification of this is possible by measuring amylase isoenzymes, either electrophoretically[82,83] or by selective inhibition of the salivary gland component.[84] In rare cases, an elevated pleural fluid amylase level is associated with either primary or metastatic carcinoma of the lung. When the isoamylase levels are measured in such cases, the predominant fraction is the salivary isoenzyme.

In malignant pleural effusions, levels of *lactic dehydrogenase* (LD) are higher than in simultaneously measured serum or benign effusions.[85,86] Elevated LD levels have also been noted in inflammatory processes, especially when the effusions are highly cellular. In patients with rheumatoid arthritis and SLE, LD activities are moderately elevated but are consistently higher in the RA.[74]

It was initially predicted that LD isoenzyme identification would be of great assistance in the differential diagnosis of pleural effusions. Subsequent reports, however, have been inconsistent and highly misleading. Some studies have shown that the number of the slower-moving bands LD_4 and LD_5 is increased in malignant effusions, while benign fluid samples have patterns similar to those of normal serum, with LD_1 and LD_2 predominating.[87,88] Other studies, how-

ever, have shown diametrically opposed patterns for malignant effusions.[89,90] This confusion may be the result of both an inadequate pathologic interpretation of the primary lesions and a mistaken enzyme pattern of the primary tumor cell, which may be superimposed on secondary cellular elements that alter the measured isoenzyme pattern.[91] A recent report clarifies these problems to some extent. Vergnon et al[92] measured the relative value of each LD isoenzyme in specimens of serum and pleural fluid from 100 patients. They found that in patients with congestive heart failure, the LD isoenzymes were similar in the serum and the pleural fluid. In patients with empyema, the serum LD isoenzyme patterns were usually normal unless there was a marked leukemoid reaction, while the pleural fluid isoenzyme values increased progressively from LD_1 to LD_5.[92] The predominance of LD_5 appeared to be due to the numerous granulocytes in the fluid. In patients with ordinary inflammatory effusions (pulmonary embolism, SLE, parapneumonic effusion, and trauma), the values of the five isoenzymes were normal.[92] With malignant effusions, however, an elevation of isoenzyme LD_5 was seen in most cases—except for patients with lymphoma and oat cell carcinoma.[92]

Alkaline phosphatase activity has been measured in the pleural fluid of patients with a variety of conditions. Feldstein et al[93] concluded in 1963 that the activity of this enzyme was of no diagnostic value in differentiating between neoplastic and non-neoplastic disorders. Alkaline phosphatase levels have since, however, been reported to be consistently elevated in pleural effusions associated with pulmonary infarction.[94]

Creatine kinase isoenzyme BB (CK-BB) has been identified in the serum samples of patients with various types of cancer. It has been suggested that this isoenzyme represents a tumor-associated marker, particularly for adenocarcinoma of the prostate gland.[95] Effusions caused by this tumor have demonstrated the presence of the BB isoenzyme. Other tumor types (adenocarcinoma and anaplastic carcinoma of the lung) have, however, also been associated with an elevated pleural fluid CK-BB level.[96] In these cases, there was also an elevated ratio of pleural-fluid-to-plasma CK-BB (>3.7), while patients with benign effusions had ratios of 1.6 or less.[96]

Lysozyme (muramidase) in normal serum is primarily derived from decomposed neutrophilic leukocytes and monocytes and is widely distributed in body fluids and tissues. Klockars et al[97,98] have shown that the activity of this enzyme in tuberculous exudates is significantly greater than that in effusions associated with carcinoma, connective tissue disorders, nonspecific pleurisy, or heart failure. Tuberculous patients also demonstrated a significantly higher ratio of pleural fluid to serum lysozyme than did the other patients. Asseo et al[99] found that this ratio was higher than 1.0 in all patients with tuberculous pleurisy, while it was lower than 1.0 in all but three nontuberculous cases, one of which involved a patient with sarcoidosis.

Adenosine deaminase is another enzyme that might be helpful in evaluating possible tuberculous exudates. In a study involving 368 effusions, the mean adenosine deaminase activity in tuberculous effusions was 92.11 units/L, compared with means of 23.23 units/L in metastatic malignant tumors, 34.86 units/L in mesotheliomas, and 23.81 units/L in pulmonary embolism.[100] Adenosine deaminase values in lymphoproliferative disorders were intermediate (mean, 64.30 units/L).[100] Parapneumonic effusions, on the other hand, gave values essentially identical to those of the tuberculous effusions.[100]

Two other enzymes, galactosyltransferase and angiotensin-converting enzyme, have been recently evaluated in pleural effusions.[101,102] However, neither currently appears to be a clinically useful indicator.

pH, Acid-Base

The pH of normal pleural fluid is reported to be 7.64.[70] When a pleural effusion develops, the pH approaches that of blood (7.40). Recent studies have advocated the measurement of pleural fluid pH whenever a diagnostic thoracentesis is performed. The specimen should be aspirated anaerobically into a syringe rinsed with heparin and transported to the laboratory immersed in ice. In one study, 183 patients had simultaneous blood and pleural fluid pH determinations; 36 were transudates and 147 were exudates.[70] In 46 cases, all of which were exudates, the pH was less than 7.30. A pleural fluid pH of less than 7.30 was consistently seen in association with one of the following diagnoses: empyema, malignant disorders,

collagen disorders, tuberculosis, esophageal rupture, or hemothorax.[70] Other reports on this subject are in general agreement with these findings,[71–73] although some exceptions have been noted.

A pleural fluid pH of 7.3 to 7.4 usually indicates a benign condition and resolves spontaneously. While malignant effusions may occasionally be associated with a low pH value, values are usually greater than 7.40.[71] Most collagen vascular diseases have effusions characterized by low pH values. This is particularly true in rheumatoid arthritis, in which pH levels are consistently below 7.30 and usually less than 7.20.[74] On the other hand, patients with SLE usually have a pleural effusion pH of 7.35 or more.[74]

In effusions associated with pneumonia (parapneumonic effusions), the measurement of the pH may have some predictive value for the course of the effusion.[72,73] Parapneumonic effusions with a pH greater than 7.20 to 7.30 usually resolve completely with appropriate antibiotic therapy and without tube drainage. Conversely, effusions with a pH below 7.20 to 7.30 tend to loculate and do not completely resolve unless drainage is also carried out. In parapneumonic effusions, there is a strong correlation between the pleural fluid pH and glucose level.[75]

The diagnosis of esophageal rupture usually poses no clinical problem. However, in those atypical cases where a diagnosis may be difficult to make, the measurement of pleural fluid pH may be helpful in that a pH of less than 6.0 is highly suggestive of esophageal rupture.[76]

In contrast to the measurement of the pleural fluid pH, there is usually little or no value in measuring the P_{CO_2} and P_{O_2} in pleural fluids, since these levels are so variable.[71,77] They may, however, be of some value in determining the source of bloody pericardial fluid, which may be due to pericardial contents or intracardiac blood.[78] In one study that analyzed several specimens of bloody pericardial fluid, the P_{CO_2} was substantially increased and the P_{O_2}, pH, and bicarbonate level were decreased when compared with those of the intracardiac (and presumably arterial) aspirates.[78] On the basis of pericardiocentesis samples from 13 patients, a "classification" of pH in pericardial fluids was suggested as follows: a pH of less than 7.1 is associated with connective tissue diseases and bacterial infection; a pH of 7.2 to 7.4 is associated with neoplasms, idiopathic disorders, and tuberculous or uremic pericarditis; and a pH greater than 7.4 is associated with postcardiotomy states and hypothyroidism.[79]

Other Biochemical Measurements

Zinc, copper, and iron have been measured in pleural fluids in both benign and malignant processes.[103] These determinations have, however, no current clinical usefulness.

Large amounts of such acid mucopolysaccharides as hyaluronic acid have been described in pleural and peritoneal fluid specimens from patients with mesotheliomas.[104] Glycosaminoglycan electrophoresis of papain-digested mesothelioma material has revealed elevated hyaluronic acid levels.[105]

Hyaluronic acid levels are not, however, elevated in all cases of mesothelioma. In a study of 165 patients with elevated pleural fluid hyaluronic acid levels, agarose gel electrophoretic studies showed that 66% of patients with levels between 5 and 50 mg/L and 82% of those with levels over 50 mg/L had mesothelioma.[106] Other tumors, such as adenocarcinoma of the lung and Wilms' tumor, may also be associated with elevated hyaluronic acid levels.

The measurement of pleural fluid lactic acid has been evaluated and levels have been found to be much higher in bacterial and tuberculous pleural infections (mean, 81 mg/dL; range, 45 to 200 mg/dL) than in effusions caused by heart failure, hepatic cirrhosis, nephrosis, trauma, or SLE (mean, 19 mg/dL; range, 6 to 47 mg/dL).[107] Moreover, the pleural fluid lactic acid level usually remains elevated for a period of time after antibiotic therapy has begun. In 15 cases of malignant effusion, lactate levels were also found to be increased, but to a lesser degree (mean, 57 mg/dL; range, 23 to 90 mg/dL).[107] A level higher than 100 mg/dL is suggestive of bacterial infection.

Immunologic Studies

Levine et al[108] reported in 1968 that the measurement of rheumatoid factor in pleural effusions by the latex fixation technique resulted in titers of 1:160 or greater in 41% of patients with bacterial pneumonia, 20% of patients with carcinoma, and 14% of patients with tuberculosis. They concluded that the occurrence of rheumatoid factor in pleural fluid could not be considered specifically related to rheumatoid disease.

Lowered complement levels have been found in pleural fluid specimens from patients with rheumatoid arthritis (RA) and SLE, although neither C4 nor C3 levels can reliably be used to distinguish between them. The complement-to-protein ratios in pleural fluid, when corrected for serum complement-to-protein ratios, revealed no difference between SLE and other exudate groups in one study.[109]

In addition to the differences in pleural fluid pH and glucose values just described, RA and SLE also differ in the levels of immune complexes. Immune complexes can be detected in all rheumatoid pleural effusions using the three-assay system: radioimmunoassay using monoclonal rheumatoid factor, the C1q component of a complement assay, and the Raji cell assay.[74] Each of these assays recognizes a different biologic property of immune complexes, and positive test results rarely occur in disorders other than RA and SLE.[74] In most of the rheumatoid pleural fluid specimens in one study, the complexes were detected with all three techniques, and the concentration levels were higher than those simultaneously measured in serum. On the other hand, immune complexes in effusion samples from patients with SLE were detected primarily by the Raji cell assay, and the pleural fluid complex concentrations were similar to those measured in serum.[74] The high concentrations found in exudates from RA suggest that these complexes are produced within the pleural cavity in this disorder, whereas in SLE the immune complexes appear to reflect the serum concentrations. These results are consistent with current theory that SLE is an intravascular immune complex disorder while RA is an extravascular one.[74]

In a study of 13 patients with lupus pleuritis, pleural fluid antinuclear antibody titers were at least 1:160 in 11 patients, and at least one typical lupus erythematosus cell was found in seven of eight pleural fluid specimens (Figure 59).[110]

Normal ranges for the pericardial fluid complement are 35 to 127 mg/dL for C3, 6.3 to 23.0 mg/dL for C4, and 1.9 to 9.1 units for the total hemolytic complement.[111] Pericardial complement levels have been reported to be lower than normal serum values in RA and SLE.[112,113]

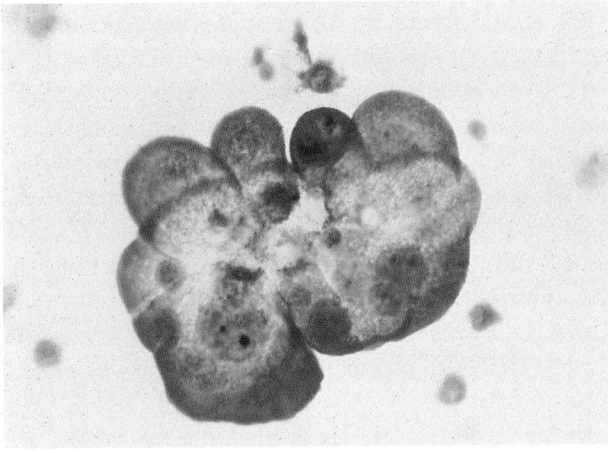

FIGURE 108. *CEA demonstrated in a clump of adenocarcinoma cells with an immuno–alkaline phosphatase technique (immuno–alkaline phosphatase stain with antibody to CEA).*

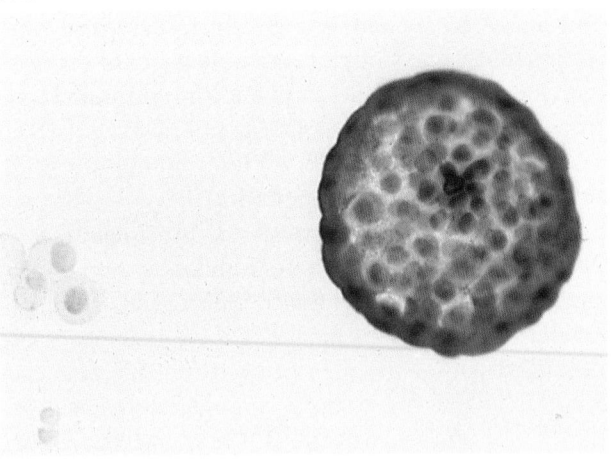

FIGURE 109. *EMA demonstrated in a clump of metastatic breast carcinoma cells (immuno–alkaline phosphatase stain with antibody to EMA). Notice negative staining in mesothelial cells.*

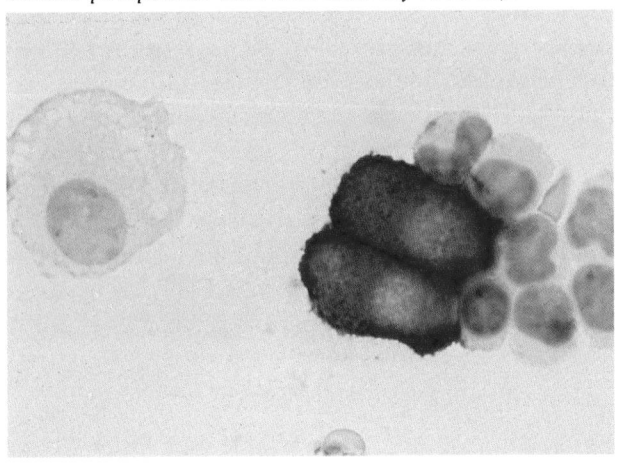

FIGURE 110. *EMA present in two tumor cells with a negative mesothelial cell and several negative lymphocytes (immuno–alkaline phosphatase stain with antibody to EMA).*

Tumor Markers

Although cytologic examination is the most specific method for identifying malignant effusions, it lacks specificity; results are positive in only 40% to 60% of confirmed cases. In recent years, however, we have seen the development of a variety of tumor markers that may serve as additional tools in differentiating between malignant and benign causes of exudative effusions.

The *carcinoembryonic antigen* (CEA) is probably the marker that to date has been most extensively studied.[114,115] Carcinoembryonic antigen is a glyco-protein component of the glycocalyx of entodermal epithelium found to be elevated in serum in a variety of tumors. It is measured with radioimmunoassay techniques, and commercial kits are available. The usefulness of CEA measurement varies according to the study: the sensitivity in different reports has varied from 20% to 60%. These results may be due to different methodologies, different patient populations, and, perhaps most important, to arbitrary cutoff values varying from 10 to 30 ng/mL.

Pleural fluid CEA has been associated with elevated levels in 50% to 60% of malignant effusions.[116,117] McKenna et al[118] concluded that measurement of pleural and plasma CEA levels in general is a poor screening test for malignant conditions. However, it may be the optimal test for adenocarcinoma (lung and breast), with a sensitivity of 91% and specificity of 92%.[118] A few cases of tuberculosis and empyema have also been associated with elevated pleural fluid CEA levels.[118]

The pleural fluid assay may also be useful in differentiating between malignant mesothelioma and metastatic carcinoma with serosal spread. In a large study,[119] all patients with mesothelioma had low levels of CEA (less than 12 ng/mL), while 50% of patients with effusions caused by metastatic carcinoma (lung, breast, kidney, gastrointestinal, or ovary) had elevated CEA levels (greater than 39 ng/mL).[119] In particular, 78.9% of patients with adenocarcinoma of the lung had markedly elevated levels.[119] Horowitz et al,[120] using cytologic examination, examined the correlation between the presence of malignant cells and the finding of elevated pleural fluid CEA levels and cytoplasmic CEA-positive cells in fluid specimens. The cytoplasmic CEA was identified by an indirect immunofluorescent technique using a specific antiserum sample to CEA.[120] Eighty-one percent of the cases (comprising breast, ovary, and lung cancers) were positive with either one or both of the markers, whereas only 54% were positive with cytologic examination alone.[120]

Using an *immunoperoxidase method* in 30 benign and 21 malignant cytologic specimens, CEA and *keratin* were studied.[121] Both mesothelial and adenocarcinoma cells showed intracytoplasmic staining with CEA, but the staining of the malignant cells was strong while the staining of the mesothelial cells was weakly positive or negative.[120] A total absence of CEA is strong evidence against a diagnosis of carcinoma (Figure 108). Keratin was not useful in differentiating between mesothelial cells and adenocarcinoma and squamous carcinoma cells.[121] In our experience, neither CEA nor keratin is useful in distinguishing between mesothelial cells and malignant cells using the immunoperoxidase method on fluid smears.

Orosomucoid (α₁-acid glycoprotein) is the main seromucoid fraction of human serum. It is an acute-phase protein, measured by radial immunodiffusion, that increases with inflammation, pregnancy, and malignant conditions. Elevated levels (greater than 100 mg/dL) were found in one study in 27 (74%) of 37 patients with malignant effusions[122]; by combining orosomucoid studies with CEA measurement, the sensitivity was increased from 36% to 86%.[122] The sensitivity of the cytologic testing alone in the same study was 46%. Measurement of α-fetoprotein and β₂-microglobulin levels has no clinical value in the diagnosis of malignant effusions, except that levels of the latter are often elevated in malignant lymphoma.[122,123]

Using an immunoperoxidase method, it has been shown that reactive mesothelial cells (exfoliated cells) consistently stain strongly with *α₁-antichymotrypsin* and have variably positive staining for *α₁-antitrypsin* and lysozyme.[124] Malignant cells (carcinoma and mesothelioma) usually have negative staining.[124] Similarly, monoclonal antibodies to human milk-fat globule (HMFG2) that is raised against epithelial cell determinants and the *epithelial membrane antigen* (EMA) react with malignant epithelial cells but not with normal or reactive mesothelial cells in smears from pleural and ascitic effusions using the immunoperoxidase techniques (Figures 109 and 110).[125,126]

Antibody to EMA, therefore, appears to be very useful in difficult cases. In addition, an antibody (T29/33) to T200, a panleukocyte antigen, is useful in distinguishing between large-cell malignant lymphoma and poorly differentiated carcinoma. This antigen is expressed on leukocytes but not in the nonlymphoid round cell tumors or in undifferentiated carcinomas. Figure 111 summarizes an approach to the use of immuno-enzymatic markers in body fluids, as follows: (1) a positive EMA with a negative α₁-antichymotrypsin test suggests a malignancy of epithelial cells; (2) a positive antitrypsin or antichymotrypsin with a negative EMA test suggests atypical mesothelial cells; (3) a negative glial fibrillary acidic protein (GFAP) and a positive EMA test together with CEA or keratin in the CSF suggests metastatic carcinoma; (4) a positive CEA with a negative or weakly positive keratin test suggests adenocarcinoma; and (5) a positive keratin test with a negative or weakly positive CEA suggests mesothelioma. It must be noted, however, that a negative EMA test does not rule out the possibility of an epithelial malignancy. In addition, the T200 antigen is absent in most plasma-cell neoplasms and may be absent in some immunoblastic lymphomas and some lymphoblastic lymphomas.

These tumor markers do not replace conventional cytologic and biopsy examinations but rather serve as additional, potentially useful tools in the diagnosis of malignant disorders.

MICROBIOLOGIC EXAMINATION

A parapneumonic effusion is one associated with a bacterial pneumonia or lung abscess. The fluid may be either turbid or clear and may be sterile. The effusion may resolve without complications following appropriate antibiotic therapy. Conversely, the fluid may be frankly purulent (empyema) and loculate in the pleural space (see under heading "Chemical Analysis," subheadings "Glucose" and "pH, Acid-Base"). The treatment for empyema consists of immediate and complete drainage of the pleural space by use of a chest tube, as well as the vigorous administration of antibiotics selected on the basis of both aerobic and anaerobic cultures and sensitivity studies.

The era of antimicrobial therapy has produced

FIGURE 111. *An approach to the use and interpretation of tumor cell markers in serous fluids containing cells that are suspicious for malignancy. EMA indicates epithelial membrane antigen; T200, panleukocyte antigen; TdT, terminal deoxynucleotidyl transferase; CALLA, common acute lymphoblastic leukemia antigen; CEA, carcinoembryonic antigen; and GFAP, and glial fibrillary acidic protein.*

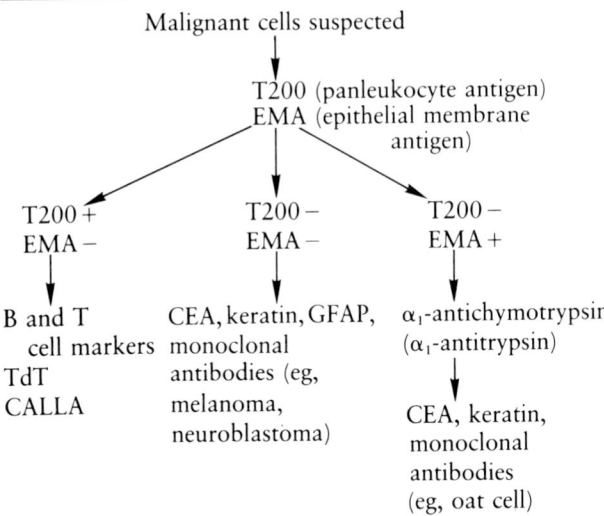

marked changes in the microbiology of empyema. *Streptococcus pneumoniae* was once the predominant pathogen. However, this organism is now seldom encountered in empyema.[127] The most common bacteria now isolated are *Staphylococcus aureus* and certain gram-negative enteric bacilli.[128] There is also a high incidence of anaerobic pleural infections in empyema. In one study, anaerobes alone were identified in 23 (35%) of 83 cases of pleural infection, and anaerobic plus aerobic bacteria were identified in an additional 34 (41%).[128] The predominant bacteria, in order of prevalence, were *S aureus, Fusobacterium nucleatum, Bacteroides melaninogenicus, Bacteroides fragilis, Clostridium* sp, *Escherichia coli*, and *Pseudomonas aeruginosa*. This study illustrates the need for careful transport and processing of the specimen to ensure recovery of oxygen-sensitive microorganisms.

A development of great interest and potential for the rapid and reliable diagnosis of empyema (or any purulent fluid) associated with anaerobic bacteria is that of gas-liquid chromatographic techniques for detecting the presence of fatty acids.[129,130] Direct analysis of purulent material showed excellent correlation between the presence of gram-negative anaerobic bacilli and that of isobutyric and butyric acids.[130]

Bacterial stains (Gram's stain, acid-fast bacilli stain, etc) are fundamental to any fluid examination. Their reliability depends primarily on the microscopic competence and experience of the laboratory worker. As with CSF, the sensitivity probably does not exceed 70% to 80% at best.

In tuberculous effusions, the staining for acid test bacilli is positive in only 5% to 20% of cases, and cultures for acid-fast bacilli are positive in only 20% to 40% of the cases.[131] The accuracy can be improved by obtaining multiple cultures, by concentrating large volumes of fluid, and by inoculation of guinea pigs. A pleural biopsy is also of recognized value and provides histologic evidence of the disease in 50% to 80% of the cases.[132] When these approaches are combined, up to 95% of the cases can be identified.[133]

On rare occasions, fungal, amebic, or echinococcal disease will be seen. In fungal disease, appropriate cultures are usually necessary for accurate diagnosis. In pleuropulmonary involvement with *Entamoeba histolytica*, there is usually an amebic hepatic cyst, and the pleural fluid may show organisms. In hydatid disease, typical hooklets and scolices are readily seen, especially in concentrated specimens.

Counterimmunoelectrophoresis and latex agglutination techniques for identification of certain bacterial antigens (eg, *S pneumoniae*) are frequently helpful and may lead to a specific diagnosis within an hour of thoracentesis. The *Limulus* lysate assay for gramnegative endotoxin is much less reliable for serous effusions than for CSF; improved techniques are needed for this procedure to yield consistently reliable results in pleural fluid. In addition, pleural fluid lactic acid levels may be useful in the diagnosis of bacterial pleuritis.

REFERENCES

1. Black LF: The pleural space and pleural fluid. *Mayo Clin Proc* 47:493–506, 1972

2. Sahebjami H, Loudon RG: Pleural effusion: Pathophysiology and clinical features. *Sem Roentgenol* 12:269–275, 1977

3. Light RW: Pleural effusions: Symposium on Pulmonary Disease. *Med Clin North Am* 61:1339–1352, 1977

4. Light RW, George RB: Incidence and significance of pleural effusion after abdominal surgery. *Chest* 65:621–625, 1976

5. Hughson WG, Friedman PJ, Feigin DS, et al: Postpartum pleural effusion: A common radiologic finding. *Ann Intern Med* 97:856–858, 1982

6. Krieg AF: Cerebrospinal fluid and other body fluids, in Henry JB (ed): *Clinical Diagnosis and Management by Laboratory Methods*, ed 16. Philadelphia, WB Saunders Co, 1979, pp 635-679

7. Melsom RD: Diagnostic reliability of pleural fluid protein estimation. *J R Soc Med* 72:823–825, 1979

8. Light RW, MacGregor MI, Luchsinger PC, et al: Pleural effusions: The diagnostic separation of transudates and exudates. *Ann Intern Med* 77:507–513, 1972

9. Peterman TA, Speicher CE: Evaluating pleural effusions: A two-stage laboratory approach. *JAMA*, 252:1051–1053, 1984

10. Teloh HA: The clinical pathology of pleural fluids. *Ann Clin Lab Sci* 3:98–107, 1973

11. Maher GC, Berger HW: Massive pleural effusion: Malignant and nonmalignant causes in 46 patients. *Am Rev Respir Dis* 105:458–460, 1972

12. Light RW, Erozan YS, Ball WC: Cells in pleural fluid: Their value in differential diagnosis. *Arch Intern Med* 854:860, 1973

13. Roy PH, Carr DT, Payne WS: The problem of chylothorax. *Mayo Clin Proc* 42:457–467, 1967

14. Dines DE, Pierre RV, Franzen SJ: The value of cells in the pleural fluid in the differential diagnosis. *Mayo Clin Proc* 50:571–572, 1975

15. Soendergaard K: On the interpretation of atypical cells in pleural and peritoneal effusion. *Acta Cytol* 21:413–416, 1977

16. Efrati P, Nir E: Morphological and cytochemical investigation of human mesothelial cells from pleural and peritoneal effusions. *Isr J Med Sci* 12:662–673, 1976

17. Spriggs AI, Boddington M: *The Cytology of Effusions,* ed 2. New York, Grune & Stratton Inc, 1968

18. Pettersson T, Klockars M, Hellström PE, et al: T and B lymphocytes in pleural effusions. *Chest* 73: 49–51, 1978

19. Domagala W, Emeson EE, Koss LG: T and B lymphocyte enumeration in the diagnosis of lymphocyte-rich pleural fluids. *Acta Cytol* 25:108–110, 1981

20. Bower G: Eosinophilic pleural effusion: A condition with multiple causes. *Am Rev Respir Dis* 95:746–751, 1967

21. Pettersson T, Riska H: Diagnostic value of total and differential leukocyte counts in pleural effusions. *Acta Med Scand* 210:129–135, 1981

22. Keshgegian AA: Lupus erythematosus cells in pleural fluid. *Am J Clin Pathol* 69:570–571, 1978

23. Light RW, Girard WM, Jenkinson SF, et al: Parapneumonic effusions. *Am J Med* 69:507–512, 1980

24. Bynum LJ, Wilson JE: Characteristics of pleural effusions associated with pulmonary embolism. *Arch Intern Med* 136:159–162, 1976

25. Sahn SA: The differential diagnosis of pleural effusions. *West J Med* 137:99–108, 1982

26. Sahn SA, Kaplan RL, Maulitz RM, et al: Rheumatoid pleurisy: Observations on the development of low pleural fluid pH and glucose. *Arch Intern Med* 140:1237–1238, 1980

27. Kaye M: Pleuropulmonary complications of pancreatitis. *Thorax* 23:297–306, 1968

28. Berger HW, Rammohan G, Neff MS, et al: Uremic pleural effusion: A study of 14 patients on chronic dialysis. *Ann Intern Med* 82:362–364, 1975

29. Galen MA, Steinberg SM, Lowrie EG, et al: Hemorrhagic pleural effusion in patients undergoing chronic hemodialysis. *Ann Intern Med* 82:359–361, 1975

30. Friedman MA, Slater E: Malignant pleural effusions. *Cancer Treat Rev* 5:49–66, 1978

31. Leff A, Hopewell PC, Costello J: Pleural effusions from malignancy. *Ann Intern Med* 88:532–537, 1978

32. Billingham ME, Rawlinson DG, Berry PF, et al: The cytodiagnosis of malignant lymphomas and Hodgkin's disease in cerebrospinal, pleural, and ascitic fluids. *Acta Cytol* 19:547–556, 1975

33. Weick JK, Kiely JM, Harrison EG, et al: Pleural effusion in lymphoma. *Cancer* 31:848–853, 1973

34. Chernow B, Sahn SA: Carcinomatous involvement of the pleura: An analysis of 96 patients. *Am J Med* 66:695–702, 1977

35. Meyer PC: Metastatic carcinoma of the pleura. *Thorax* 21:437–443, 1966

36. Sahn SA: Pleural effusion in lung cancer: Symposium on Recent Advances in Lung Cancer. *Clin Chest Med* 3:443–452, 1982

37. Gondos B, McIntosh KM, Renston RH, et al: Application of electron microscopy in the definitive diagnosis of effusions. *Acta Cytol* 22:297–304, 1978

38. Domagala W, Woyke S: Transmission and scanning electron microscopic studies of cells in effusions. *Acta Cytol* 19:214–224, 1974

39. Spriggs AI, Boddington MM: Oat cell carcinoma: Identification of cells in pleural fluid. *Acta Cytol* 20:525–529, 1976

40. Raju RN, Kardinal CG: Pleural effusion in breast carcinoma: Analysis of 122 cases. *Cancer* 48:2524–2527, 1981

41. Fentiman JS, Millis R, Sexton S: Pleural effusion in breast cancer: A review of 105 cases. *Cancer* 47:2087–2092, 1981

42. Spriggs AI, Vanhegan RI: Cytological diagnosis of lymphoma in serous effusions. *J Clin Pathol* 34:1311–1325, 1981

43. Krajewski AS, Dewar AE, Ramage EF: T and B lymphocyte markers in effusions of patients with non-Hodgkin's lymphoma. *J Clin Pathol* 35:1216–1219, 1982

44. Case records of the Massachusetts General Hospital: Case 27-1982. *N Engl J Med* 307:104–112, 1982

45. Kwee WS, Veldhuizen RW, Alons CA, et al: Quantitative and qualitative differences between benign and malignant mesothelial cells in pleural fluid. *Acta Cytol* 26:401–406, 1982

46. Boon ME, Veldhuizen RW, Ruinaard C, et al: Qualitative distinctive differences between the vacuoles of mesothelioma cells and of cells from metastatic carcinoma exfoliated in pleural fluid. *Acta Cytol* 28:443–449, 1984

47. Kwee WS, Veldhuizen RW, Golding RP, et al: Histologic distinction between malignant mesothelioma, benign pleural lesion and carcinoma metastasis: Evaluation of the application of morphometry combined with histochemistry and immunostainings. *Virch Arch (Pathol Anat)* 397:287–299, 1982

48. Chandrasekhar AJ, Buehler JH: Diagnostic evaluation of pleural effusion. *Geriatrics* 29:116–123, 1974

49. Byrd RB: Current concepts in diagnosing the cause of pleural effusion. *Geriatrics* 32:44–48, 1977

50. Frist B, Kahan AV, Koss LG: Comparison of the diagnostic value of biopsies of the pleura and the cytologic evaluation of pleural fluids. *Am J Clin Pathol* 72:48–51, 1979

51. Salyer WR, Eggleston JC, Erozan YS: Efficacy of pleural needle biopsy and pleural fluid cytopathology in the diagnosis of malignant neoplasm involving the pleura. *Chest* 67:536–539, 1975

52. King DT, Nieberg RK: The use of cytology to evaluate pericardial effusions. *Ann Clin Lab Sci* 9:18–23, 1979

53. Dewald G, Dines DE, Weiland LH, et al: Usefulness of chromosome examination in the diagnosis of malignant pleural effusions. *N Engl J Med* 295:1,494–1,500, 1976

54. Falor WH, Ward RM, Brezler MC: Diagnosis of pleural effusions by chromosome analysis. *Chest* 81:193–197, 1982

55. Shallenberger DW, Daniel TM: Quantitative determination of several pleural fluid proteins. *Am Rev Respir Dis* 106:121–122, 1972

56. Rudman D, Chawla RK, DelRio AE, et al: Orosomucoid content of pleural and peritoneal effusions. *J Clin Invest* 54:147–155, 1974

57. Agostoni A, Marasini B: Orosomucoid contents of pleural and peritoneal effusions of various etiologies. *Am J Clin Pathol* 67:146–148, 1977

58. Vladutin AO, Adler RH, Brason FW: Diagnostic value of biochemical analysis of pleural effusions. *Am J Clin Pathol* 71:210–214, 1979

59. Asseo PP, Tracopoulos GD: Orosomucoid, α_2-macroglobulin and immunoglobulins in serum and pleural effusions. *Am J Clin Pathol* 76:437–441, 1981

60. Evrin PE, Wibell L: The serum levels and urinary excretion of α_2-microglobulin in apparently healthy subjects. *Scan J Clin Lab Invest* 29:69–74, 1972

61. Riska H, Pettersson T, Froseth B, et al: Beta$_2$-microglobulin in pleural effusions. *Acta Med Scand* 211:45–50, 1982

62. Raja OG, Casson IF: Fibrinogen degradation products in pleural effusions. *Br J Dis Chest* 74:164–168, 1980

63. Seriff NS, Cohen ML, Samuel P, et al: Chylothorax: Diagnosis by lipoprotein electrophoresis of serum and pleural fluid. *Thorax* 32:98–100, 1977

64. Staats BA, Ellefson RD, Budahn LL, et al: The lipoprotein profile of chylous and nonchylous pleural effusions. *Mayo Clin Proc* 55:700–704, 1980

65. Light RW, Ball WC Jr: Glucose and amylase in pleural effusions. *JAMA* 225:257–260, 1973

66. Lillington GA, Carr DT, Mayne JG: Rheumatoid pleurisy with effusion. *Arch Intern Med* 128:764–768, 1971

67. Carr DT, Mayne JG: Pleurisy with effusion in rheumatoid arthritis, with reference to the low concentration of glucose in pleural fluid. *Am Rev Respir Dis* 85:345–350, 1962

68. Carr DT, Lillington GA, Mayne JG: Pleural fluid glucose in systemic lupus erythematosus. *Mayo Clin Proc* 45:409–412, 1970

69. Berger HW, Maher G: Decreased glucose concentration in malignant pleural effusions. *Am Rev Respir Dis* 103:427–429, 1971

70. Good JT, Taryle DA, Maulitz RM, et al: The diagnostic value of pleural fluid pH. *Chest* 78:55–59, 1980

71. Funahashi A, Sarkar TK, Kory RC: Measurements of respiratory gases and pH of pleural fluid. *Am Rev Respir Dis* 108:1266–1268, 1973

72. Light RW, MacGregor MI, Ball WC, et al: Diagnostic significance of pleural fluid pH and pCO_2. *Chest* 64:591–596, 1973

73. Potts DE, Levin DC, Sahn SA: Pleural fluid pH in parapneumonic effusions. *Chest* 70:328–331, 1976

74. Halla JT, Schrohenloher RE, Volankis JE: Immune complexes and other laboratory features of pleural effusions. *Ann Intern Med* 92:748–752, 1980

75. Potts DE, Taryle DA, Sahn SA: The glucose-pH relationship in parapneumonic effusions. *Arch Intern Med* 138:1378–1380, 1978

76. Dye RA, Laforet EG: Esophageal rupture: Diagnosis by pleural fluid pH. *Chest* 66:454–456, 1974

77. Houston MC: Pleural effusion: Diagnostic value of measurements of PO_2, PCO_2, and pH. *South Med J* 74:585–589, 1981

78. Mann W, Miller JE, Glauser FL: Bloody pericardial fluid: The value of blood gas measurements. *JAMA* 239:2151–2152, 1978

79. Kindig JR, Goodman MR: Clinical utility of pericardial fluid pH determination. *Am J Med* 75:1077–1079, 1983

80. Anderson WJ, Skinner DB, Zuidema GD, et al: Chronic pancreatic pleural effusions. *Surg Gynecol Obstet* 137:827–830, 1973

81. Sherr HP, Light RW, Merson MH, et al: Origin of pleural fluid amylase in esophageal rupture. *Ann Intern Med* 76:985–986, 1972

82. Legaz ME, Kenny MA: Electrophoretic amylase fractionation as an aid in diagnosis of pancreatic disease. *Clin Chem* 22:57–62, 1976

83. Leclerc P, Forest JC: Electrophoretic determination of isoamylases in serum with commercially available reagents. *Clin Chem* 28:37–40, 1982

84. O'Donnell MD, Fitzgerald O, McGeeney KF: Differential serum amylase determination by use of an inhibitor, and design of a routine procedure. *Clin Chem* 23:560–566, 1977

85. Wroblewski F, Wroblewski R: The clinical significance of lactic dehydrogenase activity in serous effusions. *Ann Intern Med* 48:813–822, 1958

86. Wroblewski F: The significance of alterations in lactic dehydrogenase activity in body fluids in the diagnosis of malignant tumors. *Cancer* 12:27–39, 1959

87. Richterich R, Zuppinger K, Rossi E: Diagnostic significance of heterogeneous lactic dehydrogenases in malignant effusions. *Nature* 191:507–508, 1961

88. Richterich R, Burger A: Lactic dehydrogenase isoenzymes in human cancer cells and malignant effusions. *Enzymol Biol Clin* 3:65–72, 1963

89. Frohlich C, Keller A: LDH-isoenzyme muster in pleuroergussen benigner und maligner atiolgie und ihre diagnostishe bedeutung. *Klin Wochenschr* 45:457–461, 1967

90. Light R, Ball WC Jr: Lactate dehydrogenase isoenzymes in pleural effusions. *Am Rev Respir Dis* 108:660–664, 1973

91. Griffiths JC: Oral communication, February 1978

92. Vergnon JM, Guidollet J, Gateau O, et al: Lactic dehydrogenase isoenzyme electrophoretic patterns in the diagnosis of pleural effusion. *Cancer* 54:507–511, 1984

93. Feldstein AM, Samachson J, Spencer H: Levels of calcium, phosphorus, alkaline phosphatase and protein in effusion fluid and serum in man. *Am J Med* 35:530–535, 1963

94. Doust JY, Kohout E: Alkaline phosphatase in pleural effusions. *Isr J Med Sci* 9:1588–1590, 1973

95. Silverman LM, Dermer GB, Zweig MH, et al: Creatine kinase BB: A new tumor-associated marker. *Clin Chem* 25:1432–1435, 1979

96. Pettersson T, Weber TH, Ojala K: Creatine kinase isoenzyme BB as a tumor marker in pleural effusions. *Clin Chem* 27:1147–1148, 1981

97. Klockars M, Pettersson T, Riska H: Pleural fluid lysozyme in tuberculous and non-tuberculous pleurisy. *Br Med J* 1:1381, 1976

98. Klockars M, et al: Pleural fluid lysozyme in human disease. *Arch Intern Med* 139:73–77, 1979

99. Asseo PP, Tracopoulos GD, Kotsovoulou-Fous-kaki V: Lysozyme (muramidase) in pleural effusions and serum. *Am J Clin Pathol* 78:763–767, 1982

100. Maritz FJ, Malan C, Le Roux I: Adenosine deaminase estimations in the differentiation of pleural effusion. *S Afr Med J* 62:556–558, 1982

101. Bedrossian CWM, Stein DA, Miller WC, et al: Levels of angiotensin-converting enzyme in pleural effusion. *Arch Pathol Lab Med* 105:345–346, 1981

102. Kim YD, Weber GF, Tomita JT, et al: Galactosyltransferase variant in pleural effusion. *Clin Chem* 28:1133–1136, 1982

103. Dines DE, Elvebach LR, McCall JT: Zinc, copper and iron content of pleural fluid in benign and neoplastic disease. *Thorax* 27:368–370, 1972

104. Hellstrom PE, Friman C, Teppo L: Malignant mesothelioma of 17 years' duration with high pleural fluid concentration of hyaluronate. *Scand J Respir Dis* 58:97–102, 1977

105. Waxler B, Eisenstein R, Battifora H: Electrophoresis of tissue glycosaminoglycans as an aid in the diagnosis of mesotheliomas. *Cancer* 44:221–227, 1979

106. Boersma A, Degand P, Biserte G: Hyaluronic acid analysis and the diagnosis of pleural mesothelioma. *Bull Eur Physiopathol Respir* 16:41–45, 1980

107. Brook I: Measurement of lactic acid in pleural fluid. *Respiration* 40:344–348, 1980

108. Levine H, Szanto M, Grieble HG, et al: Rheumatoid factor in nonrheumatoid pleural effusions. *Ann Intern Med* 69:487–492, 1968

109. Small P, Frank H, Kreisman H, et al: An immunological evaluation of pleural effusions in systemic lupus erythematosus. *Ann Allerg* 49:101–103, 1982

110. Good JT, King TE, Antony VB, et al: Lupus pleuritis: Clinical features and pleural fluid characteristics with special reference to pleural fluid antinuclear antibodies. *Chest* 84:714–718, 1983

111. Kinney E, Wynn J, Hinton DM, et al: Pericardial-fluid complement: Normal values. *Am J Clin Pathol* 72:972–973, 1979

112. Richards AJ, Koehler BE, Broder I, et al: Rheumatoid pericarditis: Comparison of immunologic characteristics of pericardial fluid, synovial fluid and serum. *J Rheumatol* 3:275–282, 1976

113. Goldenberg DL, Left G, Grayzel AI: Pericardial tamponade in systemic lupus erythematosus with absent hemolytic complement activity in pericardial fluid. *NY State J Med* 75:910–912, 1975

114. Rittgers RS, Loewenstein MS, Feinerman AE, et al: Carcinoembryonic antigen levels in benign and malignant pleural effusions. *Ann Intern Med* 88:631–634, 1978

115. Vladutin AO, Adler RH, Brason FW: Diagnostic value of biochemical analysis of pleural effusions: Carcinoembryonic antigen and beta$_2$-microglobulin. *Am J Clin Pathol* 71:210–214, 1979

116. Klockars M, Lindgren J, Pettersson T: Carcinoembryonic antigen in pleural effusions: A diagnostic and prognostic indicator. *Eur J Cancer* 16:1149–1152, 1980

117. DiStefano A, Tashima CK, Fritsche HA: Carcinoembryonic antigen levels in malignant pleural fluids obtained from patients with mammary cancer. *Am J Clin Pathol* 73:386–389, 1980

118. McKenna JM, Chandvasekhav AJ, Henkin RE: Diagnostic value of carcinoembryonic antigen in exudative pleural effusions. *Chest* 78:587-590, 1980

119. Faravelli B, D'Amore E, Nonseuzo M: Carcinoembryonic antigen in pleural effusions: Diagnostic value in malignant mesothelioma. *Cancer* 53:1194-1197, 1984

120. Horowitz AT, Fuks Z, Okon E, et al: The use of carcinoembryonic antigen for identification of human tumor cells in malignant effusions. *Oncology* 40:18–25, 1983

121. Walts AE, Said JW, Banks-Schlegel S: Keratin and carcinoembryonic antigen in exfoliated mesothelial and malignant cells: An immunoperoxidase study. *Am J Clin Pathol* 80:671–676, 1983

122. Vladutin AO, Wells Brason F, Adler RH: Differential diagnosis of pleural effusions: Clinical usefulness of cell marker quantitation. *Chest* 79:297–301, 1981

123. Martinez-Vea A, Gatell JM, Segura F: Diagnostic value of tumoral markers in serous effusions. *Cancer* 50:1783–1788, 1982

124. Herbert A, Gallagher PJ: Interpretation of pleural biopsy specimens and aspirates with the immunoperoxidase technique. *Thorax* 37:822–827, 1982

125. Epenetos AA, Canti G, Taylor-Papadimitriou J: Use of two epithelium specific monoclonal antibodies for diagnosis of malignancy in serous effusions. *Lancet* 2:1004–1006, 1982

126. To A, Deernaley DP, Ormerod MG: Epithelial membrane antigen: Its use in the cytodiagnosis of malignancy in serous effusions. *Am J Clin Pathol* 78:214–219, 1982

127. Light RW, Girard WM, Jenkinson SG, et al: Parapneumonic effusions. *Am J Med* 69:507–512, 1980

128. Bartlett JG, Thodepalli H, Gorback SL, et al: Bacteriology of empyema. *Lancet* 1:338–340, 1974

129. Gorbach SL, Mayhew JW, Bartlett JG, et al: Rapid diagnosis of anaerobic infections by direct gas-liquid chromatography of clinical specimens. *J Clin Invest* 5:478–484, 1976

130. Ladas S, Arapakis G, Malamou-Ladas H, et al: Rapid diagnosis of anaerobic infections by gas-liquid chromatography. *J Clin Pathol* 32:1163–1167, 1979

131. Kumar S, Seohadri MS, Koshi G, et al: Diagnosing tuberculous pleural effusion: Comparative sensitivity of mycobacterial culture and histopathology. *Br Med J* 283(6283):20, 1981

132. Berger HW, Mijia E: Tuberculous pleurisy. *Chest* 63:88–92, 1973

133. Levine H, Metzger W, Lacera D, et al: Diagnosis of tuberculous pleurisy by culture of pleural biopsy specimen. *Arch Intern Med* 126:269–271, 1970

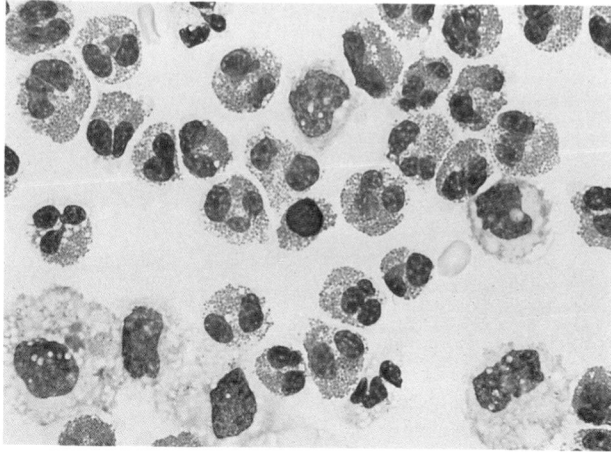

CHAPTER 4

Peritoneal Fluid

Much of the material discussed in chapter 3 on pleural and pericardial fluid also applies to the examination of peritoneal fluid.

ANATOMY AND PATHOPHYSIOLOGY

The peritoneum is a delicate, smooth serous membrane that covers the walls and viscera of the abdomen and pelvis. The peritoneum consists of two layers that are contiguous with one another, the space between them forming the peritoneal cavity. This cavity is lined by a single layer of mesothelial cells. The two layers of peritoneum are separated by a thin film of fluid that facilitates movement of the two membranes against one another. The peritoneal cavity is not a true cavity but only becomes so in the presence of disease that causes fluid to accumulate within it. The accumulation of fluid within the peritoneal cavity constitutes a peritoneal effusion, whereupon the patient

is said to have ascites. The fluid is also called ascitic fluid.

Peritoneal fluid is formed by plasma ultrafiltration. The accumulation of peritoneal fluid may result from increased hydrostatic pressure in the systemic circulation, decreased plasma osmotic pressure, increased permeability of the capillaries in the peritoneum, and decreased lymphatic absorption.

TRANSUDATES AND EXUDATES

The presence of more than 500 mL of peritoneal fluid is usually required before the effusion can be detected by roentgenography or physical examination. The major causes of peritoneal effusions are listed in Table 4–1.[1] The indications for aspiration of peritoneal fluid (by abdominal paracentesis) are ascites of unknown origin, suspected intestinal perforation, hemorrhage, or infarct, with the two most

TABLE 4–1. Causes of Peritoneal Effusions

Transudates
  Congestive heart failure
  Cirrhosis
  Hypoproteinemia

Exudates
  Infections (primary or secondary peritonitis)
  Malignant disorders
  Trauma
  Pancreatitis

Chylous effusion
  Trauma
  Carcinoma
  Lymphoma
  Tuberculosis

Note: Adapted from Krieg.[1] Used by permission.

common indications for paracentesis being complications of cirrhosis (such as spontaneous bacterial peritonitis) and a suspected intra-abdominal malignant disorder. Aspiration of peritoneal fluid may also be combined with lavage.

The laboratory criteria for separating transudates from exudates are less clearly defined with ascitic fluid than with pleural fluid. Nevertheless, the interpretation of serum-to-peritoneal fluid ratios for total protein and lactate dehydrogenase (LD), as described under "Transudates and Exudates" in chapter 3, will provide a reasonably accurate guide in many cases. During diuresis and infusion of albumin in patients with chronic liver disease, however, these ratios increase to be similar to those present in patients with exudative peritoneal effusion, making them unreliable for diagnosis. Pare et al[2] have recently shown that when either liver disease or a malignant disorder is suspected as the cause of ascitic fluid, the serum-ascites albumin concentration gradient is more reliable. This gradient is calculated by subtracting the ascitic fluid albumin concentration from the simultaneously determined serum albumin concentration. In a study involving 15 patients with malignant ascites, 14 had a gradient of less than 1.1, while one of 29 patients with ascites caused by liver disease had a gradient of less than 1.1.[1] In distinguishing between ascites caused by liver disease and that resulting from a malignant condition, therefore, the serum-ascites albumin concentration gradient was thought to be more reliable than the ascitic fluid-to-serum ratio for either total protein or LD. Rector and Reynolds[2] have more recently verified the superiority of the ascites-serum albumin gradient over the ascites total-protein concentration in differentiating between transudates and exudates. The serum-ascites albumin gradient was significantly greater in transudates (1.6 ± 0.5 g/dL) than exudates (0.6 ± 0.4 g/dL).[3] Although perfect separation did not occur, the authors recommended this method as the one of choice in the diagnostic evaluation of ascites.

PERITONEAL LAVAGE

Root[4] in 1965 first demonstrated the usefulness of peritoneal lavage in evaluating the conditions of patients with blunt trauma. Since then, the procedure has been widely accepted as an accurate, low-risk test for distinguishing between patients with significant injury and those with insignificant or no injury. It should be noted that peritoneal lavage does not detect retroperitoneal injury in blunt or penetrating trauma of the flank and back.

Peritoneal lavage consists of inserting a peritoneal dialysis catheter into the abdominal cavity through a small midline infraumbilical incision. The catheter is aspirated, and, if blood is not observed grossly, 1 L of Ringer's lactate solution is infused. The lavage fluid is immediately retrieved by gravity, and if the result is indeterminate, the catheter is left in place and the procedure repeated in one to two hours.[5] Table 4–2 lists the criteria used for interpretation of the test results.[5,6] When the lavage fluid is not grossly bloody, a sample is sent to the laboratory for RBC and WBC counts, microscopic examination, and chemical and microbiologic evaluations.[7] Peritoneal lavage using the dye-dilution technique with Evans blue human albumin complex has been recommended as a useful adjunct in the evaluation of patients with acute abdominal pain of gynecologic origin.[8] In one study, an exudate volume of more than 250 mL was highly suggestive of an intraperitoneal inflammatory process.[8]

GROSS EXAMINATION

Transudates are usually clear and pale yellow (Table 4–3). *Exudates* are cloudy or turbid due to

TABLE 4–2. Criteria for Diagnosing Blunt and Penetrating Trauma by Peritoneal Lavage Fluid Analysis

DIAGNOSIS	GROSS FINDINGS	FINDINGS ON LABORATORY ANALYSIS
Positive	Blood noted in aspirate or lavage return	RBC count >100,000/μL (>50,000/μL in cases of penetrating trauma—stab or gunshot wounds)
	Lavage fluid retrieved via Foley catheter or chest tube	WBC count >500/μL
	Evidence of food, foreign particle, or bile	Amylase level more than twice that of serum amylase level
Indeterminate	Small amount of bloody fluid noted in dialysis catheter on insertion	RBC count 50,000–100,000/μL (10,000–50,000/μL in cases of penetrating trauma)
		WBC count 100–500/μL
		Amylase level slightly higher than serum amylase level
Negative	NA*	RBC count <25,000/μL
		WBC count <100/μL
		Amylase level lower than serum amylase level

Note: Data modified from Alyono et al.[5,6] Used by permission.
*NA indicates not applicable.

large numbers of leukocytes, elevated protein levels, and, occasionally, microorganisms. Such fluids may be seen with peritonitis, perforated or infarcted intestine, and pancreatitis. Bile-stained fluid is greenish and may be seen with perforation of the gallbladder or intestine or with duodenal ulcer. Greenish fluid may also be present in cholecystitis and acute pancreatitis. The presence of bile can be confirmed with a "spot" test for bilirubin.[1]

Grossly *hemorrhagic peritoneal fluids* may be seen in trauma (ruptured spleen or liver), intestinal infarction, pancreatitis, and malignant disorders. Where pathologic hemorrhage must be distinguished from a traumatic tap, a visual quantitation of blood in the peritoneal fluid may be useful. The peritoneal lavage method is very sensitive in detecting the presence of blood. As few as eight drops of blood per liter of saline will cause pink discoloration.[9] More than 25 mL of blood per liter of lavage fluid gives a bright red, opaque appearance.[10]

True *chylous peritoneal fluid* is rare. When present, it is creamy and has the consistency of milk (Figure 112). Chylous ascites is caused by leakage of lymphatic vessels resulting from trauma, carcinoma, lymphoma, tuberculosis, and hepatic cirrhosis.[11] Malignant lymphoma and carcinoma are the two most common causes. Pseudochylous fluid, which may be associated with chronic effusions of any cause, has a milky or greenish appearance because of cellular debris and cholesterol crystals. Methods for differentiating between true chylous and pseudochylous fluids are outlined in chapter 2. In true chylous ascites, the triglyceride levels in the fluid exceed those of serum by a factor of 2 to 8.[1]

CELL COUNTS

In general, total leukocyte counts are of limited value in the differential diagnosis, although a leukocyte count higher than 300/μL is considered abnormal.[12,13] In addition, counts higher than 500/μL are considered useful in distinguishing between peritoneal transudates caused by spontaneous bacterial peritonitis and those associated with cirrhosis.[13,14] There is, however, a wide normal range for the ascitic fluid WBC count in patients with chronic liver disease because of extracellular shifts in fluid associated with ascites formation or resolution.[15] The same patients may have transudative and exudative patterns at different times. Thus, during diuresis, the WBC count may increase from less than 300/μL to more than 1,000/μL. It should be noted that the neutrophil con-

TABLE 4–3. Appearance of Peritoneal Fluid and
Associated Diseases

APPEARANCE	DISEASE
Clear, pale yellow	Cirrhosis
Cloudy, turbid	Bacterial peritonitis, pancreatitis, malignant condition
Green	Biliary tract disease, ruptured bowel
Bloody	Trauma, malignant disorder, pancreatitis, intestinal infarction
Milky	Chylous ascites caused by trauma, malignant disorder

FIGURE 112. *Chylous ascites in a patient with malignant lymphoma. Microscopic examination of this fluid revealed many lymphocytes and RBCs.*

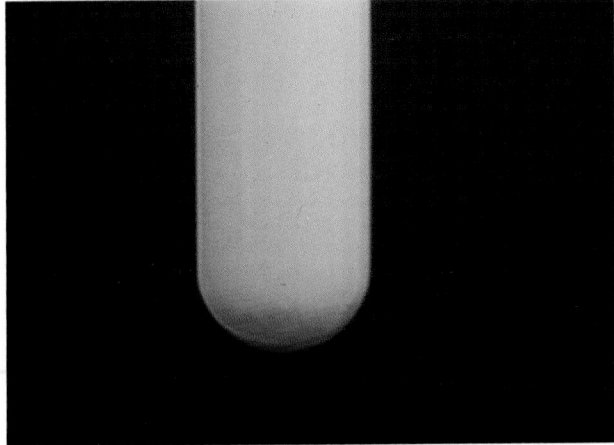

FIGURE 113. *Neutrophils in peritoneal fluid sample from a patient with bacterial peritonitis.*

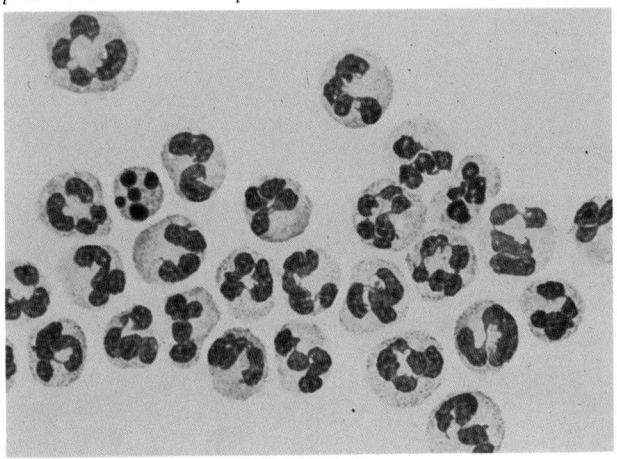

centration usually remains low and usually does not lead to confusion of cirrhosis with spontaneous bacterial peritonitis. However, in one study of ascitic fluid specimens taken from patients with alcoholic cirrhosis, the percentage of neutrophils exceeded 30% in 32% of patients.[16]

Cell counts improve the accuracy and specificity of the diagnosis in peritoneal lavage.[7] A positive result by lavage is an indication for laparotomy.[5-7] If the initial test results are indeterminate, another lavage may be indicated in one to two hours.[5] Using the criteria outlined in Table 4–2, Alyono and Perry[5] reported an accuracy of 98.6%, a sensitivity of 94.3%, and a specificity of 98.8% in a study of 1,588 patients. Peritoneal lavage has a somewhat lower accuracy in diagnosing penetrating trauma (gunshot and stab wounds) of the abdomen, with a sensitivity of 84% and a specificity of 98%.[17] In a study of patients with penetrating injury of the colon, the result by lavage was positive in 23 (70%) of 33 subjects, and false-negative results occurred in ten patients (30%).[17]

The WBC count may occasionally be elevated independently of the RBC count in penetrating abdominal trauma with visceral injury.[7] In addition, if the lavage is performed immediately after the injury occurs, the WBC count may not yet be elevated.[5]

MICROSCOPIC EXAMINATION

A differential cell count should be performed on a stained smear. The cell types encountered in the peritoneal fluid are the same as those in pleural fluid.[18] For a description of these cells, the reader is referred to chapter 3.

A differential cell count with more than 25% *neutrophils* is considered abnormal.[13] A predominance of neutrophils is suggestive of bacterial infection. An absolute neutrophil count is helpful; a count of more than 250/μL is thought to be a fairly sensitive indicator of spontaneous or secondary bacterial peritonitis[19] (Figure 113).

A predominance of *lymphocytes* is seen in transudates resulting from congestive heart failure, cirrhosis, and nephrotic syndrome. A predominance of lymphocytes may also be seen in chylous effusions, tuberculous peritonitis, and malignant disorders (Figure 114).

In contrast to pleural effusions, tuberculous peritoneal effusions may contain many *mesothelial cells.*

Peritoneal fluid *eosinophilia* is less common than pleural fluid eosinophilia. It has, however, been described in association with malignant ascites, ruptured hydatid cyst, congestive heart failure, chronic peritoneal dialysis, and vasculitis (Figure 115).[20]

As with other serous fluids, *lupus erythematosus cells* have occasionally been reported in peritoneal fluids.[21]

In addition to performing a differential cell count, it is important to examine the smear for possible *malignant cells.* When a malignant condition is suspected, a specimen should always be submitted for cytologic examination (Figures 116 through 119). With an experienced observer, a cytologic examination is extremely accurate in detecting the presence of malignant cells. The cells that are most difficult to differentiate from malignant cells are mesothelial cells (see also chapter 3) (Figure 120). Ascitic fluid associated with cirrhosis may contain highly atypical mesothelial cells (Figures 121 and 122).[18]

CHEMICAL ANALYSIS

Protein

The measurement of total protein in peritoneal fluid has generally been limited to classification of the fluid as either a transudate or an exudate. Classically, fluids containing less than 3.0 g/dL of total protein have been defined as transudates, while those having more than 3.0 g/dL have been classified as exudates. It is now well known that this is an oversimplification and that there are many exceptions. As a result, the measurement of total protein is of limited value in the assessment of peritoneal fluid. Other test values, such as those reported for pleural fluids in chapter 3, may provide more useful information in separating transudates from exudates.

Tuberculous peritonitis, pancreatic ascites, chronic renal failure, and intra-abdominal neoplasms are usually associated with fluids having protein concentrations of more than 3.0 g/dL. On the other hand, in spontaneous bacterial peritonitis, the protein concentration reportedly averages 1.8 g/dL.[22] The fractionation of peritoneal fluid proteins is of little clinical value.

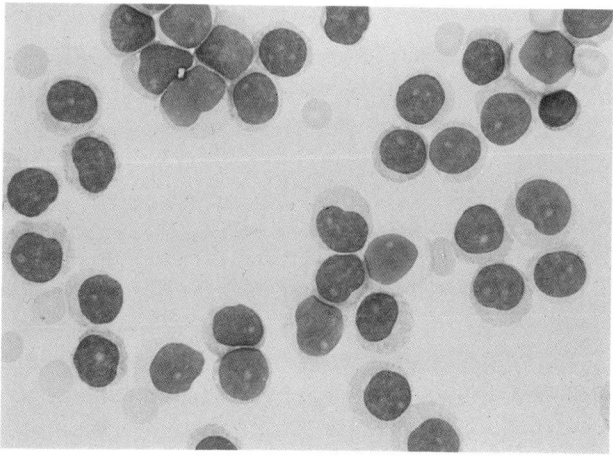

FIGURE 114. *Many lymphocytes present in ascitic fluid sample from a patient with nephrotic syndrome.*

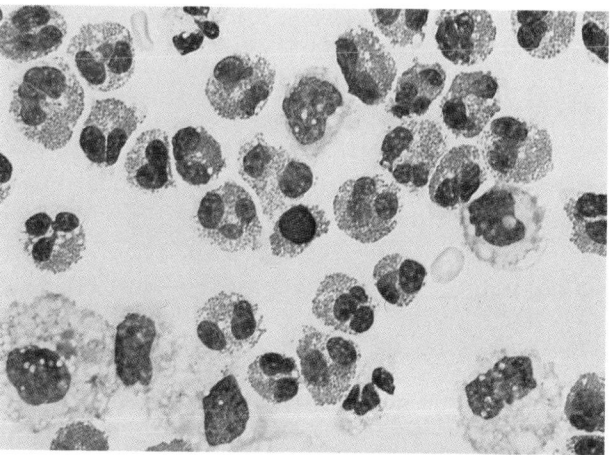

FIGURE 115. *Eosinophils and macrophages in ascitic fluid sample from a patient undergoing long-term peritoneal dialysis.*

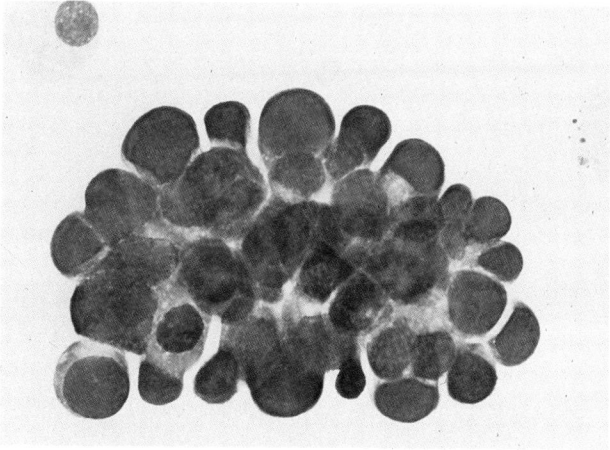

FIGURE 116. *Clump of malignant cells in ascitic fluid sample from a patient with ovarian carcinoma.*

Glucose

The measurement of glucose in peritoneal fluid may be clinically useful in selected cases. The normal levels approximate those found in serum. Unfortunately, few in-depth studies involving a wide variety of disease states have been carried out.

Ascitic fluid glucose levels are decreased in 30% to 60% of tuberculous peritonitis cases and in about 50% of abdominal carcinomatosis cases.[23,24] On the other hand, patients with cirrhosis or congestive heart failure rarely have values below normal. In one study in which patients' blood glucose levels were determined simultaneously with ascitic fluid glucose levels, the ratio of blood glucose to ascitic fluid glucose was reportedly 1.0 or greater in 80% of 15 cases with tuberculosis, while all patients with cirrhosis or congestive heart failure had ratios of less than 1.0.[23]

Enzymes

An amylase determination for a peritoneal fluid sample is often considered part of the complete laboratory examination of ascitic fluid. Elevations of amylase levels above the normal serum value occur in up to 90% of patients with acute or traumatic pancreatitis or pancreatic pseudocyst. A striking difference between the ascitic fluid and serum amylase levels is almost specific for ascites of pancreatic disease. However, in about 10% of patients with pancreatic disease, ascitic fluid and serum amylase levels may be normal.[3] Increased ascitic fluid amylase activity is not limited to pancreatic disease but has been reported in 77% of 26 patients with gastroduodenal perforation[25] and in patients with acute mesenteric venous occlusion[26] and small-bowel strangulation with or without perforation.[27]

In a study involving 1,588 patients who had suffered blunt trauma to the abdomen, routine amylase determinations for peritoneal lavage fluid specimens were elevated over serum values in only six patients.[5] Five of these six patients also had elevated WBC counts.[5] Patients with traumatic pancreatitis usually have elevated serum amylase levels.

The amylase isoenzyme pattern of fallopian tube epithelium is different from that of either the pancreas or the salivary gland, and it is possible to determine both salivary and genital isoamylase levels.[28] Patients with acute salpingitis who are undergoing laparoscopy have total peritoneal fluid amylase levels well below those seen in normal women or in those with other lower genital tract infections.[28] In addition, the isoenzyme patterns in these patients show absent or markedly decreased salivary and genital peaks by electrophoresis.[28] It has therefore been suggested that isoamylase determinations in peritoneal fluid samples obtained by cul-de-sac puncture may constitute a specific diagnostic test for acute salpingitis.[28]

Ascitic fluid *lipase* determination is considered complementary to—and perhaps more reliable than—amylase determination in the diagnosis of pancreatic ascites.[29] In a study of patients with pancreatic disease, lipase activity was significantly increased over normal serum levels and appeared to fluctuate less than amylase activity, remaining within a narrow range.[29]

Alkaline phosphatase (ALP) activity is very high in the intestinal tract. Several studies have shown that the measurement of ALP in peritoneal fluid may be helpful in evaluating the conditions of certain patients with abdominal disorders.[30-32] Patients with bowel strangulation, intestinal perforation, or traumatic hemoperitoneum may have greatly elevated peritoneal fluid ALP levels in comparison with serum ALP levels. With these conditions, the activity of other enzymes, notably LD and aldolase, is also elevated but is less specific than that of ALP for diagnosis.

In isolated traumatic liver injuries, both serum and peritoneal fluid may show pronounced elevations in levels of aspartate aminotransferase, alanine aminotransferase, and LD.

Lactate dehydrogenase (LD) levels are usually elevated in malignant abdominal effusions when compared with simultaneously determined serum levels. Benign effusions usually have values comparable to or lower than those in the serum. Ascitic fluid LD levels are increased more than 500 Sigma units in about 60% of patients with malignant effusions.[33] Ascitic fluid LD to serum LD ratios greater than 0.6 are said to increase the diagnostic sensitivity to about 80%.[33] The reverse ratio (serum LD to ascitic fluid LD) has also been used and is reported to be useful in distinguishing between ascites caused by cirrhosis and that resulting from a malignant disorder.[34]

γ-Glutamyltransferase (GGT) levels in ascitic fluid have been reported to be greatly increased in patients with primary hepatoma.[35] By comparison, peritoneal

FIGURE 117. *Adenocarcinoma of the colon in a peritoneal effusion. Note several malignant "signet-ring" cells.*

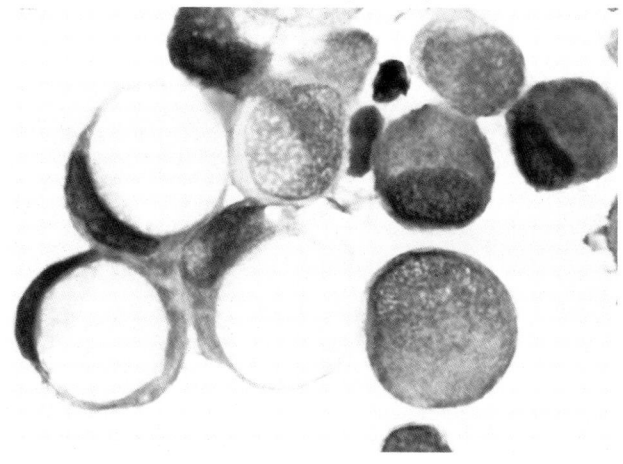

FIGURE 118. *Burkitt's lymphoma cells in peritoneal effusion. Note characteristic cells with blue, vacuolated cytoplasm, moderately clumped chromatin, and often prominent nucleoli.*

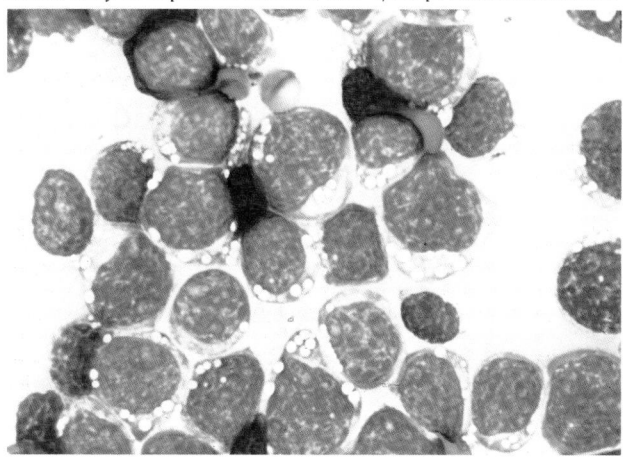

FIGURE 119. *Burkitt's lymphoma cells showing immunofluorescence with antibody to λ light chain. The presence of surface immunoglobulins is characteristic of B cells. The identification of a monoclonal B-cell population is consistent with a diagnosis of malignant lymphoma.*

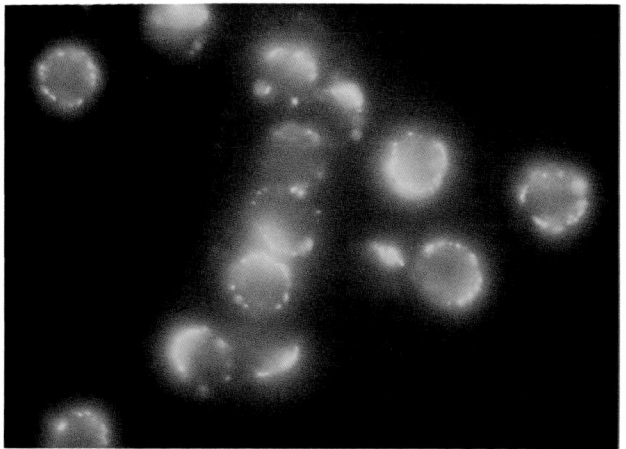

FIGURE 120. *Clump of mesothelial cells in ascitic fluid.*

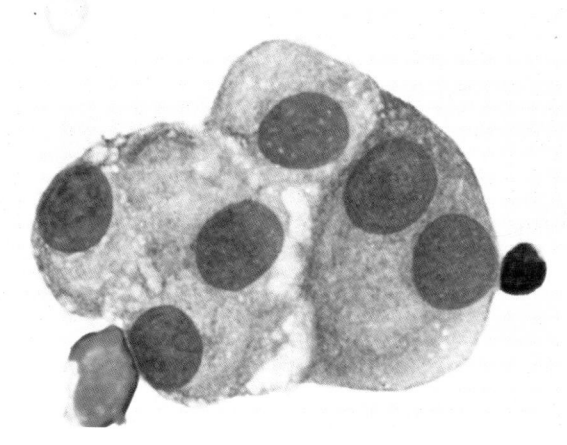

FIGURE 121. *Atypical mesothelial cells in ascitic fluid sample from patient with cirrhosis of liver.*

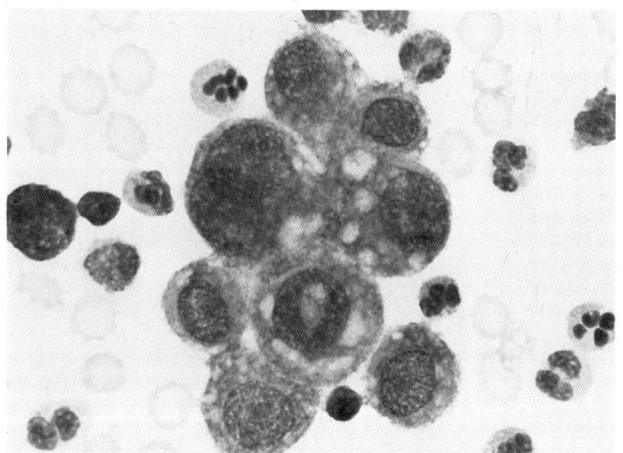

FIGURE 122. *Clumps of atypical mesothelial cells resembling malignant cells.*

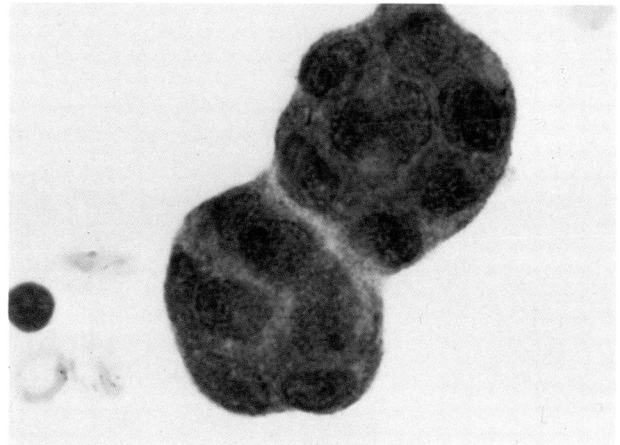

fluids from a variety of other hepatic disorders, including metastatic carcinoma, have shown greatly decreased levels. Only in cases of active cirrhosis with cellular regeneration have the GGT levels been mildly elevated, as compared with other hepatic disorders.[35] However, another study revealed no difference in peritoneal fluid GGT levels in specimens from 44 patients, including ten with hepatoma, ten with increased α_1-fetoprotein levels without evidence of hepatoma, and 24 with ordinary liver cirrhosis.[36]

Other Biochemical Measurements

Ammonia levels in peritoneal fluid have been shown to be consistently increased over plasma levels measured simultaneously in cases of ruptured appendix, perforated peptic ulcer, bowel strangulation with or without perforation, and ruptured urinary bladder with extravasation of urine.[37,38] Ammonia values are normal in patients with pancreatitis.

Blood urea nitrogen (BUN) and *creatinine* measurements are sometimes used to differentiate between peritoneal fluid and urine. Elevated levels of BUN and creatinine in the peritoneal fluid with normal serum values indicate aspiration from the urinary bladder. Elevated BUN and creatinine levels in the fluid with a high serum BUN but a normal serum creatinine level suggest rupture of the bladder.

The measurement of ascitic fluid *lactic acid* has been recommended as a reliable test for the diagnosis of bacterial peritonitis.[39] In one study, a significantly higher lactate level was seen in 24 patients with peritonitis than in 53 patients with uninfected ascites (mean, 77 mg/dL *vs* 14 mg/dL, respectively).[39] The measurement of lactate is considered to be especially useful in diagnosing spontaneous bacterial peritonitis (SBP) in patients with cirrhosis.[39]

Early diagnosis and treatment of intestinal infarction is a difficult clinical problem; the mortality approaches 90% when necrosis is extensive. It has been suggested, however, that early diagnosis is possible using the appropriate clinical techniques and with the knowledge that these patients frequently have elevated serum and peritoneal fluid phosphorus levels, metabolic acidosis, and leukocytosis.[40]

More recently, the value of *serum inorganic phosphate* concentration in the diagnosis of ischemic bowel disease was evaluated in a retrospective study involving 24 patients.[41] Only 25% of the patients had elevations of serum phosphate levels (greater than 5.5 mg/dL), but these patients had a combination of extensive bowel injury, acute renal insufficiency, and acidosis.[41] Although the serum phosphate level was not a sensitive indicator of ischemic bowel disease, elevations did predict extensive injury and a poor prognosis.[41]

Several studies have shown that the "boardlike" abdomen characteristic of peptic ulcer perforation is not caused by acid peritonitis. The *pH* of the peritoneal fluid following perforation is actually alkaline in nearly all cases because of rapid neutralization of the liberated gastric acid.[42,43] As a result, pH measurements in ascitic fluid have little diagnostic value in these cases. On the other hand, a recent report[44] indicates that an ascitic fluid pH of less than 7.31 is useful in the diagnosis of SBP in alcoholics with cirrhosis and in the absence of systemic acidosis. The mechanism for the low pH in patients with SBP is unknown. Although increased lactate production is believed to be one reason for these low pH values, it does not appear to be the only one.[44]

Tumor Markers

The diagnostic value of *carcinoembryonic antigen* (CEA) measurements in ascitic fluid has been demonstrated.[45] In "benign" ascites, the levels were consistently lower than 10 ng/mL. Fluid specimens with CEA levels higher than 10 ng/mL were considered to represent malignant effusions.[45] Using these criteria, CEA measurements accurately detected 14 of 29 malignant effusions, while a cytologic examination detected only 12.[45] The combined use of cytologic examination and CEA measurements resulted in an accurate diagnosis in 20 of 29 cases.[45]

There is evidence that CEA is synthesized by tumor cells and subsequently released into the ascitic fluid and the circulation. In a study of 56 patients with histologically confirmed advanced ovarian cancer, 32 (57%) showed a positive CEA result in serum, while 44 (78%) had a positive result in ascitic fluid.[46] In most patients, CEA levels were much higher in ascitic fluid than in serum.[46] Aspiration of fluid via the cul-de-sac is thought to provide another source of fluid samples for CEA measurements.

In addition to measuring tumor antigens in the

fluid, *immunocytochemical methods* have recently become available for demonstrating a variety of cell and tissue antigens in serous effusions. These techniques may be very useful in cases where a definitive diagnosis cannot be made on morphologic grounds alone. With the immunoperoxidase technique using the avidin-biotin complex or the immunoalkaline phosphatase procedure, a panel of monoclonal antibodies has been studied.[47] These include antibodies to common leukocyte antigen, CEA, human milk-fat globule membrane, epithelial membrane antigen (EMA), keratin, and several intermediate filament antigens, among others. The method of preparation involves fixing cytocentrifuge slide preparations with acetone or alcohol or storing air-dried smears unfixed, then wrapping them in aluminum foil at −20 °C and subsequently fixing them.

Carcinoembryonic antigen has been demonstrated on malignant cells in serous effusions from adenocarcinomas of the breast, ovary, lung, stomach, and colon (Figure 109).[48] Weak or moderate staining is seen in mesothelial cells. Keratin staining does not differentiate between mesothelial cells or between adenocarcinoma and squamous cell carcinoma. The anti–human milk-fat globule membrane and EMA have been demonstrated on malignant cells in carcinomas of breast, ovary, lung, and colon (Figures 109 and 110). In our experience, EMA is not usually seen on mesothelial cells, making the antibody to EMA very useful in distinguishing between atypical mesothelial cells and malignant cells (Figure 111). The T29/33 antibody, an antibody to the pan-leukocyte antigen T200, is useful in distinguishing between large cell lymphomas and poorly differentiated carcinoma, neuroblastoma, Wilms' tumor, and Ewing's sarcoma. However, T200 may be absent from some immunoblastic lymphomas and most plasma cell neoplasms.

It should be noted that immunochemical evaluation does not replace the need for routine cytologic examination, but it does provide a valuable means of verifying the accuracy of the cytologic diagnosis. It may also increase the diagnostic accuracy of cytologic examination. In a recent study of 41 patients with a variety of malignant effusions, 12 cases had positive immunocytochemical staining with negative cytologic test results.[48]

MICROBIOLOGIC EXAMINATION

The diagnosis of *tuberculous peritonitis* is often difficult to make and frequently overlooked, since the classic features of prolonged fever—weight loss, exudative ascites, and a positive PPD test result—may not always be present. Of assistance in these cases is the fact that, in tuberculous peritonitis, ascitic fluid protein levels usually exceed 3.0 g/dL and glucose values are lower than 60 mg/dL or the simultaneous blood glucose–to–ascitic fluid glucose ratio is 1.0 or greater.[23] When either or both of these findings are present, appropriate cultures for tubercle bacilli should be requested. Acid-fast stain and culture may be positive in only 25% to 50% of tuberculous effusions. Concentrating large amounts of fluid increases the sensitivity. A peritoneal biopsy may be of diagnostic significance.

Spontaneous bacterial peritonitis (SBP) is a relatively common disease, and in patients with cirrhosis, the mortality is high (80% to 95%).[13] The ascitic fluid is cloudy, and the WBC count (predominantly polymorphonuclear) is usually above 1,000/μL. A Gram stain of the centrifuged specimen is helpful but is only positive in about 30% of cases. In about two thirds of these cases, gram-negative bacilli *(Escherichia coli)* are present, while pneumococci account for most of the remaining cases. In contrast to tuberculous peritonitis, the protein content in ascitic fluid specimens from patients with SBP is usually less than 3.0 g/dL.

In a recent evaluation of patients with ascites caused by either SBP or gastrointestinal tract perforation, neither clinical signs nor symptoms were helpful.[14] However, all patients with perforation peritonitis fulfilled at least two of the following criteria: ascitic fluid total protein level higher than 1.0 g/dL, glucose level lower than 50 mg/dL, and LD activity greater than 225 mU/mL.

The measurement of lactic acid and pH in peritoneal fluid may also be helpful in the diagnosis of SBP, as described under "Other Biochemical Measurements" in this chapter. A pH of less than 7.35, an arterial-ascitic fluid pH difference of more than 0.10, an ascitic fluid lactate level higher than 25 mg/dL, and an arterial-ascitic fluid lactate difference of at least 20 mg/dL are predictive values favoring the diagnosis of bacterial peritonitis.[49] The most reliable discriminatory test result, however, is thought to be an ascitic fluid polymorphonuclear leukocyte count of more than 500/dL.

Counterimmunoelectrophoresis for bacterial antigens may be extremely useful, just as it is for other body fluids. On the other hand, *Limulus* lysate assays are less reliable for peritoneal fluid than for CSF. Further studies and improved techniques are needed before the latter procedure becomes routine with peritoneal or pleural fluids (see chapter 1).

Organic acid measurements by gas-liquid chromatography may prove to be a specific and useful method for the rapid detection of fecal anaerobes in patients with intra-abdominal infections.[50] One report showed that succinic acid was present in peritoneal fluid in 32 of 33 culture-positive cases, while the volatile propionic, isobutyric, butyric, and isovaleric acids were present in 13, 10, 11, and 11, respectively, of the 33 culture-positive cases. The volatile acids (excluding acetic acid) were uniformly absent in culture-negative cases, while succinic acid was present in only seven of 44 culture-negative cases.[50]

Analysis of peritoneal fluid is useful in differentiating between *gastrointestinal tract perforation* and SBP.[14] In perforation peritonitis, the peritoneal fluids have significantly higher total protein and LD levels and lower glucose concentrations.[14] The WBC and neutrophil counts, however, do not appear to be significantly different enough to be useful in distinguishing between these two entities.[14] In a study of 32 patients with spontaneous bacterial peritonitis and six patients with bacterial peritonitis caused by gastrointestinal tract perforation, the latter group had at least two of three diagnostic findings: total protein level higher than 1 g/dL, glucose level lower than 50 mg/dL, and LD level higher than 225 mU/mL.[14] With SBP, such values were found in only two patients.[14]

REFERENCES

1. Krieg AF: Cerebrospinal fluid and other body fluids, in Henry JB (ed): *Clinical Diagnosis and Management by Laboratory Methods*, ed 16. Philadelphia, WB Saunders Co, 1979, pp 635–679

2. Pare P, Talbot J, Hoets JC: Serum-ascites albumin concentration gradient: A physiologic approach to the differential diagnosis of ascites. *Gastroenterology* 85:240–244, 1983

3. Rector WG, Reynolds TB: Superiority of the serum-ascites difference over the ascites total protein concentration in separation of "transudative" and "exudative" ascites. *Am J Med* 77:83–85, 1984

4. Root HD, Hauser CW, McKinley CR, et al: Diagnostic peritoneal lavage. *Surgery* 57:633–637, 1965

5. Alyono D, Perry JF: Value of quantitative cell count and amylase activity of peritoneal lavage fluid. *J Trauma* 21:345–348, 1981

6. Alyono D, Morrow CE, Perry JF: Reappraisal of diagnostic peritoneal lavage criteria for operation in penetrating and blunt trauma. *Surgery* 92:751–757, 1982

7. Vij D, Horan P, Obeid FN, et al: The importance of WBC count in peritoneal lavage. *JAMA* 249:636–638, 1983

8. Shapira SC, Weiss DB, Yersky Y: Quantitative peritoneal lavage in evaluating acute abdominal pain of gynecological origin. *Int Surg* 68:171–173, 1983

9. Parvin S, Smith DE, Ascher M, et al: Effectiveness of peritoneal lavage in blunt abdominal trauma. *Ann Surg* 181:255–261, 1975

10. Olsen WR, Redman HC, Hidreth DH: Quantitative peritoneal lavage in blunt abdominal trauma. *Arch Surg* 104:536–543, 1972

11. Lesser GT, Bruno MS, Enselberg K: Chylous ascites. *Arch Intern Med* 125:1073–1077, 1970

12. Kline MM, McCallum RW, Guth PH: The clinical value of ascitic fluid in alcoholic liver disease. *Gastroenterology* 70:408–412, 1976

13. Conn HO: Spontaneous bacterial peritonitis: Multiple revisitations. *Gastroenterology* 70:455–457, 1976

14. Runyon BA, Hoefs JC: Ascitic fluid analysis in the differentiation of spontaneous bacterial peritonitis from gastrointestinal tract perforation into ascitic fluid. *Hepatology* 4:447–450, 1984

15. Hoefs JC: Increase in ascites white blood cell and protein concentrations during diuresis in patients with chronic liver disease. *Hepatology* 1:249–254, 1981

16. Wilson JAP, Suguitan EA, Cassidy WA: Characteristics of ascitic fluid in the alcoholic cirrhotic. *Dig Dis Sci* 24:645–648, 1979

17. Obeid FN, Sorensen V, Vincent G, et al: Inaccuracy of diagnostic peritoneal lavage in penetrating colonic trauma. *Arch Surg* 119:906–908, 1984

18. Spriggs AI, Boddington MM: *The Cytology of Effusions*, ed 2. New York, Grune & Stratton Inc, 1968

19. Jones SR: The absolute granulocyte count in ascitic fluid: An aid to the diagnosis of spontaneous bacterial peritonitis. *West J Med* 126:344–346, 1977

20. Adams HW, Mainz DL: Eosinophilic ascites. *Am J Dig Dis* 22:40–43, 1977

21. Mertzger AL, Coyne M, Lee S: In vivo LE cell

formation in peritonitis due to SLE. *J Rheumatol* 1:130, 1974

22. Conn HO, Fessel JM: Spontaneous bacterial peritonitis in cirrhosis: Variations on a theme. *Medicine* 50:161–197, 1971

23. Polak M, Torres Da Costa AC: Diagnostic value of the estimation of glucose in ascitic fluid. *Digestion* 8:347–352, 1973

24. Brown JD, An ND: Tuberculous peritonitis. *Am J Gastroenterol* 66:277–282, 1976

25. Amerson JR, Howard JM, Vowles KDJ: The amylase concentration in serum and peritoneal fluid following perforation of gastroduodenal ulcers. *Ann Surg* 147:245–250, 1958

26. Gray EB Jr, Amador E: Acute mesenteric venous thrombosis simulating acute pancreatitis: The value of peritoneal fluid analysis. *JAMA* 167:1734–1736, 1958

27. Mansberger AR Jr: The diagnostic value of abdominal paracentesis with special reference to peritoneal fluid ammonia levels. *Am J Gastroenterol* 42:150–161, 1964

28. Westrom L, Skude G, Mardh PA: Amylases of the genital tract: II. Peritoneal fluid isoamylases in acute salpingitis. *Am J Obstet Gynecol* 126:657–660, 1976

29. Sileo AV, Chawla SK, LoPresti PA: Pancreatic ascites: Diagnostic importance of ascitic lipase. *Dig Dis Sci* 20:1110–1114, 1975

30. Lee YN: Alkaline phosphatase in intestinal perforation. *JAMA* 208:361, 1969

31. Rush BF Jr, Host WR, Fewel J, et al: Intestinal ischemia and some organic substances in serum and abdominal fluid. *Arch Surg* 105:151–157, 1972

32. Delaney HM, Moss CM, Carnevale N: The use of enzyme analysis of peritoneal blood in the clinical assessment of abdominal organ injury. *Surg Gynecol Obstet* 142:161–167, 1976

33. Boyer TD, Kahn AM, Reynolds TB: Diagnostic value of ascitic fluid lactic dehydrogenase, protein and WBC levels. *Arch Intern Med* 138:1103–1105, 1978

34. Greene LS, Levine R, Gross MJ, et al: Distinguishing between malignant and cirrhotic ascites by computerized step-wise discriminant functional analysis of its biochemistry. *Am J Gastroenterol* 70:448–454, 1978

35. Peters TJ, et al: Gamma-glutamyltransferase levels in ascitic fluid and liver tissue from patients with primary hepatoma. *Br Med J* 1:1516, 1977

36. Cortes-Ruis M, Escoda J, Fuste L, et al: Gamma-glutamyltransferase in ascitic fluid in primary hepatoma. *Br Med J* 2:1435, 1978

37. Mansberger AR Jr: The value of peritoneal fluid ammonia levels in the differential diagnosis of the acute abdomen. *Ann Surg* 155:998–1010, 1962

38. Mansberger AR Jr: The diagnostic value of abdominal paracentesis with special reference to peritoneal fluid ammonia levels. *Am J Gastroenterol* 42:150–161, 1964

39. Brook I, Altman RS, Lachman WW, et al: Measurement of lactate in ascitic fluid: An aid in the diagnosis of peritonitis with particular relevance to spontaneous bacterial peritonitis of the cirrhotic. *Dig Dis Sci* 26:1089–1094, 1981

40. Sawer BA, Jamieson WG, Durand D: The significance of elevated peritoneal fluid phosphate level in intestinal infarction. *Surg Gynecol Obstet* 146:43–45, 1978

41. May LD, Berenson MM: Value of serum inorganic phosphate in the diagnosis of ischemic bowel disease. *Am J Surg* 146:266–268, 1983

42. Moretz WH, Erickson WG: Neutralization of hydrochloric acid in the peritoneal cavity. *Arch Surg* 75:834–837, 1957

43. Howard JM, Singh LM: Peritoneal fluid pH after perforation of peptic ulcers. *Arch Surg* 87:483–484, 1963

44. Gitlin N, Stauffer JL, Silvestri RC: The pH of ascitic fluid in the diagnosis of spontaneous bacterial peritonitis in alcoholic cirrhosis. *Hepatology* 2:408–411, 1982

45. Loewenstein MS, Rittgers RA, Feinerman AE, et al: Carcinoembryonic antigen assays of ascites and detection of malignancy. *Ann Intern Med* 88:635–638, 1978

46. Khoo SK, Hill R, Daunter B, et al: Carcinoembryonic antigen in ovarian cancer: Correlation of concentrations in tumor tissue, cyst fluid, ascitic fluid and peripheral blood. *Aust NZ J Obstet Gynecol* 22:65–70, 1982

47. Ghosh AK, Spriggs AI, Taylor-Papadimitriou J, et al: Immunocytochemical staining of cells in pleural and peritoneal effusions with a panel of monoclonal antibodies. *J Clin Pathol* 36:1154–1164, 1983

48. Ghosh AK, Mason DY, Spriggs AI: Immunocytochemical staining with monoclonal antibodies in cytologically 'negative' serous effusions from patients with malignant disease. *J Clin Pathol* 36:1150–1153, 1983

49. Garcia-Tsao G, Conn HO, Lerner E: The diagnosis of bacterial peritonitis: Comparison of pH, lactate concentration, and leukocyte count. *Hepatology* 5:91–96, 1985.

50. Spiegel CA, Malangoni MA, Condon RE: Gas-liquid chromatography of rapid diagnosis of intra-abdominal infection. *Arch Surg* 119:28–32, 1984

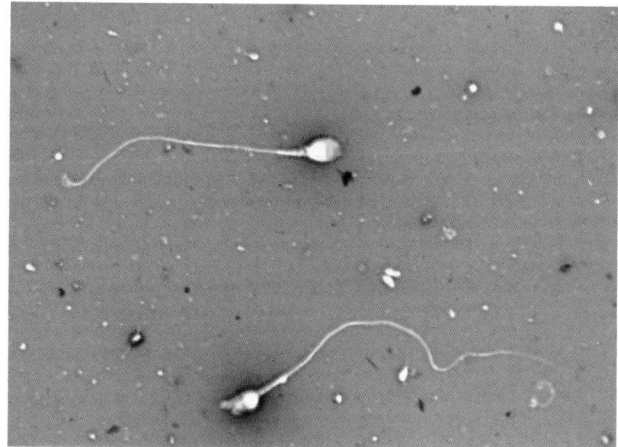

CHAPTER 5

Seminal Fluid

Written by Ronald Urry, PhD
University of Utah School of Medicine

ANATOMY AND PHYSIOLOGY

Semen is a biochemically complex solution consisting of fluid contributed or modified by the testicle, epididymis, seminal vesicles, prostate gland, Cowper's glands, Littre's glands, and perhaps the vasa deferentia. Despite its biochemical complexity, the main function of human semen appears to be to transport the spermatozoa to female cervical mucus. After deposition in the female genital tract, sperm appear to remain in the seminal plasma for only a short period while they enter the mucus. Contributions of the various organs to semen are as follows.

Spermatozoa, which make up only a small part of the volume of the ejaculate, exit the *testicle* with a small amount of fluid through the ductuli efferentia. The fluid from the testicle also contains many other compounds, including steroids, the principal ones

being testosterone and dihydrotestosterone. Androgen-binding protein is also found in the ejaculate[1] but in decreased amounts in vasectomized patients, indicating that this protein has a mostly testicular or epididymal origin. Other proteins (including many enzymes) and some lipids and electrolytes are also present in the semen. A portion of these compounds is probably contributed by the fluid that comes from the testicles. The function of many of the constituents of semen, including many of those from the testis, remains uncertain.

The contribution of the *epididymis* to the seminal plasma remains unclear even though something is known of the modifications that occur in semen during its passage through this structure.[2] The epididymis picks up carnitine from the blood and contributes it, along with acetylcarnitine and glycerylphosphorylcholine, to the seminal plasma. The role of these compounds in the function of spermatozoa remains unclear, but it has been suggested that carnitine and acetylcarnitine enable the spermatozoa to metabolize fatty acids and may have other useful roles.[3] They have been shown to be altered in concentration in infertile men and are related to sperm motility defects.[4,5] Since the capability for sperm motility develops in the epididymis, this could be an important observation. It remains difficult, however, to evaluate the role of these compounds in semen.

The epididymis takes up androgens from the fluid that enters from the testicle and metabolizes them. These androgens, together with peripheral androgens, play an important role in the functions of the epididymis.[6] Sperm passage through at least half to two thirds of the length of the human epididymis is necessary for spermatozoa to gain the ability to move and to fertilize the egg.[6] The epididymis also plays an important role in absorbing spermatozoa after vasectomy by moving WBCs into the lumen to phagocytose spermatoza. Some WBCs that are found in the semen and are thought to come from the prostate may originate in the epididymis.

The majority of the seminal fluid originates in the *seminal vesicles*. Seminal fluid has a high flavin content, which imparts a cream color to the fluid and is responsible for the fluorescence of semen under ultraviolet light. It also has a high fructose content that may serve as a sperm nutrient. Fructose may form tight bonds with certain proteins that are also of vesicular origin and that may contribute to semen coagulation.

Semen contains a variety of prostaglandins—which were incorrectly named when it was assumed that they were of prostatic origin.[7] The bulk of the prostaglandins appears to originate in the fluid from the seminal vesicles,[7] although it is uncertain what role these compounds play in the semen. The concentration of some types of seminal prostaglandins may correlate with the numbers and quality of spermatozoa present in the ejaculate.[8] It remains unclear, however, whether alterations in prostaglandin levels play a role in various types of fertility defects. One of the functions of seminal prostaglandins may be to influence the female response to the deposition of semen in the female tract. When semen is deposited directly into the uterus through artificial insemination, some women experience severe cramping due to uterine muscle contractions induced by seminal prostaglandins.

The *prostate* contributes 20% to 25% of the volume of the ejaculate. This fluid is rich in citric acid, which is the major anion in semen. Many enzymes are contributed by the prostate, including acid phosphatase. The proteins and enzymes from the prostate, together with those in the fluid from the seminal vesicles, participate in the regulation of semen coagulation and liquefaction.[9]

The prostate is also a major contributor of zinc to the ejaculate, with additional quantities of zinc contributed by testicular fluid and spermatozoa. Magnesium, too, is found in the fluids from the prostate and the seminal vesicles, although the role of zinc and magnesium remains unclear. Many reports have attempted to link diminished zinc levels in seminal fluid to increased numbers of WBCs in the seminal fluid and/or to infections.[10] It is also thought by some that chronic prostatitis can be diagnosed by the finding of decreased levels of zinc in the seminal fluid[11]; hence there have been attempts to use seminal zinc levels to determine the need for treatment.[11]

Only a small amount of fluid is contributed by *Cowper's glands* and *glands of Littre,* and little is known of the biochemical role or significance of the fluid from these glands in the function of spermatozoa.

SPECIMEN COLLECTION

The main indication for seminal fluid examination is infertility. Other indications include evaluating the quality of semen from donors to artificial insemination programs, determining the completeness of vasectomy, and medicolegal indications.

To evaluate semen properly, at least two or preferably more samples must be analyzed from an individual. The samples should be collected in a comfortable, private room near the laboratory, if possible, in a container provided by the laboratory. Although many laboratories share the common misconception that only glass containers can be used, sterile plastic containers, similar to those used for urine collection, are not detrimental to sperm function and can be used for semen collection.[12] The sample must be collected in a clean container that is free of chemical or soap residues. If the sample will not be examined within

30 minutes of collection, it should be kept warm at approximately 37 °C. It should be examined within one to two hours of collection. If the patient delivers the sample to the laboratory from home, he should be instructed to collect the whole sample in a clean container, wrap the container in a dry towel or washcloth to keep it warm, put it in a bag with the lid tightly closed, and deliver it to the laboratory within one hour of collection.

To obtain an accurate motility determination, semen should be observed within 1½ to two hours of collection. Although a three- to five-day period of sexual abstinence prior to collection of the sample is often recommended, a 48-hour period is probably satisfactory. The period should not exceed five days. It would probably be best if the time period coincided with the normal pattern of the couple's sexual activity. The patient should be told to abstain from all sexual activity, not just intercourse, prior to collection of the sample. Occasionally a patient will not be able, for one reason or another, to collect a sample by masturbating into a container; the laboratory must then provide him with a nonspermicidal condom, as ordinary condoms are spermicidal and cannot be used to collect semen for analysis. The patient should be questioned to be certain that the sample was collected directly into the container brought to the laboratory and not in a regular condom first and then transferred into the container. Lubricants of any kind should be avoided, since most have spermicidal properties.

GROSS EXAMINATION

Recently ejaculated semen is highly viscid, but within ten to 20 minutes the coagulum will spontaneously liquefy to form a translucent, turbid, viscous fluid. The specimen should be allowed to sit for one half to one hour after collection before observation begins. If the sample is collected near the laboratory, it should be placed in an incubator at 37 °C and allowed to liquefy for 30 minutes. If the sample is brought to the laboratory from the outside and is more than 30 minutes old, it should be evaluated immediately upon arrival.

The *color* of the semen should be observed and noted if it is different from the normal gray-white to translucent pattern of semen. If there is any degree of

brown or red coloring, there may be blood in the semen. This may be seen in prostatitis. A yellow color may indicate prostatovesiculitis, urine in the semen, or the use of certain oral antibiotics or medications. A dense white, turbid appearance can be caused by large numbers of leukocytes associated with inflammation in the urethra or in one of the ejaculatory glands.[13] The color of semen may also be altered by the length of sexual abstinence, with shorter intervals yielding more transparent semen and longer periods yielding semen that is more yellow.[13] Semen has a distinctive musty odor, but this may vary with medical conditions such as seminal infection.

Seminal *volume* should be measured to the nearest 0.1 mL. The normal seminal volume per ejaculation averages 2 to 5 mL. A correlation between sexual abstinence and seminal volume will not be seen in every man, but usually the volume increases as frequency of intercourse decreases.[14,15] When the seminal volume is consistently less than 1.0 mL, one should suspect problems with fertility. On the other hand, it is doubtful that a large ejaculate volume will have a detrimental effect on fertility if the rest of the seminal examination, including sperm count, is normal.

The various events participating in the coagulation and liquification of semen are beyond the scope of this chapter. However, the person analyzing semen specimens should be able to recognize abnormal seminal *viscosity*. Semen should normally be liquified at the end of 30 minutes. When incomplete liquification occurs, it can take two forms. One form is liquid viscosity, in which the liquid portion remains more viscous than normal for more than one hour after collection. Liquid viscosity can be evaluated with an ordinary Pasteur pipette. At least one half hour after collection, semen is drawn into the pipette and then slowly expelled. If the semen does not form normal, discrete droplets, it is rated on a viscosity scale as "minor," "moderate," or "severe," depending on the relative thickness of the fluid.

The second type of viscosity is particulate viscosity, wherein the particles in the semen are also rated on a three-point scale as minor, moderate, or severe, depending on the number and size of undissolved particles. It should be noted that a normal man may have increased seminal viscosity from time to time. Increased viscosity may only pose a problem to an individual's fertility if it is consistently abnormal from

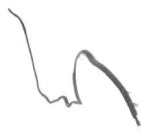

sample to sample and if it is associated with decreased sperm motility.

MICROSCOPIC EVALUATION

The tests described in the following sections are listed in the order in which they are usually performed. Since motility and viability decrease with time, the time of both collection and observation should be recorded. The sample must be observed within 1½ to two hours of collection if an accurate measurement of motility is to be obtained.

Agglutination

A drop of semen is placed on a microscope slide, coverslipped, and observed for the presence of sperm agglutination. Agglutination is seen when spermatozoa display a definite association pattern, such as head-to-head, head-to-tail, or tail-to-tail.[12] Several high-power fields should be observed to determine if such patterns of sperm association can be detected. The amount of sperm agglutination, if any, should be rated as slight, moderate, or severe. Sperm clumping is different from sperm agglutination in that no consistent pattern, as previously described, is observed. Spermatozoa may also overlap one another in any fashion. It is not unusual periodically to find clumping of spermatozoa in an otherwise normal specimen.

Consistent sperm agglutination, observed in several semen samples from one man, should be studied further. The patient should be investigated for chronic prostatitis, and the seminal plasma and serum should be evaluated for sperm-agglutinating antibodies.

Sperm-agglutinating antibodies can be measured by both macroscopic and microscopic techniques. A popular method is the Kibrick[16] macroagglutination technique, in which serum and sperm-free seminal plasma are added to a donor's sperm sample with a gelatin-buffer mixture. When antibodies are present, the fluids (serum or seminal plasma) will cause the donor's sperm to clump, forming a white, flocculent precipitate. Antibody titers higher than 1:4 to 1:16 are considered significant.[16]

Sperm Motility

Sperm motility should be evaluated within one half to one hour after collection. The time of sample collection and the time of observation should be recorded. The percentage of spermatozoa moving with normal, progressive motility (in a more or less straight line at reasonable speed) is noted. In addition, the percentage of spermatozoa observed with significant immobilizing motion (fast or slow in-place motion without forward progression) should be recorded. We recommend a reproducible system that has worked well to record sperm motility for all different types of sperm movement[12,17] and that compares favorably with more complex photographic methods used to evaluate and quantitate sperm motility. (The technique is described in detail in Appendix B.) Basically, it consists of observing a drop of coverslipped, unstained semen under the microscope and estimating how many spermatozoa are motile using a semiquantitative (0 to 4) estimation of sperm motility. With this method, at least 40% of the spermatozoa should be observed with progressive motility.

A laboratory performing semen analyses should report at least the percentage of sperm with progressive motility and note any significant increase in abnormal movement, including immobilizing-type motion. The latter type of motility is an indication for analysis of serum and seminal fluid specimens for sperm-immobilizing antibodies.

Sperm-immobilizing antibodies can be measured using the Isojima[18] immobilization test. Donor semen is incubated with the fluid to be tested (serum or sperm-free seminal plasma), along with complement. If antibodies are present, disruption of the spermatozoa membrane will occur, along with loss of sperm motility and cell death. These effects are observed microscopically.[18] Observing sperm motility provides information that can help determine the chances of the spermatozoa reaching the site of fertilization. It may also have some correlation with the ability of the spermatozoa to penetrate the ovum.

Sperm motility observations made on a single specimen at intervals throughout the day provide meaningless information because of the decline in sperm motility while spermatozoa remain in the semen specimen in the laboratory.[12] After deposition, the spermatozoa quickly move into the female cervical mucus, leaving the seminal fluid after only a short time.

Viability

The viability of spermatozoa can be determined by staining the spermatozoa and counting the number that are alive and the number dead (Figures 123 and 124).[17-19] Normally, 50% or more of the spermatozoa should be viable (Appendix B). The results should be correlated with the results of the motility study.[17]

Morphology

The morphologic characteristics of sperm can be evaluated by performing differential cell counts of normal- and abnormal-appearing spermatozoa on stained smears. One to two smears should be made, using a technique similar to that used to prepare slides for blood films.[17] Several different stains may be used for morphologic examination. The Papanicolaou technique is popular and, although somewhat complex and time-consuming, provides an attractive specimen to evaluate. We use a hematoxylin-eosin stain that is easy to perform and provides slides of good quality (Appendix B).[12] This stain enables an experienced observer to differentiate between WBCs and immature spermatozoa. For the observer who is less experienced, a peroxidase stain may be used to differentiate among leukocytes present in the ejaculate.

Spermatozoa should be examined under high magnification (usually 1,000×, oil-immersion objective), and at least 200 to 300 spermatozoa should be counted. The morphologic types are usually divided into those with normal heads (Figure 125), large heads (Figure 126), small heads (Figure 127), tapered heads (Figure 128), immature heads (Figures 129 and 130), and duplicate heads (Figure 131) and amorphous spermatozoa (Figures 132 and 133), which encompass all other types.[12,17,20] Many other shapes have been described, but identification of these categories is sufficient.

In general, more than 60% of the spermatozoa should have a normal appearance (Appendix B). Increases in the number of tapered spermatozoa (more than 20% to 30%) often signify a varicocele.[21] Patients with a varicocele may also have an increase (more than 20%) in the number of immature spermatozoa (Figures 129 and 130). An increase in both tapered and immature spermatozoa is referred to as a "nonspecific stress pattern." Such increases may be seen in patients with a varicocele or may occur in patients who seem to be under increased stress. Most types of morphologic abnormalities, however, cannot be attributed to any specific type of defect. A careful study of sperm morphology is important in fertility

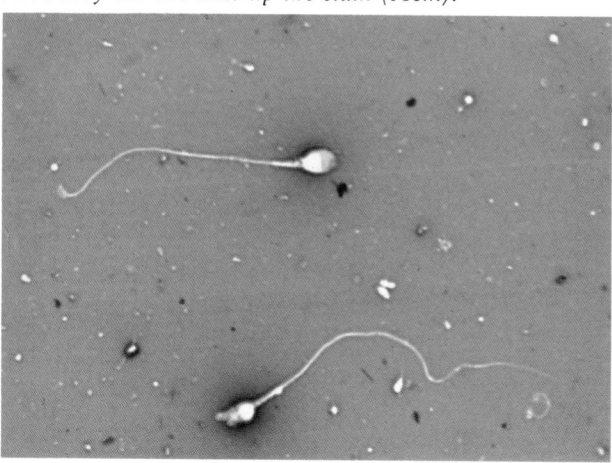

FIGURE 123. *Live spermatozoa having white appearance since they did not take up the stain (eosin).*

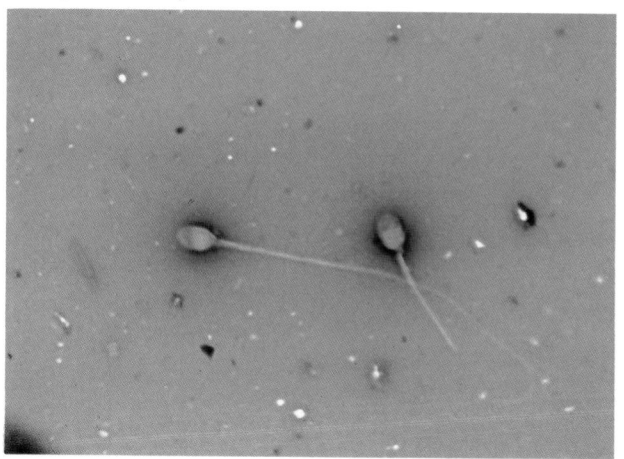

FIGURE 124. *Dead spermatozoa having orange-red appearance (eosin stain).*

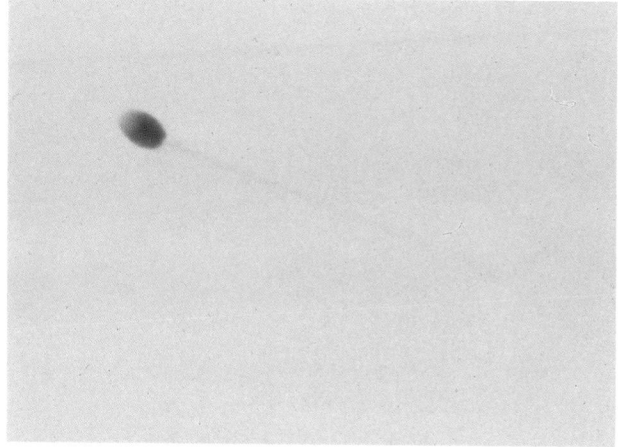

FIGURE 125. *Spermatozoon with normal, oval-shaped head (hematoxylin-eosin stain).*

FIGURE 126. *Spermatozoon in the center with large head (hematoxylin-eosin stain).*

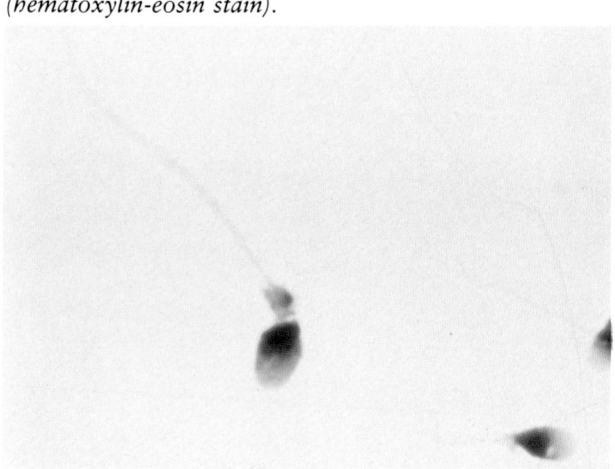

FIGURE 127. *Spermatozoon with small head (hematoxylin-eosin stain).*

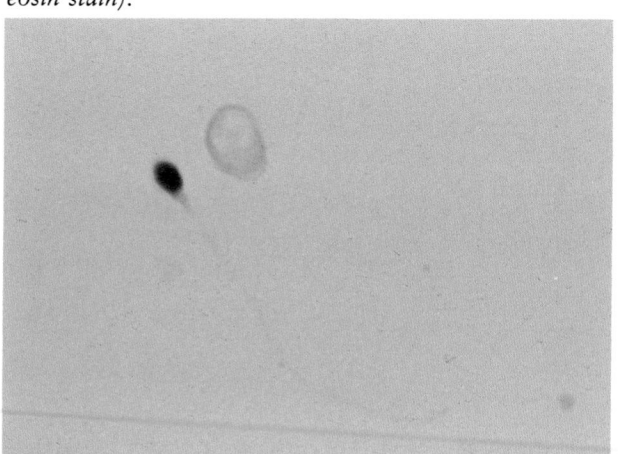

FIGURE 128. *Spermatozoon with tapered or elongated head (hematoxylin-eosin stain).*

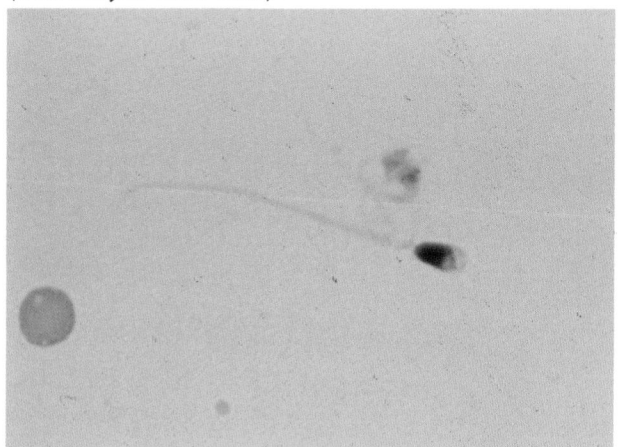

FIGURE 129. *Immature spermatozoon with tail coiled around its head (hematoxylin-eosin stain).*

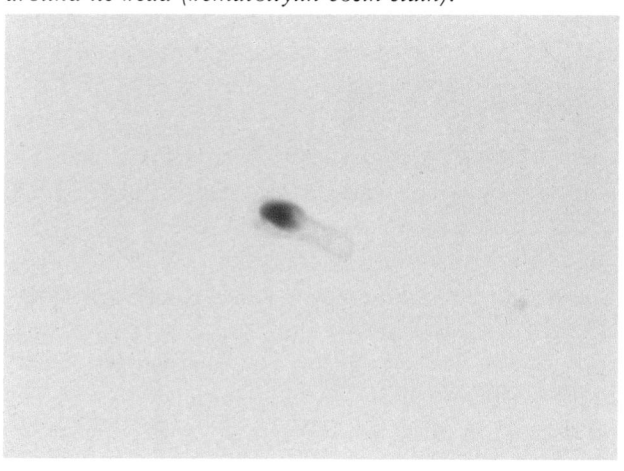

FIGURE 130. *Immature spermatozoon with a coiled tail (hematoxylin-eosin stain).*

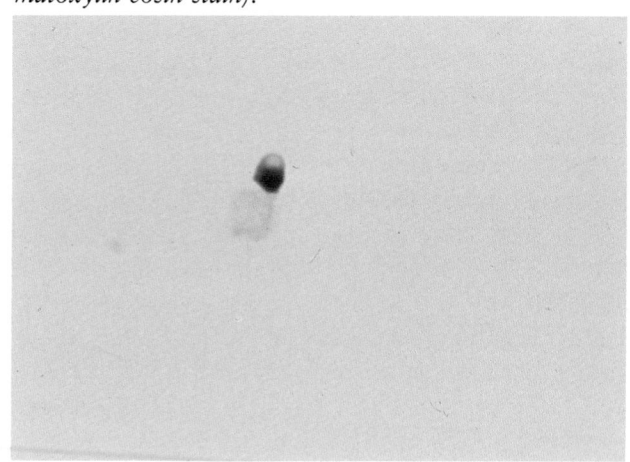

FIGURE 131. *Spermatozoon with duplicate heads (hematoxylin-eosin stain).*

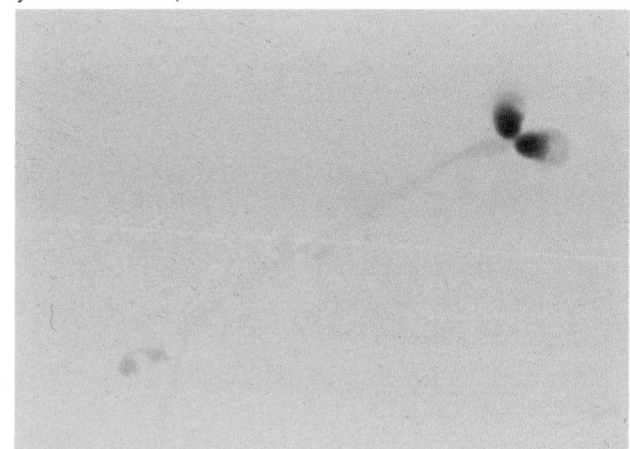

evaluation since it seems to be a good method of determining the ability of spermatozoa to fertilize an ovum.

Seminal Infection

In addition to morphologic characteristics of the sperm, the presence of RBCs, leukocytes, or bacteria in the semen should be noted. The observer should be careful not to mistake debris in the sperm sample for bacteria. Cultures for a variety of organisms should be obtained but will not usually be positive.[22,23] *Mycoplasma* cultures and routine treatment of infertile men with antibiotics effective against mycoplasma (such as tetracycline) have not been shown to be effective in significantly improving pregnancy rates in couples with infertility. Donor samples should be cultured for *Neisseria gonorrhoeae*, and all samples should be observed for *Trichomonas* organisms.

Sperm Count

The sperm count, once thought to be the most critical part of the analysis, is probably not as important as previously thought. Spermatozoa can be counted in a hemacytometer chamber following initial dilution with a WBC or RBC pipette (Appendix B).[11] If the semen sample is markedly viscous, an accurate count may be difficult to obtain and it may be necessary to add α-amylase to make the semen less viscous and the sperm count more precise.[24] Technical errors in sperm counts vary by as much as 10% to 25%. A normal count is approximately 10 to 20 × 10^6 spermatozoa per milliliter. A sperm count of less than 10 million per milliliter is considered abnormal, although not necessarily synonymous with infertility. Sperm counts increase with abstinence for up to a ten-day period[15] and do not change appreciably with the age of the individual. Fructose should be measured in all samples that are azoospermic to verify the integrity of the vas deferens and seminal vesicles (Appendix B).

ADDITIONAL TESTS

Normal seminal *pH* ranges from 7.5 to 8.0. Low pH values may help to identify semen that is composed mainly of prostatic secretion resulting from congenital aplasia of the vasa deferentia and seminal

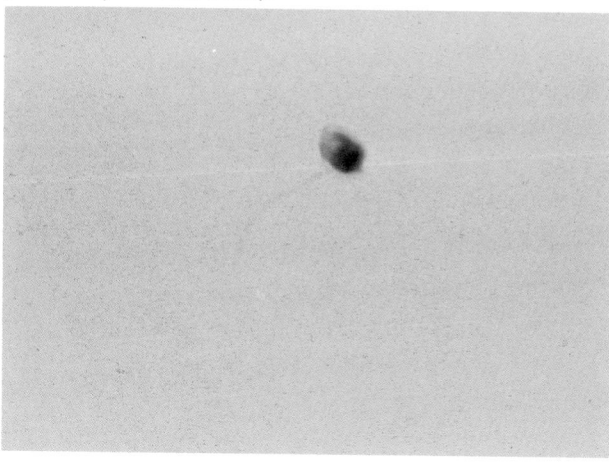

FIGURE 132. *So-called amorphous-shaped spermatozoon (hematoxylin-eosin stain).*

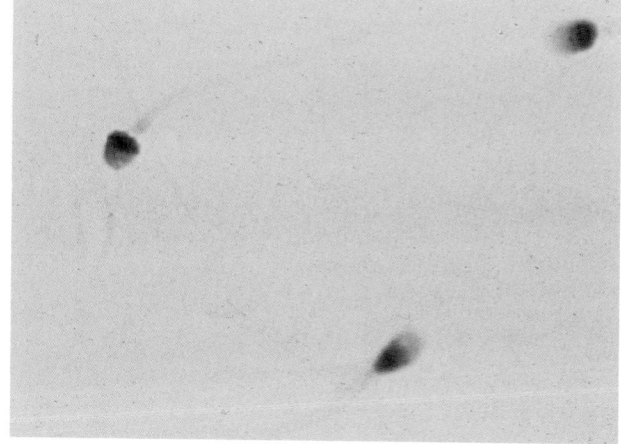

FIGURE 133. *Amorphous spermatozoa with "acorn"-shaped heads (hematoxylin-eosin stain).*

vesicles or from blockage of the ejaculatory ducts due to inflammation. Low pH may also occur with increased frequency in men with chronic prostatitis or other semen-associated infections. In general, however, determination of semen pH is rarely useful in evaluating semen for its fertility potential.

A carefully conducted semen analysis should give information about the ability of sperm to get from the site of deposition in the vagina to the site where fertilization takes place. In addition to the studies described previously, *cervical mucus-sperm compatibility tests* may be useful. There are several ways to evaluate mucus-sperm compatibility. One method is to aspirate cervical mucus at a given period (usually two to four hours) after intercourse and study the mucus under the microscope. Normally, five to eight motile spermatozoa should be seen per high-power field. Another useful way to test mucus-sperm compatibility is to aspirate cervical mucus near ovulation and study it under the microscope, together with semen from a donor and the husband. A drop of the donor's semen is placed on one side of the mucus-covered slide, and a drop of the husband's semen is put on the other side. The slide is then coverslipped, and the penetration of the spermatozoa from the two different sperm samples into the cervical mucus is observed at 20- to 30-minute intervals for 90 to 120 minutes. The type of motility of the spermatozoa that penetrate into the mucus is compared with the motility of the spermatozoa remaining outside the mucus.

While the ability of spermatozoa to get to the ovum can be estimated by semen analyses and cervical mucus-spermatozoa interaction tests, the ability of the spermatozoa to penetrate the ovum can best be determined by the *zona-free hamster ovum–human spermatozoa penetration assay*. This assay uses hamster ova obtained through supraovulation of sexually mature female hamsters, induction of ovulation, recovery of the ova, and dispersion of the ova by hyaluronidase.[25] The zona pellucida is then dissolved by trypsin, and the zona-free ova are added to preincubated human spermatozoa for four to six hours. At the end of the incubation period, the ova are examined to determine the percentage that has been penetrated by spermatozoa. At least one ovum should be penetrated.

CLINICAL CORRELATIONS

The correlation of semen analysis results with fertility is variable. The best correlation with fertility may be the hamster egg penetration assay just described. In our studies, favorable results from sperm morphologic analysis and the hamster-ova penetration assay correlate best with the ability of human ova to be fertilized in vitro or with the ability of fertilized ova to divide into embryos.

EXAMINATION FOR MEDICOLEGAL PURPOSES

In cases of alleged rape or suspected sexual assault in association with homicide, the clinical pathology laboratory may be requested to examine material from the victim's vagina and stains on clothes, skin, or hair for the presence of semen. When handling such specimens, it is essential to identify them properly (with the patient's name and type of specimen, the physician's initials, and the date and time the specimen is collected) and to maintain security of all specimens. Careful receipts should be kept to establish a chain of evidence.

Specimen Collection

It is recommended that evidence to be collected from rape victims during the physical examination include clothing (depending on the circumstances of the case); foreign material such as soil, plant material, extravaginal blood and semen stains, and saliva traces; pubic hair combings; specimens for motile sperm; vaginal swabs and smears; and swabs and smears from other areas, such as the rectum and mouth, if indicated.[26] Samples of unaffected pubic hair, head hair, blood, and saliva are taken for reference standards. It may be more useful to examine clothing and bedding for semen, saliva, and feces or blood stains than biologic specimens taken during the physical examination. A specimen from the vagina is obtained by aspiration of secretions and/or by saline lavage performed by a physician; this specimen must be examined immediately for sperm motility. Prior to this, however, direct smears from the vagina should be made for Papanicolaou staining.

The direct smears and the dried smear from the

aspiration specimen should also be stained with nuclear-fast red-picroindigocarmine.[26] It has been recommended that the swabs be dried and/or frozen for best preservation of the material.[26] The swabs may be placed upright on a stand in front of a small fan to dry.[26]

As seminal fluid exhibits a green-white fluorescence under ultraviolet light, a scan of the clothing, skin, and hair may be helpful in detecting specific sites requiring further studies. A 1-sq-cm piece of stained fabric should be cut out and soaked in 1 to 2 mL of physiologic saline for approximately one hour. This fluid is then further tested for semen. As a control, a similar piece of material, cut from a site remote to the stained area, is studied in the same manner. Similarly, stains on skin or hair can be removed with a small piece of gauze moistened in saline.

Smears for microscopic examination are prepared from the aspirate lavage or from washings of fabric, skin, or hair stains. The lavage and washings are concentrated by centrifugation and a smear is prepared from either this sediment or from that obtained by cytocentrifugation. Spermatozoa can be identified in the vagina for 24 to 72 hours after intercourse and have been recognized in exhumed bodies if they have been properly embalmed.[27] However, it should be pointed out that the sperm-detection method for determining the time lapsed between intercourse and examination is subject to considerable disagreement.[27] The presence of motile spermatozoa may suggest recent intercouse, but its absence does not mean that intercourse has not taken place. In addition, spermatozoa can survive in the vagina for two to three days; it is therefore essential to inquire about consensual intercourse that may have occurred up to 72 hours before the assault.

Acid Phosphatase Test

Seminal fluid contains about 2,500 King-Armstrong units/mL of acid phosphatase, while the concentration in other fluids is less than 5 units/mL. Acid phosphatase should be measured in the vaginal aspirate or in any wash fluid from stains. The measurement of acid phosphatase is a highly sensitive method for identification of semen.[27] Acid phosphatase disappears from vaginally deposited semen with-

in 24 to 48 hours, although it can be determined in the wash fluid from stains that are several weeks old.[28,29] Levels above 300 IU/L are considered positive for detection of semen or recent coitus.[28]

The method used for determining acid phosphatase levels should have a high specificity for prostatic acid phosphatase. When *p*-nitrophenylphosphate substrate (pH 5.5 at 25 °C) is used, the mean level of activity in semen-free vaginal swabs is approximately 0.025 units per swab,[26] and statistical studies of vaginal swab acid phosphatase indicate a 99.9% threshold value of about 0.355 units per swab.[26] Hence specimens from rape victims that show a greater enzyme activity are considered semen-positive.[26] By 12 hours, however, 50% of the acid phosphatase swab values may be below the threshold value, rendering the test invalid at that point.

Test for Male-Specific Semen Protein

The usefulness of the acid phosphatase test is limited in some cases where the vaginal fluid and female urine contain higher-than-usual levels of acid phosphatase. Although this acid phosphatase is biochemically and immunologically indistinguishable from prostatic acid phosphatase, the presence of an apparently male-specific semen glycoprotein of prostatic origin, designated "p30," can be used to establish that semen is present in the vaginal fluid.[30] The p30 antigen is found in seminal fluid from both normal and vasectomized men and is also a marker for male urine.[30] There is a linear decline on a log scale for the presence of this antigen that becomes undetectable within 48 hours after intercourse.[30]

The p30 antigen can be measured with an enzyme-linked immunosorbent assay (ELISA). The specimen may be obtained on swabs and, once dried, can be stored in a freezer or transported at ambient temperature.[30]

Genetic Typing

A, B, or H blood group substances can be found in the semen of 80% of males who are secretors. Detection of blood group substances can be made in semen specimens from the vagina or wash fluid. The method is based on the ability of semen to neutralize the agglutinating activity of a specific antiserum sample partially or completely. On occasion, it may be possible by this method to show that the seminal fluid of a suspect differs from that recovered from the victim.

The enzyme markers peptidase A (Pep A) and phosphoglucomutase (PGM), present in vaginal fluid and semen, have been shown by conventional electrophoresis to consist of three phenotypes. With more sophisticated electrophoretic analysis, however, PGM can be divided into ten phenotypes[26]; Pep A variants have been detected electrophoretically only in blacks. Combined ABO typing and PGM subtyping permit a random pair of individuals to be differentiated genetically about 90% of the time.[26]

Unfortunately, the PGM enzyme marker is quite labile and usually disappears six hours after intercourse; Pep A disappears within three hours.[26] The most useful evidence for genetic markers may be stained material from clothing or bedding. The markers are stable when dried, and activity may be retained for months in frozen dried swabs.[26]

Immunologic Test

A precipitin test may be used to identify semen of human origin and may permit positive identification of semen stains on clothing. Specific antiserum is obtained by immunizing suitable animals with human semen. The test is performed as a capillary tube precipitin reaction by overlaying the antiserum sample with wash fluid from the stain.

Absence of Semen

The absence of detectable semen, however, should not be interpreted as evidence that rape has not occurred. Semen may not be detectable if more than 24 hours have passed since the assault.[26] Moreover, the absence of ejaculation is quite common among sex offenders.[31]

References

1. Plymate SE, Fariss BL, Smith ML, et al: Seminal fluid androgen binding protein. *Andrologia* 13:308–313, 1981

2. Turner TT, Howards SS: Sperm maturation, transport and capacitation, in Cockett ATK, Urry RL (eds): *Male Fertility*. New York, Grune & Stratton Inc, 1977, pp 29–51.

3. Golan R, Setchell BP, Burrow PV, et al: A comparative study of carnitine and acetylcarnitine concentration in semen and male reproductive tract fluids. *Comp Biochem Physiol* 72:457–460, 1982

4. Kohengkul S, Tanphaichitr B, Muangman N, et al: Levels of L-carnitine and L-O-acetylcarnitine in normal and infertile human semen: A lower level of L-O-acetylcarnitine in infertile semen. *Fertil Steril* 28:1333–1338, 1977

5. Sane SP, Patel KL, Pillai KBO, et al: Evaluation of glycerylphosphocholine in semen of normal and infertile men. *J Reprod Fertil* 66:525–527, 1982

6. Crabo BG, Hunter AG: Sperm maturation and epididymal function, in Sciarra JJ, Markland C, Speidel JJ (eds): *Control of Male Fertility*. New York, Harper & Row Publishers Inc, 1975, pp 2-25.

7. Gerozissis KP, Jouannet P, Soufir JC, et al: Origin of prostaglandins in human semen. *J Reprod Fertil* 65:401–404, 1982

8. Schlegel W, Rotermund S, Farber G, et al: The influence of prostaglandins on sperm motility. *Prostaglandins* 21:87–99, 1981

9. Montagron D, Clavert A, Cranz C: Fructose, proteins and coagulation in human seminal plasma. *Andrologia* 14:434–439, 1982

10. Wood BJ, Lawrence DM, McGarrigle HHG: Similar zinc levels in seminal fluid from normospermic, oligospermic and azoospermic men. *Clin Chim Acta* 123:329–332, 1982

11. Eliasson R: Seminal plasma, accessory genital glands and infertility, in Cockett ATK, Urry RL (eds): *Male Fertility*. Grune & Stratton, 1977, pp 189–204.

12. Amelar R, Dubin L: Semen analysis, in Amelar R, Dubin L, Walsh P (eds): *Male Fertility*. Philadelphia, WB Saunders Co, 1977, pp 105–140.

13. Van Zyl JA: The infertile couple: II. Examination and evaluation of semen. *S Afr Med J* 57:485–491, 1980

14. Schwartz D, Lapslanche A, Jouannet P, et al: Within subject variability of human semen in regard to sperm count, volume, total number of spermatozoa and length of abstinence. *J Reprod Fertil* 57:391–395, 1979

15. MacLeod J, Gold R: The male factor: Fertility and infertility: Vl. Semen quality and certain other factors in relation to ease of conception. *Fertil Steril* 5:217–223, 1954

16. Kibrick S, Belding DL, Merrill B: Methods for the detection of antibodies against mammalian spermatozoa: I. A modified macroscopic agglutination test. *Fertil Steril* 3:419–426, 1952

17. Cockett ATK, Netto ICV, Dougherty KA, et al:

Semen analysis: A review of samples from 225 men seen in an infertility clinic. *J Urol* 114:560–563, 1975

18. Isojima S, Li TS, Ashitaka Y: Immunologic analysis of sperm-immobilizing factor found in sera of women with unexplained sterility. *Am J Obstet Gynecol* 101:677–679, 1968

19. Williams WW, Pollak OJ: Study of sperm vitality with the aid of eosin-nigrosin stain. *Fertil Steril* 1:178–181, 1950

20. Freund M: Standards for the rating of human sperm morphology: A cooperative study. *Int J Fertil* 11(suppl):1–9, 1966

21. Cockett ATK, Urry RL, Dougherty KA: The varicocele and semen characteristics. *J Urol* 121:435–436, 1979

22. McGowan MP, Burger HG, Baker HWG et al: The incidence of non-specific infection in the semen in fertile and sub-fertile males. *Int J Androl* 4:657–662, 1981

23. Lewis RW, Harrison RM, Domingue GJ: Culture of seminal fluid in a fertility clinic. *Fertil Steril* 35:194–198, 1981

24. Dougherty KA, Cockett ATK, Urry RL: Effect of amylase on sperm motility and viability. *J Urol* 120:425–426, 1978

25. Urry RL, Carrell DT, Hull DB, et al: Penetration of zona-free hamster ova to bovine cervical mucus by fresh and frozen human spermatozoa. *Fertil Steril* 39:690–694, 1983

26. Sensabaugh GF, Bashinsky J, Blake ET: The laboratory's role in investigating rape. *Diagnostic Med* 8:46–53, 1985

27. Soules M, Pollard A, Brown K, et al: The forensic laboratory evaluation of evidence in alleged rape. *Am J Obstet Gynecol* 130:142, 1978

28. Schuman GB, Badawy S, Peglow A, et al: Prostatic acid phosphatase: Current assessment in vaginal fluid of alleged rape victims. *Am J Clin Pathol* 66:944, 1976

29. Dahlke MB, Cooke C, Cunnane M, et al: Identification of semen in 500 patients seen because of rape. *Am J Clin Pathol* 68:740, 1977

30. Graves HCB, Sensebaugh GF, Blake ET: Postcoital detection of a male-specific semen protein. *New Engl J Med* 312:338–343, 1985

31. Groth AW, Burgess AW: Sexual dysfunction during rape. *N Engl J Med* 297:764–766, 1977

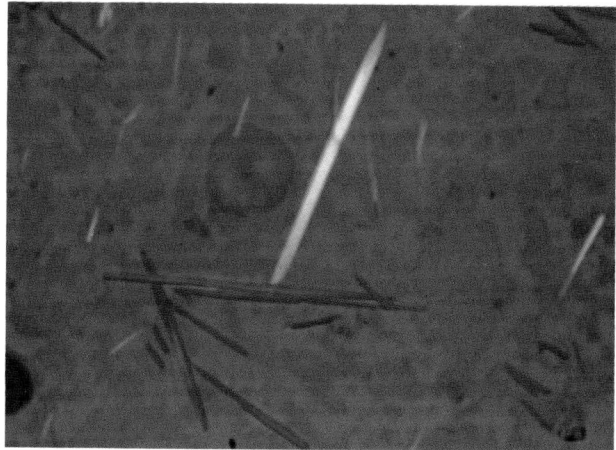

CHAPTER 6

Synovial Fluid

ANATOMY AND PATHOPHYSIOLOGY

Diarthrodial joints are lined at their margins by a synovial membrane (synovium), with synovial cells lining the joint space (Figures 134 and 135). These cells have the capacity for protein synthesis and phagocytosis. The underlying connective and adipose tissues are supplied by a rich vascular network.

Synovial fluid is basically an ultrafiltrate of the plasma combined with a mucopolysaccharide (hyaluronate) that is synthesized by the cells of the synovial membrane.[1] The functions of the synovial fluid are to lubricate the joint space and transport nutrients to the articular cartilage. The protein and immunoglobulin levels of the synovial fluid are approximately one fourth those of plasma, while the glucose and uric acid concentrations are the same as those of the blood.

Immunologic, mechanical, chemical, or bacteriologic damage may alter the permeability of the membranes and capillaries to produce varying degrees of inflammatory response (Figure 136). Various disorders produce changes in the chemical constituents of the joint fluid and in the type of cell population present.

Analysis of synovial fluid plays a major role in the diagnosis of joint disease. When infective arthritis and crystal-induced synovitis are suspected, examination of the synovial fluid may produce a definitive diagnosis. These two conditions, therefore, are the most compelling indications for arthrocentesis and synovial fluid analysis. With other diseases, a diagnosis may not be possible from synovial fluid examination alone. However, the common joint diseases can usually be categorized on the basis of synovial fluid analysis. Thus the results may indicate whether an effusion is inflammatory or noninflammatory and whether hemarthrosis is present. Normal adult reference values for the components of synovial fluid are presented in Table 6–1.[2]

Through clinical and laboratory examination of the

FIGURE 134. *Schematic drawing showing anatomic relationship of parts in a diarthrodial joint. Cutaway view.*

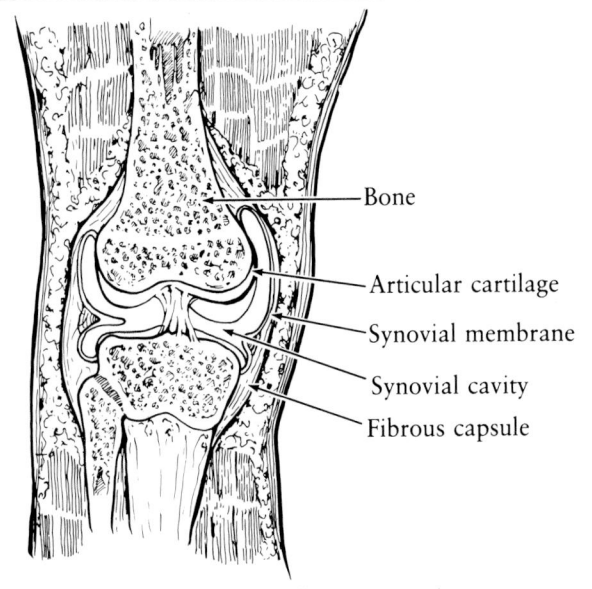

- Bone
- Articular cartilage
- Synovial membrane
- Synovial cavity
- Fibrous capsule

FIGURE 135. *Histologic section showing synovial membrane with layer of synovial cells that resemble mesothelial cells (hematoxylin-eosin stain).*

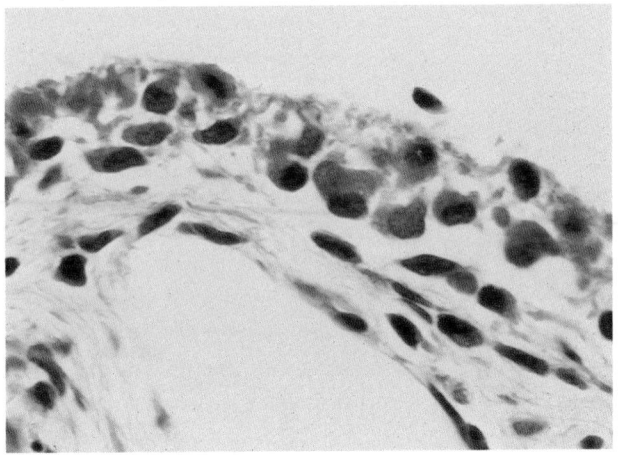

synovial fluid, joint disorders can be divided into five categories (Table 6–2). This classification is useful as long as one realizes that there may be considerable overlap in synovial fluid findings among the different groups. In addition, there may on occasion be more than one diagnosis possible. It is important, therefore, that the laboratory results be carefully correlated with the clinical history, physical examination findings, and roentgenograms. The five major disease categories are as follows: group I, noninflammatory; group II, inflammatory; group III, infectious; group IV, crystal-induced; and group V, hemorrhagic.[3]

Impaired function of the synovial fluid with age or disease may play a role in the development of degenerative joint disease (osteoarthritis). Inflammatory joint fluids contain lytic enzymes that produce depolymerization of hyaluronic acid, which greatly impairs the lubricating ability of the fluid.

SPECIMEN COLLECTION

There are no absolute contraindications to joint aspiration. The incidence of septic complications is exceedingly low when the procedure is performed by an experienced practitioner using aseptic precautions. Relative contraindications are the presence of local sepsis, such as cellulitis, bacteremia, and a congenital or acquired bleeding tendency. The technique of aspiration has been well described in recent reports.[1,4]

For routine examination, the syringe used for removing the fluid should be moistened with an anticoagulant (approximately 25 units of sodium heparin per milliliter of synovial fluid).[5] Oxalate, powdered ethylenediaminetetraacetic acid (EDTA), and lithium heparin should not be used because they can produce artifacts in the microscopic examination for crystals. Ideally, when adequate fluid is available, it should be divided into three samples. Five to 10 mL is collected in a sterile tube for microbiologic examination; 5 mL is collected in an anticoagulated tube (heparin or liquid EDTA) for microscopic examination; and the remainder is placed in a plain (no anticoagulant) tube and allowed to clot (normal fluid does not clot.) The specimen is then centrifuged to remove all cells. Cells in the synovial fluid may alter the chemical composition of the fluid; therefore, centrifugation should not be delayed. This is particularly important when complement levels are to be determined. The supernatant can be used for assays of rheumatoid factor, antinuclear antibody, and complement levels and for various biochemical procedures. It is important that, for complement determinations, the test be performed within two to three hours after collection of the specimen since complement is heat-labile. If the specimen cannot be examined immediately, the fluid should be frozen and stored at −70 °C until examined.

When the synovial fluid is unusually viscid, it may be difficult to perform several tests. As a remedy, the fluid may be digested with hyaluronidase for several hours prior to the analysis (Appendix A).[6]

If arthrocentesis results in a dry tap, there may still be a few drops of fluid in the needle that can be used for a culture or microscopic examination. One should not, therefore, discard the needle but leave it on the syringe and transport it to the laboratory inserted into a sterile cork.

Routine examination of synovial fluid should include (1) a description of color and clarity, (2) microbiologic studies, (3) WBC and differential cell counts, and (4) polarizing light microscopy for crystals. In addition, other procedures (to be described) may under certain circumstances help in the diagnosis.

When only a small amount of fluid is obtained during arthrocentesis, it may be difficult to decide whether it represents synovial fluid, fluid from subcutaneous tissue, or the local anesthetic. Testing for mucin formation and metachromatic staining are two methods used for detecting as little as 0.5 mL of synovial fluid.[7] The mucin clot test consists of precipitating any mucin present with a 2% acetic acid solution, followed by an examination for the presence of turbidity or a mucin clot.

The metachromatic staining procedure consists of spotting filter paper with synovial fluid and then staining with a few drops of a 0.2% aqueous toluidine blue solution. Metachromasia of the synovial fluid spots is seen after a few seconds. The metachromatic staining procedure is probably the most sensitive method but is not suitable for analysis of fluid that has been in contact with heparin, as heparin staining is strongly metachromatic with toluidine blue.

GROSS EXAMINATION

The analysis of synovial fluid starts with the recording of the volume and the gross appearance of

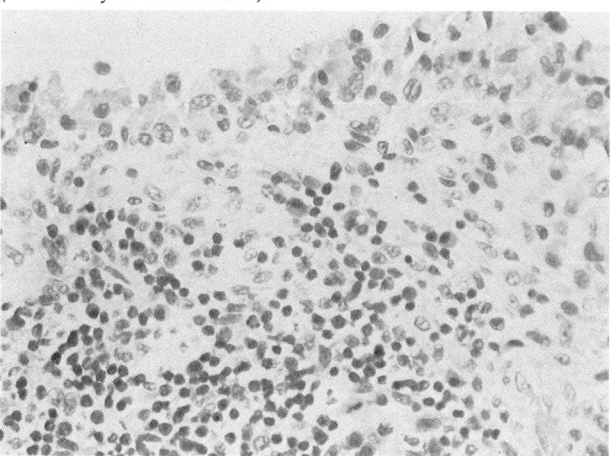

FIGURE 136. *Histologic section of synovial membrane in a patient with rheumatoid arthritis. There is hyperplasia of the synovial lining cells and a dense lymphocytic infiltrate (hematoxylin-eosin stain).*

TABLE 6–1. Normal Adult Reference Values for Synovial Fluid

COMPONENT	CONVENTIONAL UNITS	SI UNITS
Glucose level (blood–synovial fluid difference)	0–10 mg/dL	<0.55 mmole/L
Leukocyte count	0–200/μL	0–0.20 × 10⁹/L
Neutrophils	<25%	<0.25
Protein level	1–3 g/dL	10–30 g/L

Note: Adapted from Krieg.[2] Used by permission.

the removed fluid. Effusions of all arthritides produce variable volumes of synovial fluid. An aspirated volume of more than 3.5 mL from the knee is considered abnormal. There is, however, little correlation between the volume and the origin or severity of the joint disease.

Normal fluid is light yellow and clear and does not clot. Hemorrhagic fluid is homogeneously bloody. Streaks of blood are seen in a traumatic aspirate. Centrifugation of the fluid may be necessary to differentiate between a traumatic tap and hemarthrosis. Xanthochromia of the supernatant usually indicates that blood has been present in the synovial fluid for some time. Xanthochromia may, however, be difficult to interpret because of the normally light yellow appearance of synovial fluid. A dark red or brown supernatant in the presence of grossly observed blood suggests hemarthrosis rather than a traumatic tap. Turbidity usually indicates leukocytosis and increases with the degree of inflammation. Other factors that may produce a turbid fluid include cartilage debris and the presence of crystals. Fluid from a joint with crystal-induced synovitis (gout and pseudogout) may be purulent and milky and occasionally greenish. The presence of many so-called rice bodies, products of degenerating proliferative synovial lining cells or of microinfarction of the synovium, may cause the fluid to resemble pus on gross examination.[8] Cloudy, fatty fluid usually indicates the presence of cholesterol crystals, often seen in chronic arthritides. Droplets of free-floating fat, on the other hand, frequently occur in trauma with or without fracture. The presence of clear, pale-yellow, viscous fluid usually indicates a noninflammatory disease from group I. Fluid from group II patients (those with inflammatory diseases) is frequently turbid and yellow and clots while stand-

ing. Fluid from a patient with group III (infectious) disease will be grossly purulent.

As previously noted, normal synovial fluid does not clot. However, with inflammatory conditions, fibrinogen and other coagulation factors are present and clot formation does occur.

CELL COUNTS

The reported upper limit of normal for the leukocyte count in synovial fluid varies from less than 200/μL to less than 750/μL.[2] However, most authors consider 200/μL to be the upper limit of normal. The leukocyte count may be performed in a standard hemacytometer or in a Fuchs-Rosenthal chamber. Electronic counting equipment may also be used. It should be noted, however, that automated counters may give spuriously high cell counts by also counting extracellular material (eg, crystals and fat globules).

Unless the leukocyte count is very high (more than 50,000/μL), the total count can be performed with undiluted fluid.[2] Physiologic saline should be used as a diluent instead of one containing acetic acid, as the latter will precipitate hyaluronic acid and produce cell clumping. It is important that the fluid be properly agitated before being added to the counting chamber. This can be done with a bench vibratory mixer.[2] When the fluid is highly viscous, it may need to stand in the hemacytometer for more than 30 minutes before the cells settle and can be counted.[2] The addition of a solution of 0.05% hyaluronidase in phosphate buffer reduces the viscosity of the synovial fluid, making it easier to pipette and allowing a more even cell distribution in the counting chamber.

The total leukocyte count can be performed using either a phase-contrast microscope or a standard light

TABLE 6-2. Classification of Arthritides

GROUP I (NONINFLAMMATORY)	GROUP II (INFLAMMATORY)	GROUP III (INFECTIOUS)	GROUP IV (CRYSTAL-INDUCED)	GROUP V (HEMORRHAGIC)
Osteoarthrosis	Rheumatoid arthritis	Bacterial	Gout	Traumatic arthritis
Traumatic arthritis	Lupus erythematosus	Mycobacterial	CPPD* crystal deposition disease	Hemophilic arthropathy
Osteochondritis dissecans	Reiter's syndrome	Fungal		Anticoagulation
Osteochondromatosis	Rheumatic fever		Apatite-associated arthropathy	Pigmented villonodular synovitis
Neuropathic osteoarthropathy	Ankylosing spondylitis			Neuropathic osteoarthropathy
Pigmented villonodular synovitis	Regional enteritis			Synovial hemangioma
	Ulcerative colitis, psoriasis			

Note: Adapted from Rippey.[3] Used by permission.
*CPPD = calcium pyrophosphate dihydrate.

microscope. When the latter is used, a 0.1% methylene blue dye is helpful in identifying the leukocytes.[1,2] When the fluid is heavily contaminated with blood, the RBCs should be lysed using a diluent such as the absolute basophil diluent or hypotonic saline (Appendix A). The RBCs should also be counted, however, unless it is clear that they originate from a traumatic tap.

The total leukocyte count is of some use in categorizing the fluid into one of the five disease groups described previously (Table 6–3). For example, in septic arthritis, the leukocyte count is almost always greater than 50,000/μL. It should be noted, however, that there may be considerable overlap in all ranges and that a high leukocyte count in synovial fluid is not diagnostic by itself.[9] For example, in the early phase of bacterial infection the leukocyte count may be normal. In addition, fluid samples from occasional cases of gout or rheumatoid arthritis (RA) may demonstrate leukocyte counts in the range usually associated with septic arthritis.[9] There have also been occasional reports of acute gout and acute pseudogout without synovial fluid leukocytosis, which suggests an alternative inflammatory mechanism.[10]

MICROSCOPIC EXAMINATION

Differential Cell Count

The differential cell count can be made by phase-contrast microscopy at the time of the leukocyte count, although a more accurate one is obtained by using a Wright's stained smear of concentrated (centrifuged) synovial fluid. It is important that the smears be made as soon as possible after receiving the specimen. Also, the smears should be as thin as possible, since staining of the mucopolysaccharide and mucoproteins in the synovial fluid may obscure the cell structure.[1]

Normal synovial fluid contains approximately 65% mononuclear phagocytes (monocytes and histiocytes), a variable number of lymphocytes, and less than 25% neutrophils.[5] No cartilaginous or inclusion-bearing cells are normally seen, and polarized light microscopic examination usually reveals no crystals. The number of RBCs varies; increases may result from a traumatic tap.

A high percentage of neutrophils (more than 80%) is highly suggestive of septic arthritis, regardless of the magnitude of the total leukocyte count. When the percentage of neutrophils is markedly elevated, a Gram stain and a search for intracellular bacteria are essential.

In one study, 70% of patients with culture-proven infectious arthritis had synovial fluid leukocyte counts higher than 50,000/μL, while 12.5% of patients with gout, 10% of those with pseudogout, and 4% of those with RA also had leukocyte counts in this range.[9] In one fourth of the fluid specimens containing monosodium urate crystals and one third of those with calcium pyrophosphate crystals, the leukocyte counts

TABLE 6–3. Synovial Fluid Findings by Disease Category

FINDING	NORMAL	CATEGORY				
		GROUP I (NONINFLAMMATORY)	GROUP II (INFLAMMATORY)	GROUP III (INFECTIOUS)	GROUP IV (CRYSTAL-INDUCED)	GROUP V (HEMORRHAGIC)
Appearance	Yellow, clear, or slightly cloudy	Yellow or clear	Yellow, cloudy, turbid, or bloody	Yellow, green, or milky	Yellow or turbid	Red-brown or xanthochromic
WBCs/μL	0–200 (0–0.2 × 10^9/L)	0–5,000 (0–5 × 10^9/L)	2,000–200,000 (2–200 10^9/L)	50,000–200,000 (50–200 × 10^9/L)	500–200,000 (0.5–200 × 10^9/L)	50–10,000 (0.05–10 × 10^9/L)
Polymorphonuclear leuko-cytes (%)	<25	<30	>50	>90	<90	<50
Crystals present	No	No	No	No	Yes	No
RBCs present	No	No	No	Yes	No	Yes
Blood glucose to synovial fluid glucose ratio (mg/dL)	0–10 (0–0.56 mmole/L)	0–10 (0–0.56 mmole/L)	0–40 (0–2.22 mmole/L)	20–100 (1.11–5.55 mmole/L)	0–80 (0–4.44 mmole/L)	0–20 (0–1.11 mmole/L)
Culture	Negative	Negative	Negative	Often positive	Negative	Negative

Note: Adapted from Krieg[2] and Rippey.[3] Used with permission. Values in parentheses are SI units.

were below 2,555/μL.[9] This study emphasizes the need for a careful search for crystals in fluid specimens with high as well as low leukocyte counts. It is also important to note that septic arthritis can coexist with other types of arthritis such as gout, pseudogout, systemic lupus erythematosus, and RA.[2]

Lymphocytes, including transformed lymphocytes (immunoblasts), are the predominant cell type in the early stages of RA, but later there may be a predominance of neutrophils.[9,11] A predominance of monocytes may be seen in arthritis associated with serum sickness and certain viral infections (hepatitis and rubella).[12] Synovial fluid eosinophilia has been observed in chronic urticaria and angioedema, rheumatic fever, parasitic infestation, metastatic disease, and rheumatoid arthritis and with arthrography and radiation therapy.[13,14]

Cell Morphology

The types of cells that may be seen on microscopic examination of abnormal synovial fluid include neutrophils, lymphocytes, plasma cells, monocytes, eosinophils, macrophages, synovial lining cells, and lupus erythematosus cells. Neutrophils and lymphocytes generally show a morphologic structure identical to that of the corresponding cells of the blood (Figures 137 and 138). The *neutrophils* may contain vacuoles, fat droplets, bacteria, or crystals. It is common for the nuclei to show pyknosis and karyorrhexis (Figure 138). The *mononuclear phagocytes*, which include monocytes, macrophages, and histiocytes (Figure 140), may be similar to blood monocytes but often show a variable morphologic structure and may be difficult to distinguish from the *synovial lining cells* (Figures 141 and 142). These latter cells also resemble mesothelial cells (Figure 143). The presence of synovial lining cells does not appear to have any specific diagnostic significance.[1]

So-called *Reiter's cells* are vacuolated macrophages containing either neutrophilic or basophilic globular material or both (Figure 144).[15] Such cells, however, are not specific indicators for Reiter's disease. *Ragocytes,* or *RA cells,* are neutrophils containing small, dark cytoplasmic granules that are best identified with phase-contrast microscopy.[1,4,5] Immunofluorescent techniques have shown that these granules consist of such immune complexes as IgG, IgM, complement, and rheumatoid factor. The RA cells, however,

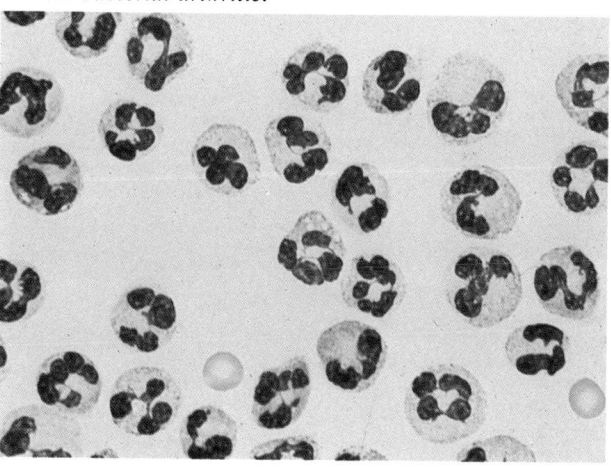

FIGURE 137. *Numerous neutrophils in synovial fluid, as seen in bacterial arthritis.*

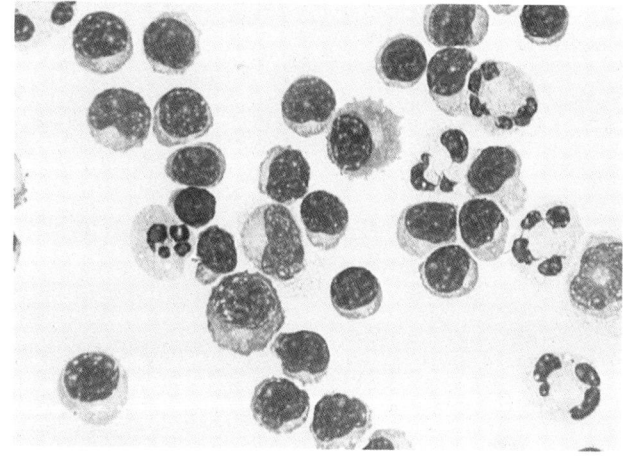

FIGURE 138. *Spectrum of small and transformed lymphocytes with occasional neutrophils in synovial fluid sample from a patient with rheumatoid arthritis.*

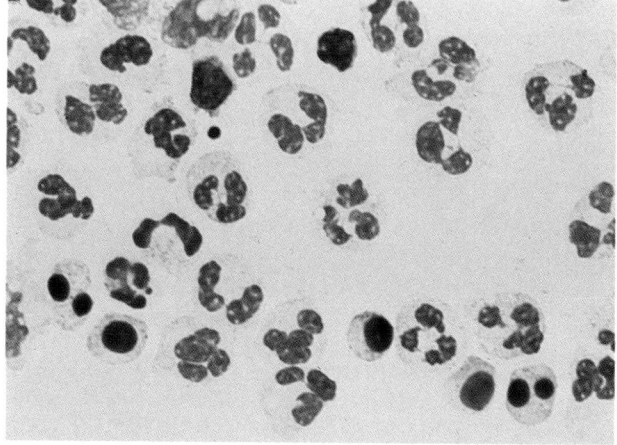

FIGURE 139. *Pyknosis and karyorrhexis of neutrophils in synovial fluid sample from a patient with gout.*

FIGURE 140. *Histiocytes, monocytes, and many neutrophils in synovial fluid sample from a patient with lupus erythematosus.*

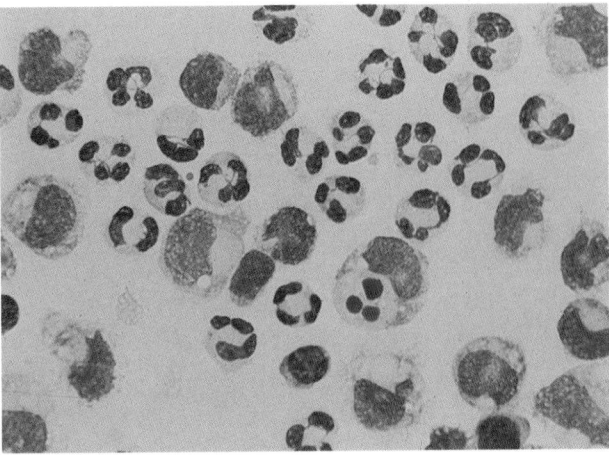

FIGURE 141. *Synovial lining cell.*

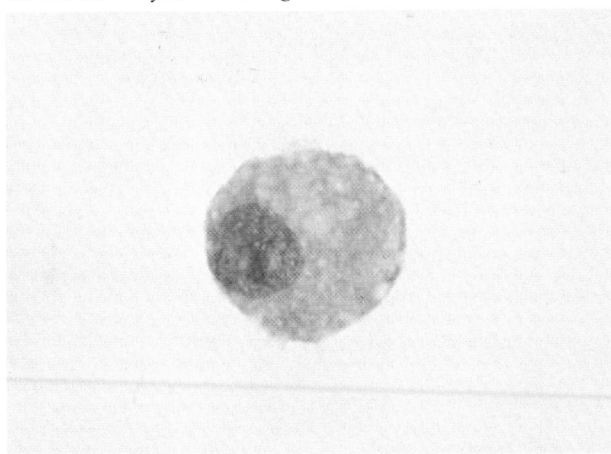

FIGURE 142. *Multinucleated synovial cell.*

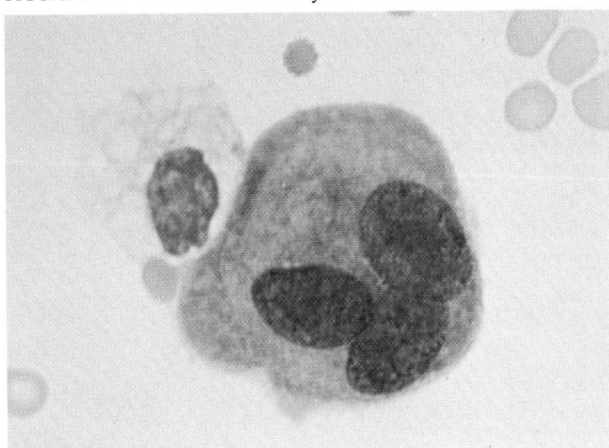

are not specific indicators for RA and may also be seen in gout and septic arthritis.[9] Occasionally, *lupus erythematosus (LE) cells* may be seen in synovial fluid samples from patients with LE, and some cases have been reported in which LE cells are initially present in the synovial fluid and not in the peripheral blood (Figure 145). Some LE cells may also be seen in synovial fluid samples from patients with RA.[2]

Giant multinucleated *cartilage cells* are typically seen in the synovial fluid of patients with osteoarthritis, but isolated cartilage cells may appear in a number of arthritides.[5,16] In pigmented villonodular synovitis, the presence of papillary aggregates of synovial cells is a characteristic finding, and hemosiderin is often found within synovial cells. Many multinucleated, foreign-bodied giant cells may also be seen.[5] In ochronosis, which refers to the accumulation of melanin-like pigment in connective tissues of persons with alkaptonuria, one may see synovial fluid speckled with dark particles resembling ground pepper. Microscopic examination of this fluid has revealed fragments of pigmented cartilage.[17]

Lipid droplets may be seen in leukocytes or lying free in the fluid and are, when present with hemorrhagic fluid, associated with trauma. The lipid droplets cause an inflammatory reaction. The presence of fat cells together with bone marrow spicules indicates that a fracture has occurred.[18]

Crystals

Examination of synovial fluid for crystals using polarized light should be done routinely. Specimens with or without anticoagulants may be used. However, as mentioned previously, powdered EDTA, oxalate, or lithium heparin should not be used as an anticoagulant, since each may be associated with crystal formation. Ideally, a wet preparation of the fluid should be examined immediately to demonstrate intracellular crystals. Birefringent crystals are also readily demonstrated in thin, dried smears when many crystals are present, as may be seen in acute gout.

The identification of crystals is one of the few pathognomonic tests in the study of arthritides. It is, therefore, important to have a polarizing microscope of good quality to examine the specimen properly. This is particularly true with calcium pyrophosphate crystals, which are weakly birefringent and may be missed unless the polarizing equipment is adequate.

Polarized light, using a polarizer and an analyzer, allows one to make a diagnosis of crystal-induced arthritis. However, the definitive identification of the type of crystal—eg, urate and/or calcium pyrophosphate dihydrate—requires the addition of a first-order red compensator (Figure 146). The red compensator is a retardation plate that alters the passage of light into slow and fast components. When inserted between the polarizer and analyzer, it retards the polarized light so that the field background becomes red instead of black[1,2,19–21] (Appendix A).

The types of crystals that may be seen in synovial fluid include monosodium urate, calcium pyrophosphate dihydrate, cholesterol, steroid, and apatite.

The presence of *monosodium urate crystals* is usually diagnostic of gout.[22] The crystals may be intracellular, extracellular, or both. They are needle-like with pointed ends and measure 1 to 30 μm in length (Figure 147). The presence of intracellular crystals should be noted in the laboratory report, since it indicates the acute stage of gout (Figure 148). Monosodium urate crystals are seen in approximately 90% of patients during acute attacks of gout. Between acute attacks, they may be seen in approximately 75% of patients.[2] In a small number of patients, even during acute attacks, monosodium urate crystals may not be found at all.[23,24] The reasons for this include aspiration from the wrong site, loculation within the joint, crystal dissolution, examiner inexperience, and insufficient search for crystals (Figure 149).[24] Therefore, repeated examinations for monosodium urate crystals may be required occasionally for a definitive diagnosis.

Under polarized light, monosodium urate crystals are strongly birefringent, that is, they appear bright against a dark, fully polarized background (Figure 150). With a red compensator, they appear yellow when their longitudinal axis is parallel to the slow component of the compensator (Figure 151). The crystals are then considered negatively birefringent.[1,2,19,20] The crystals appear blue when they are perpendicular to the axis of the compensator (see Appendix A).

Following recurrent attacks of acute gout arthritis, chalky deposits of urates known as "tophi" develop in articular and periarticular tissues (joint capsule, cartilage, and bone). The urates become surrounded by chronic inflammatory cells, foreign-body giant cells, and fibrosis (Figures 152 through 154). Destruc-

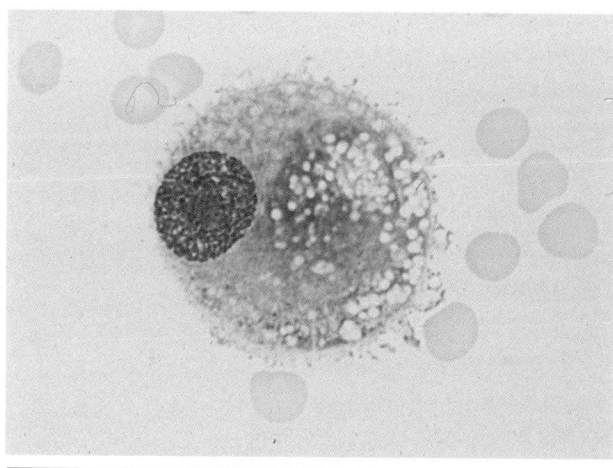

FIGURE 143. *Synovial lining cell resembling a mesothelial cell.*

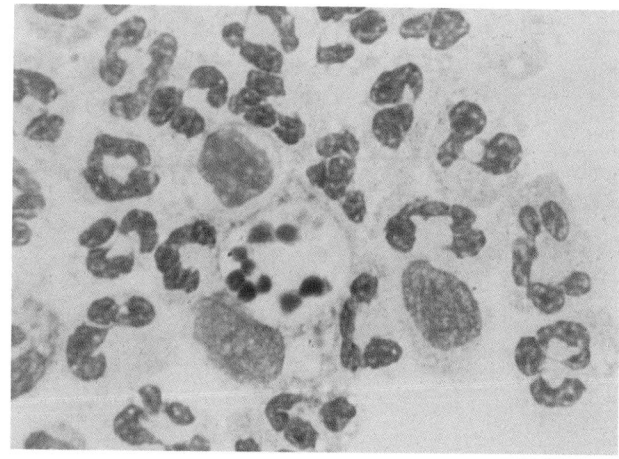

FIGURE 144. *So-called Reiter's cell in synovial fluid. Bluish intracytoplasmic inclusion in macrophage probably represents a phagocytosed neutrophil and is not a specific indicator for Reiter's disease. Traumatic arthritis.*

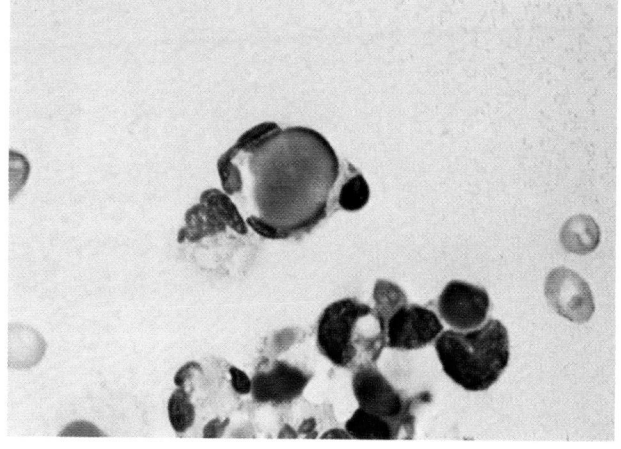

FIGURE 145. *Lupus erythematosus cell in synovial fluid sample from a patient with lupus erythematosus.*

FIGURE 146. *Schematic drawing of microscope to illustrate position of polarizer, analyzer, and compensator.*

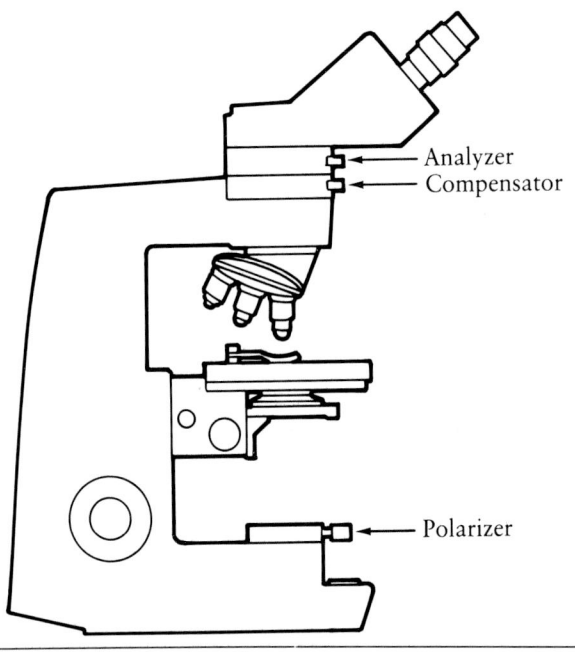

FIGURE 147. *Many typical needle-shaped monosodium urate crystals in gout seen with polarized light.*

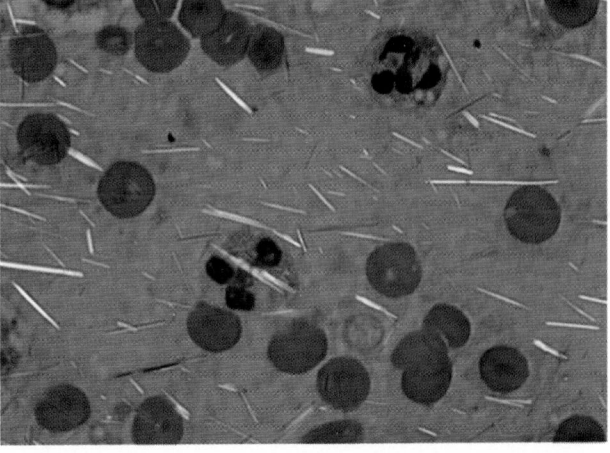

FIGURE 148. *Intracellular monosodium urate crystals seen with polarized light with red compensator.*

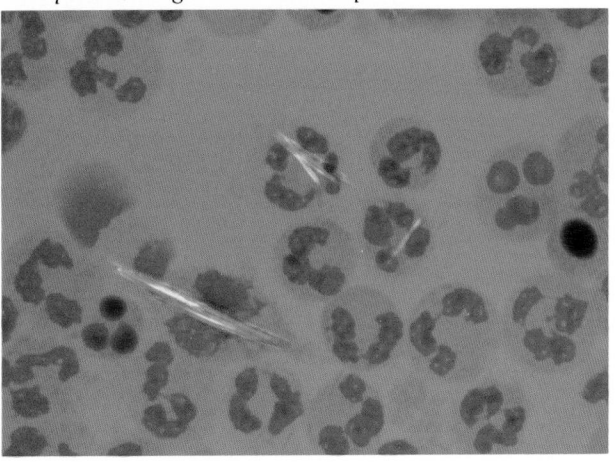

tion of the capsular tissue and bone eventually may lead to deforming chronic arthritis if the patient is not treated.

The presence of *calcium pyrophosphate dihydrate* (CPPD) *crystals* is characteristic of a group of disorders collectively called "CPPD crystal deposition disease."[25] Other terms that have been used are "pseudogout" and "chondrocalcinosis." These crystals are most commonly seen in synovial fluid samples from patients with degenerative arthritis but may also be seen in hereditary forms of pseudogout, in arthritides associated with metabolic diseases such as hyperparathyroidism, hypothyroidism, diabetes mellitus, and hemachromatosis, and occasionally together with monosodium urate crystals in gout.[25]

The clinical features of calcium pyrophosphate deposition disease are extremely variable and may mimic many different types of disorders.[26] Approximately one half of these patients have a clinical picture similar to that of osteoarthritis, with progressive degeneration of many joints, particularly the knees, wrists, metacarpal-phalangeal joints, hips, shoulders, elbows, and ankles (in order of frequency). Other patients may initially be seen with clinical features resembling gout—hence the term pseudogout. These patients experience acute or subacute attacks of arthritis, often involving one joint at a time. Septic arthritis must always be ruled out in these cases. Yet another group, comprising a small number of patients, displays clinical features resembling rheumatoid arthritis.

Calcium pyrophosphate dihydrate crystals are rodlike, plate-like, or rhomboid. The crystals appear pale against the dark background of polarized light; ie, they are weakly birefringent and may be overlooked by the inexperienced observer (Figure 155). They may also appear as needles and be mistaken for monosodium urate crystals. When a red compensator is used, calcium pyrophosphate crystals appear blue when their longitudinal axis is parallel to the slow component of the compensator. They are then considered to be positively birefringent. The crystals appear yellow when they are perpendicular to the axis of the compensator (Figure 156; see Appendix A).

The histologic changes in CPPD crystal deposition disease are similar to those seen in gout. After a time, crystalline deposits occur in articular tissue, surrounded by chronic inflammatory cells, giant cells, and fibrosis (Figures 157 and 158).

Leukocyte counts of 65,000 to 100,000/μL with more than 90% neutrophils have been found in synovial fluid samples from patients with gout and CPPD deposition disease, so that these conditions may be confused with infectious arthritis. It is, therefore, important that all synovial fluid specimens be examined for crystals.[9]

Cholesterol crystals usually have the appearance of rectangular, notched plates (Figures 159 and 160), but occasionally they may appear as long, birefringent needles or as rhomboids, resembling monosodium urate or calcium pyrophosphate crystals (Figures 161 through 164).[27,28] They are considered to be nonspecific and are sometimes seen in chronically inflamed joints—such as those associated with RA—and, occasionally, in osteoarthritis.[29]

Hydroxyapatite (HA) crystals are usually too small to be identified with the light microscope but may be seen as "shiny coins" with a phase microscope (3 to 65 μm in diameter) or as purple inclusions with Wright's stain when aggregates of crystals are present.[30–33] The crystals are nonbirefringent. Electron microscopy and electron probe analysis are required for definitive identification of HA crystals.[32] Three major syndromes have been associated with HA crystals[30,34]: In acute calcific periarthritis, in which there is periarticular inflammation and transient calcification in the vicinity of the joint, HA crystals are seen in the calcific deposits. In the second syndrome, acute (calcific) arthritis associated with calcification in and/or around the joint, HA crystals are found in synovial fluid and calcific deposits. Finally, HA crystals may be seen in synovial fluid samples from patients with subacute to chronic arthritis resembling osteoarthritis. The term "apatite-associated arthropathy" has been suggested to describe these heterogeneous disorders.[35]

A number of refractile *artifacts* may be mistaken for the crystals described previously. However, if the observer is familiar with the size, appearance, brightness, and optic signs of monosodium urate and CPPD crystals, these artifacts should not cause any difficulty in the examination. Crystals tend to have sharp, clearly defined edges and straight sides, in contrast to the indistinct forms of many artifacts. Calcium oxalate

FIGURE 149. *Monosodium urate crystals trapped in fibrin clot seen with polarized light. In this case, several preparations of same fluid revealed no crystals.*

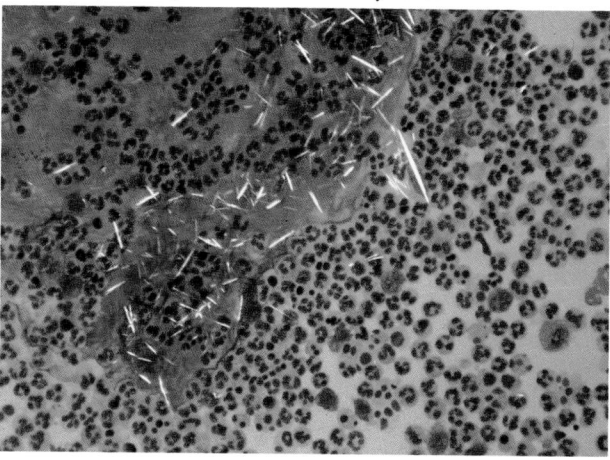

FIGURE 150. *Numerous monosodium urate crystals in synovial fluid seen with polarized light.*

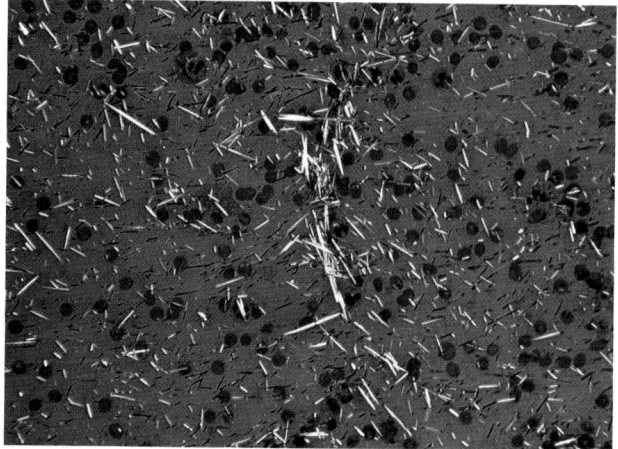

FIGURE 151. *Several monosodium urate crystals as seen with polarized light and red compensator. Color of crystals (blue or yellow) depends on orientation of crystals in relation to axis of compensator.*

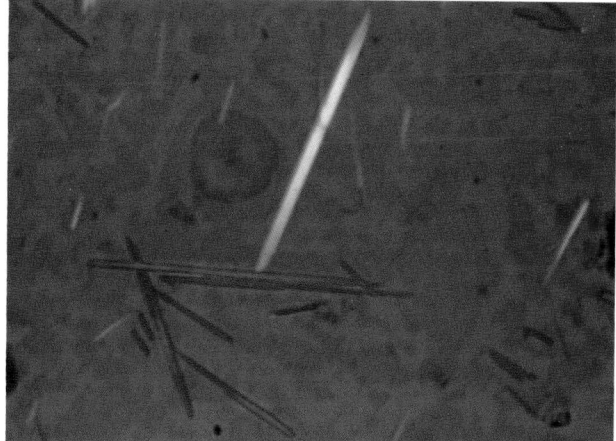

FIGURE 152. *Histologic section of synovial tissue from patient with gout showing tophus containing clusters of monosodium urate crystals and chronic inflammatory cells and giant cells (hematoxylin-eosin stain).*

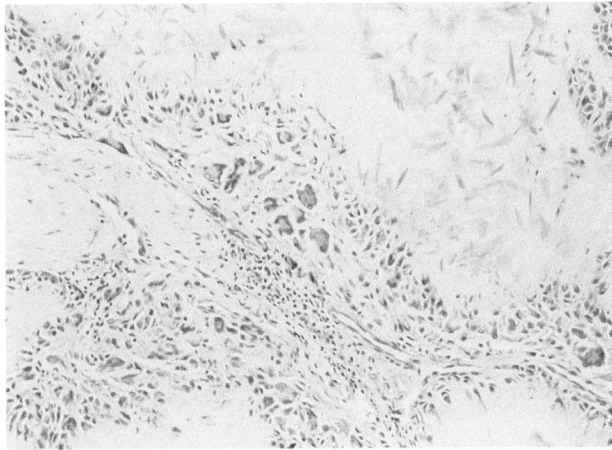

FIGURE 153. *Numerous crystals seen by polarized light in the same tissue illustrated in Figure 152.*

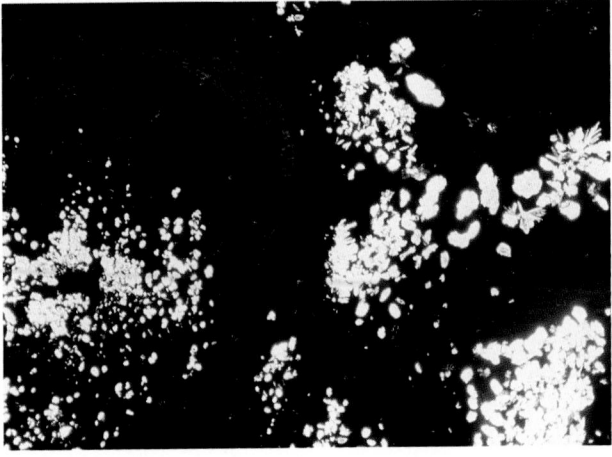

FIGURE 154. *Curious collection of monosodium urate crystals in same tissue as Figure 152. Polarized light and red compensator.*

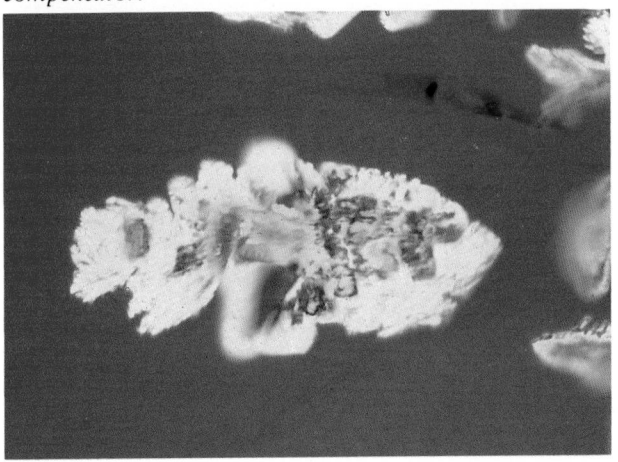

FIGURE 155. *Calcium pyrophosphate crystals in synovial fluid as seen under polarized light of Wright's stained smear. Rhomboid-shaped crystal in center is easily recognized, but other crystals are less distinct.*

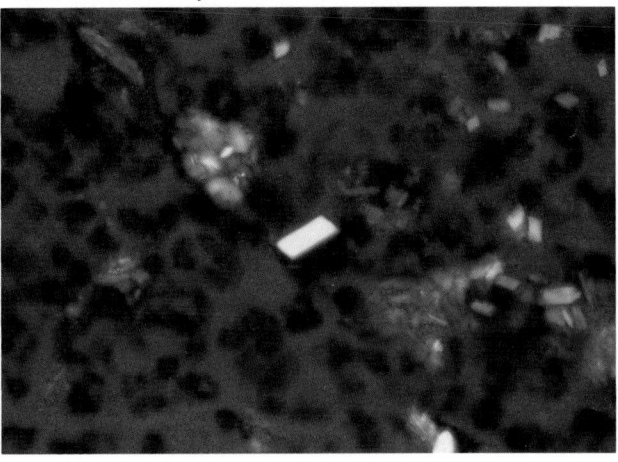

FIGURE 156. *The color of the calcium pyrophosphate crystal, as seen under polarized light with red compensator, depends on the crystal's orientation in relation to the axis of the compensator.*

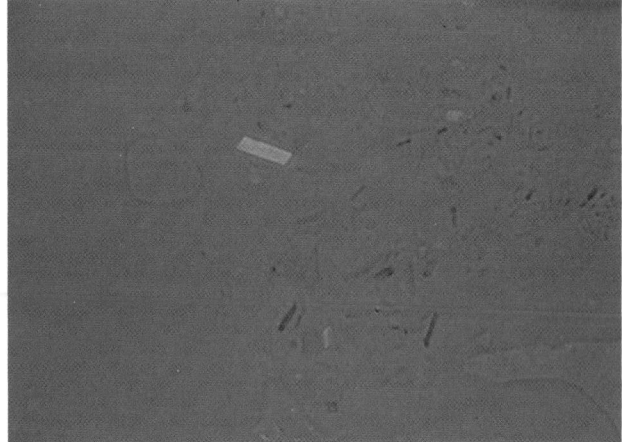

FIGURE 157. *Histologic section of synovium from patient with calcium pyrophosphate dihydrate crystal deposition disease. Dark purple area represents calcium. Surrounding tissue shows chronic inflammation and fibrosis (hematoxylin-eosin stain).*

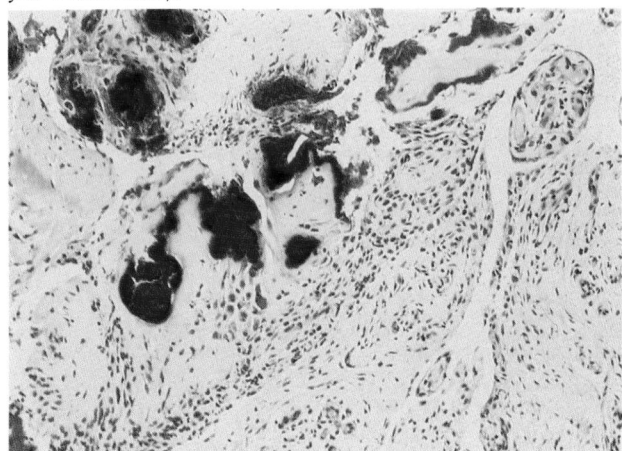

FIGURE 158. *Many calcium pyrophosphate crystals seen under polarized light with red compensator in same tissue illustrated in Figure 157.*

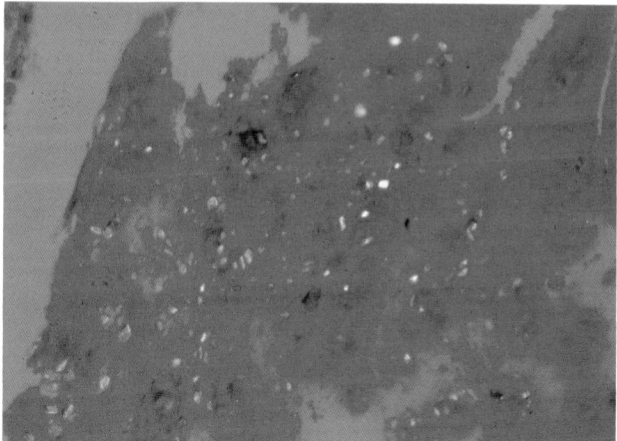

FIGURE 161. *Many vacuolated histiocytes (macrophages) in synovial fluid sample from a patient with numerous atypical cholesterol crystals illustrated in Figures 162 through 164.*

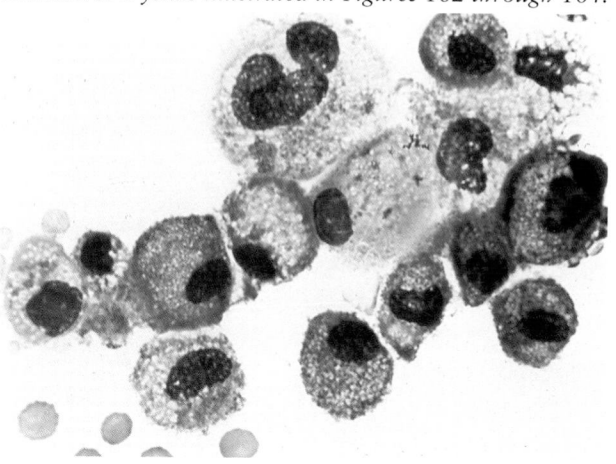

FIGURE 159. *Numerous cholesterol plate-like crystals in synovial fluid seen with polarized light.*

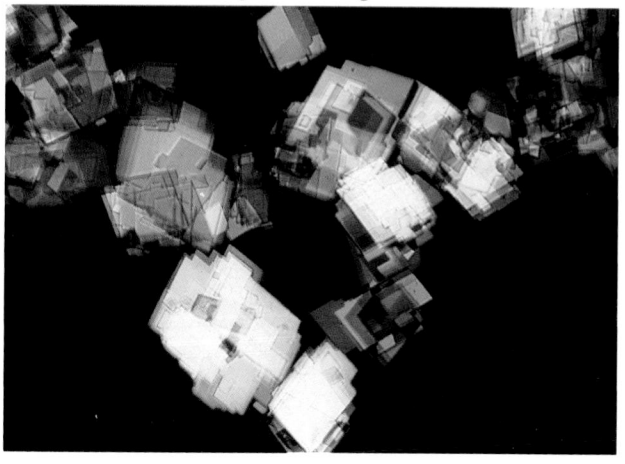

FIGURE 162. *Rectangular cholesterol crystals in synovial fluid (polarized light) resembling calcium pyrophosphate crystals.*

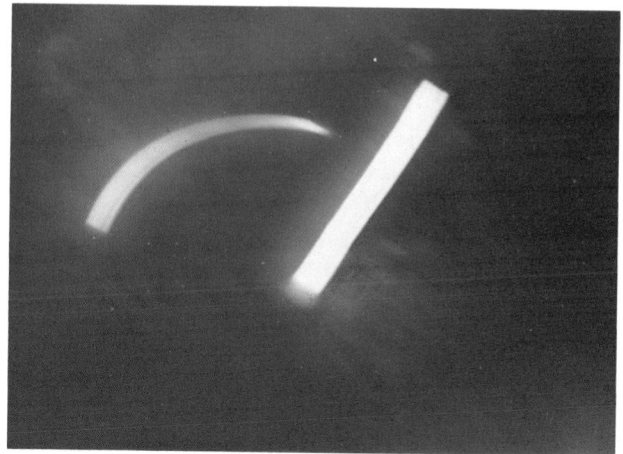

FIGURE 160. *Same specimen as in Figure 159 seen with a red compensator.*

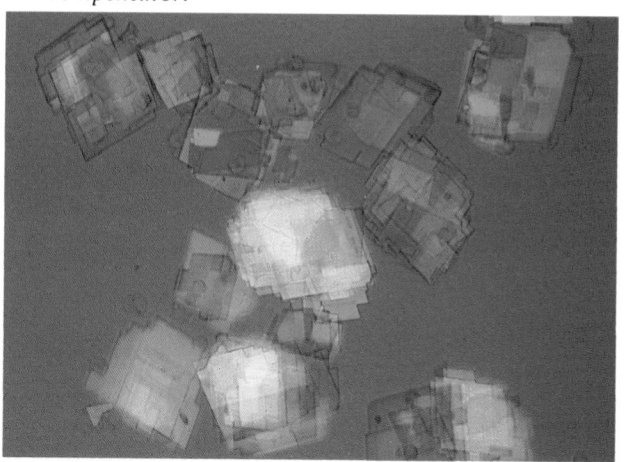

FIGURE 163. *Ring-shaped cholesterol crystals in synovial fluid (polarized light).*

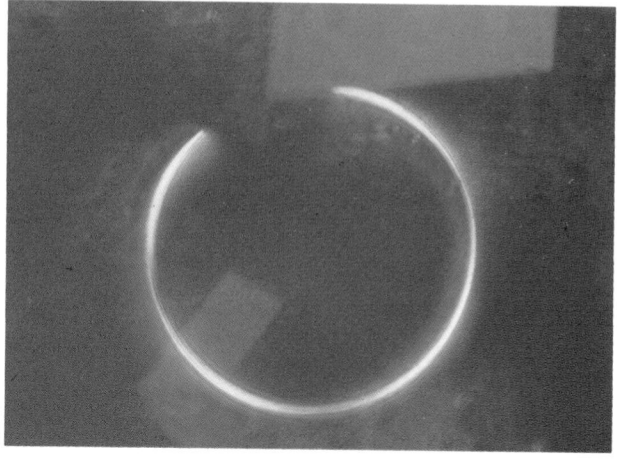

FIGURE 164. *Plate-like (blue) and needle-shaped (yellow) cholesterol crystals in synovial fluid. The latter may be mistaken for monosodium urate crystals (polarized light with red compensator).*

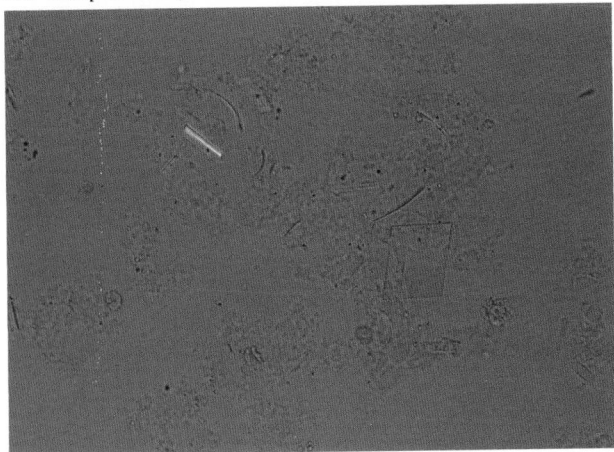

FIGURE 165. *Talcum particles in synovial fluid.*

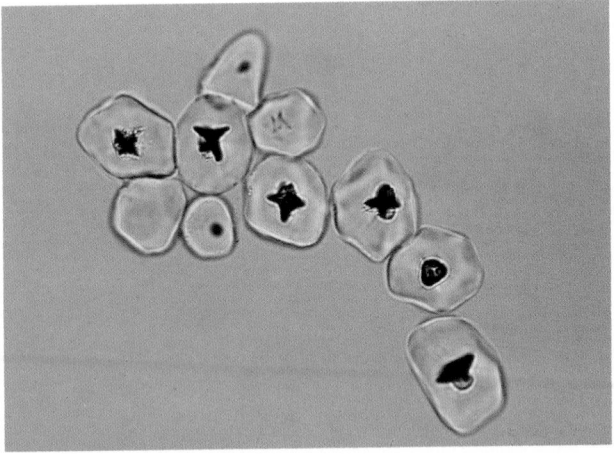

FIGURE 166. *Talcum particles as seen with polarized light appearing as bright Maltese crosses.*

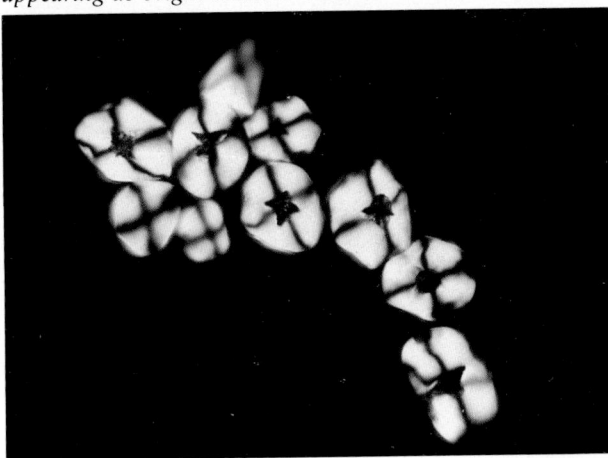

and lithium heparin, when used as anticoagulants, may crystalize in synovial fluid. Calcium oxalate crystals are usually cuboidal and of variable brightness. Lithium heparin crystals are small (2 to 5 μm) and of variable shape (sodium heparin does not form crystals). Both types of crystals may be phagocytosed by polymorphonuclear leukocytes. Talcum powder from surgical gloves may sometimes be seen in the synovial fluid as bright Maltese crosses when the fluid is polarized (Figures 165 through 167). A more common artifact is *corticosteroid* crystals, which may be seen several weeks or months after an intra-articular injection.[36] They may be similar in size and shape to monosodium urate or CPPD crystals. Plastic materials from joints containing a prosthesis are birefringent. Nail polish, which is used to seal the coverslip for a wet preparation, may be seen as bright refractile rods at the coverslip margin.[21] Similarly, dust and fibers from lens paper are refractile, and immersion oil may contain birefringent crystals (Figure 168). Finally, refractile collagen fibrils may be mistaken for crystals by the inexperienced observer.[21]

CHEMICAL ANALYSIS

In the past, the chemical analysis of synovial fluid, if performed at all, consisted of measuring glucose and, occasionally, total protein. Other tests that are rough indicators of disease and still frequently performed are the mucin and fibrin clot evaluations.[2] The mucin clot test essentially determines the state of the hyaluronic acid–protein complex and hence is related to viscosity. Both mucin clot formation and hyaluronic acid concentration are generally decreased in inflammatory conditions. The fibrin clot test is simply the observation of the fluid sample for spontaneous clotting. Normally, synovial fluid does not clot, since fibrinogen and other clotting factors are absent. Inflammatory and bloody fluids both produce spontaneous clotting.

Considerably more diagnostic information is now available on the chemical and immunologic composition of synovial fluid. Although much of this information has little clinical significance, there are several new tests available that can be helpful in selected patients. Most of the chemical and immunologic tests carried out on serum can be applied with equal utility to synovial fluid. If viscosity presents a technical problem, it can usually be overcome by appropriate dilution of the specimen or by prior sonication; pretreatment with the enzyme hyaluronidase is also effective (0.9 mL of synovial fluid incubated for four hours at 37 °C with 0.1 mL of bovine testicular hyaluronidase).

Hyaluronic Acid

Hyaluronic acid, a copolymer of glucuronic acid and N-acetyl-glucosamine, is secreted by the synovial lining cells and imparts to the fluid its stickiness and high viscosity. The normal mean concentration is about 0.41% (g/dL), which is considerably greater than the mean of 0.24% obtained from fluid at postmortem examination.[37] Both of these values are significantly greater than those found in synovial fluid samples from patients with osteoarthritis (0.12%), rheumatoid arthritis (0.07%), or traumatic arthritis (0.11%).[37] The mean hyaluronic acid concentration in synovial fluid samples from patients with gout, local synovitis, and ankylosing spondylitis is also less than that of postmortem specimens.[37] In addition, its concentration is decreased in the elderly.[37] However, there appears to be little correlation between hyaluronic acid concentration and the severity of the disease process. As a result, its specific routine measurement has no clinical significance.

Protein

The normal synovial fluid protein concentration is approximately one third that of serum, with an average of about 2.0 g/dL.[2] Levels higher than 3.0 g/dL suggest an inflammatory or hemorrhagic exudate. The quantitative methods used for measuring total serum protein are satisfactory for measuring synovial fluid. The protein concentration of synovial fluid depends on the synovial membrane permeability, the synovial fluid resorption by lymphatics, the molecular weight of the various protein molecules, and local synthesis.[2] Increased levels are routinely seen in RA, gout, septic arthritis, SLE, the inflammatory arthropathies accompanying Crohn's disease, and in Reiter's disease, ankylosing spondylitis, psoriasis, and ulcerative colitis. Most of these proteins are derived from plasma because of increased vascular permeability. There is also local immunoglobulin synthesis.

Clinically, the finding of an elevated total protein level merely confirms the presence of an inflammatory

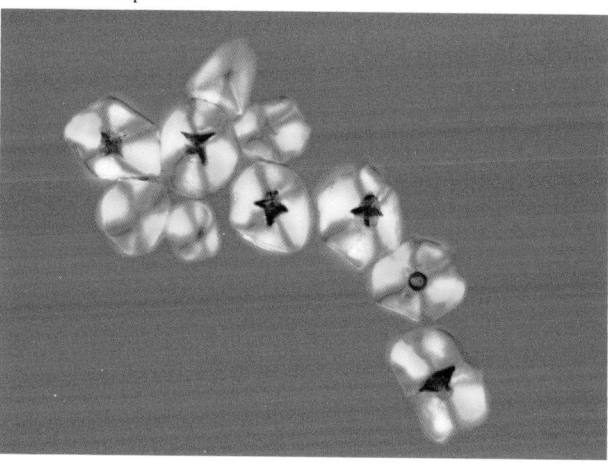

FIGURE 167. *Talcum particles as seen with polarized light and red compensator.*

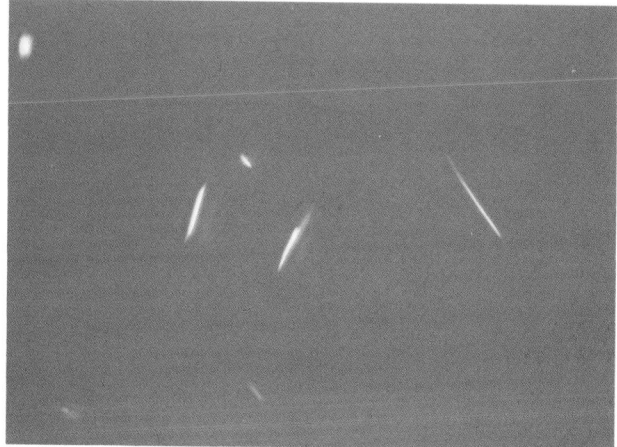

FIGURE 168. *Dust particles resembling monosodium urate crystals (polarized light).*

process, which is usually determined from other observations. The electrophoretic distribution of the protein fractions is unlike that of serum. Moreover, some differences in this distribution exist among the major groups of pathological joint fluids.[37] For example, fluid specimens removed at postmortem examination exhibit a significantly increased relative concentration of the α_1-*globulins* and a decreased relative concentration of the α_2-*globulins*.[38] As a result, the normal α_1-α_2 *ratio* in synovial fluid (mean, 1.0) is about twice that found in serum.[38] This is a consequence of the greatly increased concentration of α_1-acid glycoprotein and a significant decrease in the relative concentration of haptoglobin and the 19 S α_2-macroglobulins.[38] *Albumin* concentrations are relatively increased over those of serum, but to a lesser degree than are α_1-acid glycoprotein concentrations.[38]

The low molecular-weight (11,700) protein β_2-*microglobulin* is present in low concentrations in normal serum and urine, and levels have been noted to be increased in patients with renal tubular disorders and in renal transplant recipients, particularly at the time of rejection.[39,40] With the use of radioimmunoassay, levels of this protein have also been shown to be considerably increased in the synovial fluid of patients with both RA and Sjögren's syndrome, when compared with other inflammatory nonrheumatoid arthritides and with noninflammatory joint disease.[41] In a study involving eight patients with RA, the mean β_2-microglobulin level was 6.21 μg/mL, compared with 3.30 μg/mL for the inflammatory nonrheumatoid group and 2.55 μg/mL for the noninflammatory joint-disease group.[41] A more recent report, in which the β_2-microglobulin level, WBC count, total protein concentration, acid phosphatase level, and total hemolytic complement were compared in 12 patients with RA and ten with other arthropathies, showed that only the β_2-microglobulin level was significantly higher in cases of RA when compared with the non-RA cases.[42] These observations must be further expanded so that the role of β_2-microglobulin in the differential diagnosis of arthritis may be more fully appreciated.

Fibronectin is a high molecular-weight glycoprotein found in body fluids, the connective tissue matrix, and basement membranes. Although it is produced by many types of cultured cells, fibroblasts are particularly prominent producers.[43] Vartio et al[44] have measured fibronectin in synovial fluid samples from patients with RA. In a study involving 51 patients with RA and related disorders (eg, juvenile RA and ankylosing spondylitis), synovial fluid fibronectin concentrations were 445 ± 103 μg/mL (mean ± SD), as compared with normal plasma levels of about 300 to 350 μg/mL.[45] Immunofluorescence staining showed a prominent increase of fibronectin in the proliferating synovial connective tissue in RA, as compared with that in patients with normal synovial membranes.[45] This suggests that the local production of this glycoprotein is increased in rheumatoid synovial tissue. The routine laboratory measurement for fibronectin, however, must await further clinical and laboratory studies before its diagnostic value can be evaluated.

Glucose

The measurement of synovial fluid glucose may be of clinical value but abnormal levels are not a specific indicator for any disease process. Like CSF glucose, synovial fluid levels are interpreted along with serum values. Ideally, to establish an equilibrium, the synovial and serum levels are obtained six to eight hours postprandially, but this is usually impossible from a practical standpoint. The synovial fluid glucose level is normally equal to or slightly lower than (within 10 mg/dL) the serum level. In general, patients with noninflammatory joint disorders (degenerative joint disease, neuropathic osteoarthropathy, pigmented villonodular synovitis, trauma, and so forth) have glucose levels lower than 20 mg/dL below the serum levels measured simultaneously. Patients with inflammatory joint diseases (rheumatoid arthritis, rheumatic fever, SLE, and Reiter's disease, among others) have levels that are more than 25 mg/dL lower than the serum levels. In cases of septic arthritis, the synovial fluid glucose level is often more than 40 mg/dL lower than the serum concentration (Table 6–3).[3] There is, however, considerable overlap of levels in noninflammatory joint disorders and septic arthritis.

Uric Acid

Although the diagnosis of gout can usually be made by synovial fluid crystal identification, misinterpretations may occur. This is particularly true when the examiner is relatively inexperienced or the proper polarizing equipment is not available.

The quantitation of synovial fluid uric acid levels will not only verify the presence of monosodium urate crystals but may even be diagnostically significant when no crystals are found. It has been suggested that the synovial fluid uric acid concentration is a better single diagnostic factor than the serum level.[46] Normally, however, serum and synovial fluid uric acid levels are correlated positive indicators; that is, the serum uric acid concentration reflects the uric acid level in synovial fluid.[47] A synovial fluid uric acid concentration that is significantly higher than the normal serum level is probably diagnostic of gout.[6] In untreated gout, both synovial fluid and serum levels of uric acid are usually elevated. It should be mentioned, however, that some investigators believe that the measurement of uric acid in synovial fluid has little or no diagnostic value.[2,4]

Enzymes

Many enzymes have been studied in synovial fluid, including lactate dehydrogenase (LD), aspartate aminotransferase, acid and alkaline phosphatase, muramidase (lysozyme), β-acetyl-glucosaminidase, and 5'-nucleotidase, among others.

In one study, synovial fluid but not serum LD levels were shown to be increased in patients with RA, infectious arthritis, and gout.[48] The LD activity is normal, however, in synovial fluid samples from patients with osteoarthritis. Isoenzyme patterns of synovial fluid in patients with RA, infectious arthritis, and gout showed a predominance of LD_5.[48] This isoenzyme is probably derived from neutrophils that are usually abundant in all of these disorders, especially during the acute phase. On the other hand, AST (GOT) levels were normal in all cases in the same study.[48]

Considerable interest has been expressed in the action of acid hydrolases as destructive agents in rheumatoid joint disorders. Studies of both acid phosphatase and β-acetyl-glucosaminidase levels in patients with these disorders have been carried out,[48–51] showing elevations of both enzymes, with the highest values being seen in RA. Nevertheless, increased activity is not a specific indicator for this disorder. It may be

that the acid phosphatase originates from polymorphonuclear leukocytes. Alkaline phosphatase activity, although present in synovial fluid, is not elevated in any of the inflammatory arthropathies. Enzyme activity appears to be related primarily to the degree of synovial inflammation.

To date, the measurement of enzymes adds no additional useful clinical information that is not obtained from more routine examinations.

Organic Acids

Several publications[52–58] have established that synovial fluid lactic acid levels are increased in patients with monoarticular septic arthritis when compared with those of patients with nonseptic monoarticular arthritis. Although reference lactic acid intervals for normal fluid have not been established, it is assumed that they would be similar to those found in blood and spinal fluid of normal individuals—9 to 29 mg/dL and 0.98 to 3.7 mmole/L, respectively.[59,60] The lactate level in synovial fluid is slightly increased in most cases of monoarticular arthritis. In septic arthritis, notably elevated levels are usually seen. In one study involving 27 cases of nongonococcal septic arthritis with both gram-positive cocci and gram-negative rods, the mean synovial fluid lactate concentration was 1,170 mg/dL, while in 45 cases of inflammatory and degenerative arthritis, the mean was 34 mg/dL.[52] Interestingly, in 12 cases of gonococcal arthritis, the mean lactate value was only 27 mg/dL.[52] The finding of relatively low lactate values in gonococcal arthritis has been confirmed by several authors,[53,54,60] but not by all.[55] Although Borenstein et al[57] reported overall lactate concentrations lower than 27 mg/dL in all categories, they suggested that septic arthritis could be diagnosed in almost all cases where the synovial fluid lactate level exceeded 250 mg/dL. Since lactic acid levels can be determined in less than 30 minutes, the method would appear to be particularly valuable for rapid diagnosis.

The reasons for increased synovial fluid lactate levels in infected joints are uncertain. Although small amounts of lactate are undoubtedly produced by the neutrophilic leukocytes and bacteria that are present, the major contributor is probably the synovial tissue. It has been suggested that the increased metabolic demand in the inflamed synovium leads to hypoxia, resulting in the synovial tissue conversion from aerobic to anaerobic glycolysis, in which lactic acid is the end product.[61]

There are four primary limitations that one should take into consideration in interpreting synovial fluid lactate levels. First, intermediate values may neither confirm nor exclude infection. Second, in gonococcal arthritis, the levels are usually low but not invariably so. Third, lactate levels may be elevated in nonseptic arthritis, particularly RA.[58] Fourth, the test gives no clue to the specific nature of the infecting organism, and the physician will have to treat the patient accordingly until the culture results are known.

Using gas-liquid chromatography, it is possible to identify other organic acids that may prove helpful in differentiating between septic and nonseptic arthritis. In addition to finding elevated lactate levels in most patients studied with septic arthritis, Brook et al[53] noted two additional chromatographic peaks with retention times of 546 and 848 seconds. These two organic acids were not seen in the sterile inflammatory or degenerative arthritis cases. Presumptive evidence suggested that these compounds are *n*-valeric and *n*-hexanoic acids, respectively.[53] More recently, Borenstein et al[57] noted the presence of succinic acid, in addition to lactic acid, in all of 23 cases of septic arthritis and in only five of 57 nonseptic synovial fluid specimens. The detection of succinic acid was thought to be helpful in recognizing patients with septic arthritis who had received partial treatment.[57] If these study findings are verified further, the measurement of multiple organic acids may prove to be helpful.

Other Biochemical Measurements

Many other substances have been measured in the synovial fluid of normal and diseased joints. For example, the concentration of iron has been found to be consistently elevated in both the synovial fluid and synovial membranes of patients with RA.[62] The levels are usually greater than the corresponding serum concentrations. Increased iron deposition in the synovium also occurs in patients with hemochromatosis and pigmented villonodular synovitis. In one study, synovial fluid ferritin levels in patients with RA were compared with those in patients with osteoarthritis and found to be notably higher in the former.[63] The ferritin was presumed to be derived from the synovial reticuloendothelial cells. These same authors subsequently noted a significant association among synovial fluid ferritin concentrations, synovial immune complexes, and other local indices of inflammation, which caused them to raise the question of whether iron is an index or a cause of the inflammation in patients with RA.[64] Zinc has been found in greater concentrations in the synovial fluid of patients with RA than in their serum.[65] Although these findings may be interesting, they have little clinical usefulness.

Synovial effusions containing cholesterol crystals have been described in several types of chronic arthritis and are particularly common in RA.[66,67] These fluids are turbid and white or yellow, and have a thick consistency. Quantitative cholesterol levels of these fluids are usually considerably greater than those of the corresponding serum. The lipid levels in synovial fluid are, however, only rarely measured.

IMMUNOLOGIC STUDIES

Normal synovial fluid contains only about 10% of the *immunoglobulin* levels of normal serum, although mild increases occur in crystal synovitis and degenerative joint disease. In patients with RA and related disorders, the immunoglobulin levels approach those of the serum and may exceed the serum concentrations in some RA cases.[68] There is no apparent relationship between the immunoglobulin concentration and age, sex, duration of disease, sedimentation rate, or rheumatoid factor latex fixation titer.[68] The serum to synovial-fluid ratios for both IgG and IgM appear to exceed those theoretically calculated for their molecular weights, implying both an excessive exudation of plasma proteins to the synovial fluid and the in situ production of immunoglobulins.[68] Local production of immunoglobulins has been previously demonstrated.[69,70] In addition, the light chain ratio of IgG eluted from rheumatoid synovium has been shown to be different from that of IgG in serum; λ light chains predominate over κ light chains in most eluates.[71]

In studying classic RA with nodules, Cracchiolo and Barnet,[72] using radioimmunodiffusion, reported that the synovial fluid to serum ratios for IgG, IgA, and IgM averaged 0.7. The average ratios of those RA cases without nodules were 0.5, as were the ratios of "probable" RA cases.[72] Patients with osteoarthritis had mean ratios of 0.3.[72] In seven cases of Reiter's syndrome, the ratio of synovial fluid to serum for IgM approached 1.4, the IgA ratio averaged 1.0, and the IgG ratio averaged 0.85. This was the only disease in which the ratios consistently exceeded 1.0.[72] In a study comparing the synovial fluid immunoglobulin levels in 12 patients with ankylosing spondylitis with those in 37 patients with RA, it was found that the lymphocyte count and immunoglobulin levels in patients with ankylosing spondylitis were both significantly higher than in those with RA.[73] The synovial fluid levels for IgG, IgA, and IgM in patients with ankylosing spondylitis averaged 1,995 mg/dL, 343 mg/dL, and 64 mg/dL, respectively, as compared with concentrations of 957 mg/dL, 178 mg/dL, and 36 mg/dL in patients with RA.[73]

Rheumatoid factors are most often detected by the agglutination of sensitized sheep RBCs, bentonite, or latex particles coated with γ-globulin. These tests are semiquantitative and do not indicate the distribution of the anti-γ-globulins among the different classes. Only IgM rheumatoid factor is measured by these tests. Methods for the detection of IgG and IgA rheumatoid factors are generally considered to be research tools. The latex fixation test appears to be the most sensitive but can lead to a few false-positive results. While the sensitized sheep RBC agglutination test appears less sensitive, it may be more specific.[72] Rheumatoid factors are present in the serum of about 80% of the patients with RA and can also be detected in the synovial fluid of about 60%.[72] The rheumatoid factors have been shown by in vivo and in vitro techniques to be produced by the rheumatoid synovium.[74,75] Occasionally, patients with seronegative test results will have positive results for rheumatoid factor in synovial fluid.[72,74] Since a wide variety of other chronic inflammatory processes are characterized by persistent antigenic stimuli, false-positive results are common.[74,76,77] In general, however, assays for rheumatoid factor in synovial fluid have not been helpful for diagnosis or prognosis.[78]

Antinuclear antibodies (ANAs) are immunoglobulins with specific antibody activity against antigens in cell nuclei. They occur in all three classes of immunoglobulins and can be detected by the same methods used for serum. Nearly all patients with active SLE will have detectable ANAs in their serum samples, while 10% to 65% of the patients with RA will have ANA-positive results, depending on the sensitivity of the test used.[78] Approximately 70% of patients with SLE and about 20% of patients with RA will also have ANAs in the synovial fluid.[72] There is, however, little disease specificity associated with synovial ANAs.[77] In patients with systemic lupus erythematosus (SLE), Wright's stained smears of the joint fluid frequently show typical LE cells (Figure 143). Although this finding is not a pathognomonic indicator for SLE, the specificity of this finding probably exceeds 95% if rheumatoid arthritis can be excluded.

Complement components are a group of nonspecific serum factors that interact in a specific sequence during immunologic reactions. Within the joints of patients with RA and SLE, immune complexes activate the complement system. When so activated, the system generates biologic factors that alter blood vessel permeability and recruit neutrophilic leukocytes from the blood circulation to phagocytose the antigen-antibody complexes.[78] The neutrophils then liberate various lysosomal enzymes, which damage the articular cartilage. The most frequent measurement for complement is that for the total hemolytic complement (CH_{50}), which is a measurement of the ability of the fluid to lyse 50% of a standard suspension of sheep erythrocytes coated with rabbit antibody. Assays for the various separate complement components (C3, C4) are also available. Synovial fluid complement levels correlate well with total protein concentration, so that interpretation depends not only on the total complement level but also on the total protein concentration. Bunch et al[80] reported the values given in Table 6–4.

From this information, appropriate interpolations can be made for other protein-complement values. It should be noted that in the report of Bunch et al, the normal serum range was reported as 40 to 90 CH_{50} units/mL. In another study, the reference level of synovial total complement suggested that normal values are more than 30% of the simultaneous serum value.[77] It is possible that the C4 value is a more sensitive index than is the total complement value.[81]

Total synovial fluid complement values are normal in traumatic or degenerative joint disease. However, decreased levels are usually seen in SLE, RA, and bacterial synovitis. Levels may be elevated in Reiter's disease.[15] Serum complement levels are usually decreased in SLE, particularly in patients with renal disease, and are normal or increased in RA (Table 6–5). Panush et al[82] have reported a linear relationship be-

TABLE 6–4. Correlation of Protein and Complement Levels in Normal Synovial Fluid

Total Protein (mg/mL)	Complement (CH$_{50}$ UNITS/mL)
20	8–38
30	11–42
40	15–46
50	19–50

Note: From Bunch et al.[80] Used with permission.

TABLE 6–5. Complement Levels in Patients With Joint Disease

Disease	Serum Levels	Synovial Fluid Levels
Rheumatoid arthritis	Normal or increased	Normal or decreased
Systemic lupus erythematosus	Normal or decreased	Decreased
Reiter's disease	Increased	Increased
Gout	Increased	Increased

tween elevated serum or synovial-fluid IgG and IgM anti–γ-globulin levels and lowered serum or synovial fluid complement. Hence, an elevation of serum and synovial fluid levels for complement and rheumatoid factor may occasionally be helpful in difficult or unusual cases. Earlier studies seemed to be in general agreement that the measurement of synovial fluid complement levels was clinically useful, both in the evaluation of the patient with RA having seronegative test results and in predicting the severity and prognosis of this disease (association of low synovial fluid complement and/or rheumatoid factor levels with severe disease).[83] However, more recent studies of synovial fluid CH$_{50}$ measurements suggest that this test may be of little use in making a diagnosis and in measuring the disease activity of RA.[84,85]

The percentage of *T-lymphocytes* is higher in synovial fluid than in blood, while the percentage of *B-lymphocytes* is lower in synovial fluid than in blood.[86] Recent studies on T-lymphocyte subset populations in RA have revealed contrasting findings in blood, synovial membrane (synovium), and synovial fluid.[87,88] In patients with active RA, decreased numbers of sup-

pressor/cytotoxic T cells are found in the blood and in the synovial membrane, while normal or increased numbers are found in the synovial fluid. The numbers of helper/inducer T cells in the synovial fluid tend to be lower than those in the blood, and numerous such cells have been demonstrated in the synovium. The significance of these findings is not yet clear.

MICROBIOLOGIC EXAMINATION

Septic arthritis is the most rapidly destructive disease of joints. The routine examination of synovial fluid should, therefore, include a Gram stain and culture for microorganisms (Figure 169), even if the Gram stain is negative. Where an effusion from a joint is noted, careful consideration of the possible causes should precede aspiration. A consultation at this stage with the microbiology laboratory may prove helpful, saving a great deal of time and possibly leading to a diagnosis that otherwise might be missed. In early or mild bacterial infections, for example, the gross examination of the fluid alone may suggest a nonseptic origin; and even in cases of arthritis of presumably known, noninfectious origin, it must be kept in mind that a secondary bacterial infection is possible. Hence, failure to culture the specimen may result in a missed or delayed diagnosis, a prolonged clinical course, and possible permanent injury to the joint.

When performing the arthrocentesis, care should be taken to avoid contamination of the synovial fluid with local anesthetic, since such agents may interfere with recovery of bacteria and the interpretation of gas-liquid chromatography. The aspirated fluid must be put in a sterile container and transported to the laboratory as soon as possible.

Although viruses, tuberculosis, and fungi may all be possible causative agents, bacteria are clearly the most common infectious organisms and usually reach the synovial membrane through the bloodstream. Hence the factors determining the incidence of infectious arthritis are essentially those of bacteremia.

The age of the patient is critical in diagnosing the cause of infectious arthritis and gives important clues to the specific organism one might expect to recover.[89] In young children, systemic infections such as pneumonia or meningitis are often present with infectious arthritis. The most common organisms are *Staphylococcus aureus* (Figure 170), *Streptococcus pyo-*

genes, *Streptococcus pneumoniae,* and *Hemophilus influenzae.* The last organism is seen almost exclusively in children younger than 2 years. In children aged 2 to 15 years, *S aureus, S pyogenes,* and *S pneumoniae* account for about 85% of the cases. In patients aged 16 to 50 years, *Neisseria gonorrhoeae* accounts for 75% of the cases and *S aureus* for 15%. In patients older than 50 years, gonococci are rarely seen, and *S aureus* accounts for up to 75% of the cases; the remaining 25% are composed of a variety of different bacteria. Adults with RA are prone to development of joint infection, with 80% of cases caused by *S aureus.* The joints most commonly involved are the wrist, hip, knee, and ankle.

The enteric organisms are only occasionally isolated as causative agents. Although they are most frequently seen in patients older than 50 years, they account for no more than 10% of these cases. Microorganisms other than those already mentioned collectively account for less than 5% of the cases in any age group.

Since *N gonorrhoeae* is such an important causative agent, it is imperative that the proper media be inoculated immediately after aspiration of the fluid. Because of the fastidious nature of this organism, the appropriate prewarmed culture media should be immediately available. The Gram stain is positive in approximately 40% of proven gonococcal arthritis cases.

If tuberculosis, fungi, or anaerobic bacteria are suspected, special handling and culture media are needed. Synovial fluid smears are positive for acid-fast bacilli in about 20% of proven cases, while cultures are usually positive in about 80% of proven cases. Prior consultation with the laboratory is, again, very helpful. In the case of tuberculosis, a closed synovial biopsy specimen taken for histologic examination may provide the most rapid diagnosis.

Routine microbiologic studies frequently require several days before results are available. The Gram stain is deficient in sensitivity, and the synovial WBC count is unreliable in separating septic from other arthritides. Therefore, several new, rapid methods, which do not depend on bacterial culture, have been introduced in recent years. These include detection of microbial metabolites by gas chromatography; detection of microbial antigens by latex agglutination, radioimmunoassay and counterimmunoelectrophore-

FIGURE 169. *Gram's stain of synovial fluid showing* Neisseria gonorrhoeae.

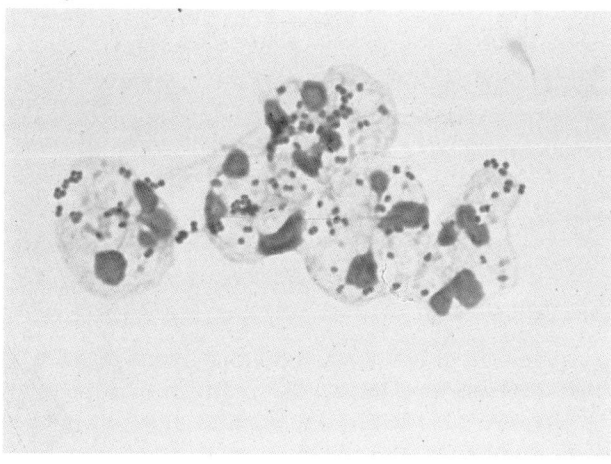

FIGURE 170. *Gram's stain of synovial fluid showing* Staphylococcus aureus.

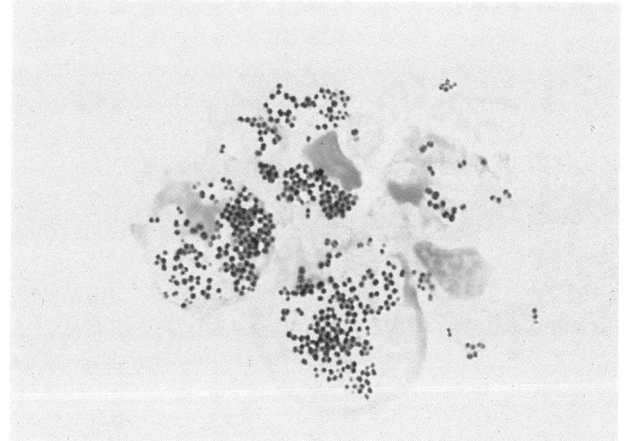

sis; and examination for endotoxin by the *Limulus* lysate assay. These procedures have been described in the chapters on CSF and pleural fluid. The measurement of lactic acid, using either gas-liquid chromatography or an ultraviolet enzyme technique, in the study of septic arthritis has been described earlier in this chapter. The *Limulus* assay for detection of bacterial endotoxin in synovial fluid lacks sensitivity but appears specific for infectious processes.[90]

REFERENCES

1. Currey HLF, Roberts BV: Examination of synovial fluid. *Clin Rheum Dis* 2:149–176, 1976
2. Krieg AF: Cerebrospinal fluid and other body fluids, in Henry JB (ed): *Clinical Laboratory Methods,* ed 16. Philadelphia, WB Saunders Co, 1979, pp 635–657
3. Rippey JH: Synovial fluid analysis. *Lab Med* 10:140–145, 1979
4. Cohen AS, Brandt KD, Krey PR: Synovial fluid, in Cohen AS (ed): *Laboratory Diagnostic Procedures in the Rheumatic Diseases.* Boston, Little Brown & Co, 1975
5. Naib AM: Cytology of synovial fluids. *Acta Cytol* 17:299–309, 1973
6. Teloh HA: Clinical pathology of synovial fluid. *Ann Clin Lab Sci* 5:282–287, 1975
7. Goldenberg DL, Brandt KD, Cohen AS: Rapid, simple detection of trace amounts of synovial fluid. *Arthritis Rheum* 16:487–490, 1973
8. Cheung HS, Ryan LM, Kozin F, et al: Synovial origins of rice bodies in joint fluid. *Arthritis Rheum* 23:72–76, 1980
9. Krey PR, Bailen DA: Synovial fluid leukocytosis: A study of extremes. *Am J Med* 67:436–442, 1979
10. Matthay M, Lindamood M, Steigerwald JC, et al: Acute pseudogout in the absence of synovial fluid leukocytes. *J Rheumatol* 4:303–306, 1977
11. Gatter RA, Richmond JD: Predominance of synovial fluid lymphocytes in early rheumatoid arthritis. *J Rheumatol* 2:340–345, 1975
12. Brawer AE, Cathcart ES: Acute monocytic arthritis. *Arthritis Rheum* 22:294–301, 1979
13. Podell TE, Ault M, Sullam P, et al: Synovial fluid eosinophilia. *Arthritis Rheum* 23:1060–1061, 1980
14. Klofkorn RW, Lehman TJA: Eosinophilic synovial effusions complicating chronic urticaria and angioedema. *Arthritis Rheum* 25:708–709, 1982

15. Pekin TJ, Malinin TI, Zvaifler NJ: Unusual synovial fluid findings in Reiter's syndrome. *Ann Intern Med* 66:677–684, 1967
16. Broderick PA, Corvese N, Pierik MG, et al: Exfoliative cytology interpretation of synovial fluid in joint disease. *J Bone Joint Surg Am* 58:396–399, 1976
17. Hunter T, Gordon DA, Ogryslo MA: The ground pepper sign of synovial fluid: A new diagnostic feature of ochronosis. *J Rheumatol* 1:45–53, 1974
18. Lawrence C, Seifo B: Bone marrow in joint fluid: A clue to fracture. *Ann Intern Med* 74:740–742, 1971
19. Phelps P, Steele AD, McCarty DJ: Compensated polarized light microscopy. *JAMA* 203:166–179, 1968
20. Yehia SR, Duncan H: Synovial fluid analysis. *Clin Orthop* 107:11–24, 1975
21. Gatter RA: *A Practical Handbook of Joint Fluid Analysis.* Philadelphia, Lea & Febiger, 1984
22. McCarty DJ, Hollander JL: Identification of urate crystals in gouty synovial fluid. *Ann Intern Med* 54:452–460, 1961
23. Romanoff NR, Rubinow A, Canoso JJ, et al: Gout without crystals on initial synovial fluid analysis. *Postgrad Med J* 54:95–97, 1978
24. Schumacher HR, Jimenez SA, Gibson T, et al: Acute gouty arthritis without urate crystals identified on initial examination of synovial fluid: Report on nine patients. *Arthritis Rheum* 18:603–612, 1975
25. McCarty DJ: Calcium pyrophosphate dihydrate crystal deposition disease: 1975. *Arthritis Rheum* 19:275–285, 1976
26. Moss EG, Solomon SD: Calcium pyrophosphate deposition disease: A commonly unrecognized entity. *Med Soc NJ* 78:369–372, 1981
27. Kitridou RC: Synovianalysis. *Am Fam Physician* 5:101–107, 1972
28. Nye WHR, Terry R, Rosenbaum DL: Two forms of crystalline lipid in cholesterol effusions. *Am J Clin Pathol* 48:718–728, 1968
29. Fam AG, Pritzker KPH, Cheng PT, et al: Cholesterol crystals in osteoarthritic joint effusions. *J Rheumatol* 8:273–280, 1981
30. Schumacher HR, Smolyo AP, Tse RL, et al: Arthritis associated with apatite crystals. *Ann Intern Med* 87:411–413, 1977
31. Fam AG, Pritzker KPH, Stein JL, et al: Apatite-associated arthropathy: A clinical study of 14 cases and of 2 patients with calsific bursitis. *J Rheumatol* 6:461–471, 1979
32. McCarty DJ, Gatter RA: Recurrent acute inflammation associated with focal apatite crystal deposition. *Arthritis Rheum* 9:804–819, 1966

33. Schumacher HR: Pathogenesis of crystal-induced synovitis, in Kelley W (ed): *Clinics in Rheumatic Diseases.* London, WB Saunders, 1977, vol 3: *Crystal Induced Arthropathies.*

34. McCarty DJ, Halverson PB, Carrera GF: "Milwaukee shoulder": Association of microspheroids containing hydroxyapatite crystals, active collagenase, and neutral protease with rotator cuff defects: I. Clinical aspects. *Arthritis Rheum* 24:464–473, 1981

35. Huskisson EC, Dieppe PA, Crocker P, et al: Apatite deposition disease: A new arthropathy. *Lancet* 1:266–269, 1976

36. Kahn CB, Hollander JL, Schumacher HR: Corticosteroid crystals in synovial fluid. *JAMA* 211:807–809, 1970

37. Stafford CT, Niedermeier W, Holley H, et al: Studies on the concentration and intrinsic viscosity of hyaluronic acid in synovial fluids of patients with rheumatic diseases. *Ann Rheum Dis* 23:152–157, 1964

38. Binette JP, Schmid K: The proteins of synovial fluid: A study of the α_1/α_2 globulin ratio. *Arthritis Rheum* 8:14–28, 1965

39. Berggard I, Bearn AG: Isolation and properties of a low molecular weight beta-2-microglobulin occurring in human biological fluids. *J Biol Chem* 243:4095–4103, 1968

40. Grey HM, Kubo RT, Starzl TE, et al: Serum β_2-microglobulin in homografted patients. *J Clin Invest* 53:30A, 1974

41. Talal N, Grey HM, Zvaifler N, et al: Elevated salivary and synovial fluid β_2-microglobulin in Sjögren's syndrome and rheumatoid arthritis. *Science* 188:1196–1198, 1975

42. Todesco S, Punzi L, Montanaro D, et al: Beta-2-microglobulin in synovial fluid of rheumatoid arthritis. *J Rheum* 7:555–558, 1980

43. Ruoslahti E, Vaheri A: Novel human serum protein from fibroblast plasma membrane. *Nature* 248:789–791, 1974

44. Vartio T, Vaheri A, Von Essen R, et al: Fibronectin in synovial fluid and tissue in rheumatoid arthritis. *Eur J Clin Invest* 11:207–212, 1981

45. Mosesson MW, Umfleet RA: The cold insoluble globulin of human plasma: I. Purification, primary characterization and relationship to fibrinogen and other cold insoluble fraction components. *J Biol Chem* 245:5728–5736, 1970

46. Reeves B: Significance of joint fluid uric acid levels in gout. *Ann Rheum Dis* 24:569–571, 1965

47. Weinberger A, Wysenbeck A, Agam G, et al: Synovial fluid urate concentration in normouricemic and hyperuricemic subjects without joint disease. *Clin Chim Acta* 11:279–280, 1981

48. Cohen AS: Lactic dehydrogenase (LDH) and transaminase (GOT) activity of synovial fluid and serum in rheumatic disease states, with a note on synovial fluid LDH isozymes. *Arthritis Rheum* 7:490–501, 1964

49. Lehman MA, Kream J, Brogna D: Acid and alkaline phosphatase activity in the serum and synovial fluid of patients with arthritis. *J Bone Joint Surg Am* 46:1732–1738, 1964

50. Caygill JC, Pitkeathly DA: A study of β-acetylglucosaminase and acid phosphatase in pathological joint fluids. *Ann Rheum Dis* 25:137–144, 1966

51. Veys EM, Gabriel P, Decrans L, et al: N-acetyl-β-D-glucosaminidase activity in synovial fluid. *Rheumatol Rehabil* 14:50–56, 1975

52. Brook I, Reza MJ, Bricknell KS, et al: Synovial fluid lactic acid: A diagnostic aid in septic arthritis. *Arthritis Rheum* 21:774–778, 1978

53. Brook I, Reza MJ, Bricknell KS, et al: Abnormalities in synovial fluid of patients with septic arthritis detected by gas-liquid chromatography. *Ann Rheum Dis* 39:168–172, 1980

54. Mossman SS, Coleman JM, Gow PP, et al: Synovial fluid lactic acid in septic arthritis. *N Z Med J* 93:115–117, 1981

55. Behn AR, Mathews JA, Phillips I: Lactate UV-system: A rapid method for diagnosis of septic arthritis. *Ann Rheum Dis* 40:489–492, 1981

56. Riordan T, Doyle D, Tabaqchali S: Synovial fluid lactic acid measurement in the diagnosis and management of septic arthritis. *J Clin Pathol* 35:390–394, 1982

57. Borenstein DG, Gibbs CA, Jacobs RP: Gas-liquid chromatographic analysis of synovial fluid. *Arthritis Rheum* 25:947–953, 1982

58. Curtis GDW, Newman RJ, Slack MPE: Synovial fluid lactate and the diagnosis of septic arthritis. *J Infection* 6:239–246, 1983

59. Knight JA, Dudek SM, Haymond RE: Early (chemical) diagnosis of bacterial meningitis-cerebrospinal fluid glucose, lactate, and lactate dehydrogenase compared. *Clin Chem* 27:1431–1434, 1981

60. Paulsen O, Berghard G: Synovial fluid lactate determinations as a diagnostic aid in cases of monoarticular arthritis. *Scand J Infect Dis* 13:239–240, 1981

61. Treuhaft PS, McCarty DJ: Synovial fluid pH, lactate, oxygen, and carbon dioxide partial pressure in various joint disease. *Arthritis Rheum* 14:475–484, 1971

62. Senator GB, Muirden KD: Concentration of iron in synovial membrane, synovial fluid, and serum in rheumatoid arthritis and other joint diseases. *Ann Rheum Dis* 27:49–53, 1968

63. Blake DR, Bacon PA, Eastham EJ, et al: Synovial fluid ferritin in rheumatoid arthritis. *Br Med J* 281:715–716, 1980

64. Blake DR, Bacon PA: Synovial fluid ferritin in rheumatoid arthritis: An index or cause of inflammation? *Br Med J* 282:189, 1981

65. Bonebrake RA, McCall JT, Hurder GG, et al: Zinc accumulation in synovial fluid. *Mayo Clin Proc* 47:746–750, 1972

66. Meyers OL, Watermeyer GS: Cholesterol-rich synovial effusions. *S Afr Med J* 50:973–975, 1976

67. Ettlinger RE, Hunder GG: Synovial effusions containing cholesterol crystals. *Mayo Clin Proc* 54:366–374, 1979

68. Pruzanski W, Russell ML, Gordon DA, et al: Serum and synovial fluid proteins in rheumatoid arthritis and degenerative joint diseases. *Am J Med Sci* 265:483–490, 1973

69. Slirvinski AJ, Zvaifler NJ: In vivo synthesis of IgG by rheumatoid synovium. *J Lab Clin Med* 76:304–310, 1970

70. Zvaifler NJ: Immunoreactants in rheumatoid synovial effusions. *J Exp Med* 134:276s–285s, 1971

71. Lindstrom FD: Kappa:lambda light chain ratio in IgG eluted from rheumatoid arthritis synovium. *Clin Exp Immunol* 7:1–10, 1970

72. Cracchiolo A, Barnett EV: The role of immunological tests in routine synovial fluid analysis. *J Bone Joint Surg Am* 54:828–840, 1972

73. Kendall MJ, Farr M, Meynell MJ, et al: Synovial fluid in ankylosing spondylitis. *Ann Rheum Dis* 32:487–492, 1973

74. Rodnap GP, Eisenbeis CH, Creighton AS: The occurrence of rheumatoid factor in synovial fluid. *Am J Med* 35:182–188, 1963

75. Cecere F, Lessard J, McDuffy S: Evidence for the local production and utilization of immune reactants in rheumatoid arthritis. *Arthritis Rheum* 25:1307–1315, 1982

76. Huskisson EC, Hart FD, Lacey BW: Synovial fluid Waaler-Rose and latex tests. *Ann Rheum Dis* 30:67–72, 1971

77. Seward CW, Osterland CK: The pattern of anti-immunoglobulin activities in serum, pleural and synovial fluids. *J Lab Clin Med* 81:230–240, 1973

78. McCarty DJ Jr: Synovial fluid, in Hollander JL, McCarty DJ Jr (eds): *Arthritis and Allied Conditions: A Textbook of Rheumatology.* Philadelphia, Lea & Febiger, 1979, pp 51–69

79. Cracchiolo A: Joint fluid analysis. *Am Fam Physician* 4:87–94, 1971

80. Bunch TW, et al: Synovial fluid complement determination as a diagnostic aid in inflammatory joint disease. *Mayo Clin Proc* 49:715–720, 1974

81. Ruddy S, Austen KF: The complement system in rheumatoid synovitis: I. An analysis of complement component activities in rheumatoid synovial fluids. *Arthritis Rheum* 13:713–723, 1970

82. Panush RS, Bianco NE, Schur PH: Serum and synovial fluid IgG, IgA and IgM antigammaglobulins in rheumatoid arthritis. *Arthritis Rheum* 14:737–747, 1971

83. Bunch TW, Hunder GG, Offord K, et al: Synovial fluid complement: Usefulness in diagnosis and classification of rheumatoid arthritis. *Am Intern Med* 81:32–35, 1974

84. Kim HJ, McCarty DJ, Kozin F, et al: Clinical significance of synovial fluid total hemolytic complement activity. *J Rheum* 7:143–152, 1980

85. Sheppard H, Lea DJ, Ward DJ: Synovial fluid total hemolytic complement activity in rheumatic diseases: A reappraisal. *J Rheum* 8:390–397, 1981

86. Bjelle A, Tärnvik A: Lymphocytes of synovial fluid and peripheral blood in reactive arthritis. *Scand J Infect Dis* 24(suppl):58–62, 1980

87. Veys EM, Hermanns P, Verbruggen G, et al: Evaluation of T cell subsets with monoclonal antibodies in synovial fluid in rheumatoid arthritis. *J Rheumatol* 9:821–826, 1982

88. Duke O, Panayi GS, Janossy G, et al: Analysis of T cell subsets in the peripheral blood and synovial fluid of patients with rheumatoid arthritis by means of monoclonal antibodies. *Ann Rheum Dis* 42:357–361, 1983

89. Parker RH: Septic arthritis, in Hoeprich PD (ed): *Infectious Diseases,* ed 2. New York, Harper & Row Publishers Inc, 1977, pp 1125–1132

90. Cesario T, Jason M, Andrew BS, et al: Limulus assay for bacterial endotoxin in synovial fluid. *Ann Rheum Dis* 42:571–574, 1983

Laboratory Methods

The methods for obtaining most extravascular body fluids are considerably more complicated than those for collecting a peripheral blood specimen. The process is sometimes potentially dangerous and usually uncomfortable for the patient. These fluids should, therefore, be handled and examined with great care.

FLUID COLLECTION

Ideally, *CSF* should be divided into three samples and placed in sterile tubes, which are labeled sequentially. Tube 1 should be used for chemical and immunologic studies, tube 2 for microbiologic examination, and tube 3 for cell count and cytologic examination. This collection sequence reduces the possibility of contamination with peripheral blood, which would otherwise invalidate the cell count.

Improper specimen handling of *serous fluids* (pleural, peritoneal, and pericardial) is frequently a major problem preventing their appropriate evaluation. Too often a large syringe or vacuum bottle filled with fluid is sent to the laboratory with a request slip for multiple tests or for a single examination (usually "cytology"). This practice frequently creates problems in the laboratory, as the specimen often has to be divided among several laboratory sections. Such practice also creates a biohazard for laboratory personnel. Serous fluid specimens, therefore, should be collected in several containers, the number depending on how many laboratory tests are to be performed. Table A–1 lists the sample volume and the appropriate containers for some of the commonly requested tests. If a microbiologic examination is indicated, the specimen must be submitted in a sterile tube.

All fluid samples should be sent to the laboratory as soon as possible and examined promptly. As lysis of cells in the CSF takes place soon after removal from the body, the CSF specimen should always be ex-

TABLE A–1. Requirements for Laboratory Evaluation of Serous Fluid Specimens

VOLUME (mL)*	ANTICOAGULANT TUBE	TESTS
3-7	EDTA	Hematology (WBC and RBC counts, differential cell count, and smear evaluation)
8-10	Heparin	Chemistry (total protein, lactate dehydrogenase, glucose, and amylase determinations)
8-10	Heparin (sterile)	Microbiology (Gram's stain, AFB stain, culture, CIE)
≥25	Heparin container	Cytology (Papanicolaou's stain, cell block)

Note: A blood specimen should be obtained simultaneously for serum total protein, lactate dehydrogenase, glucose, and amylase when indicated.

*Smaller amounts of fluid may be adequate, depending on the instruments available and the type of tests requested.

Abbreviations: EDTA = ethylenediaminotetraacetic acid; AFB = acid-fast bacilli; CIE = counterimmunoelectrophoresis.

amined immediately and handled as a "STAT" specimen. Examination of synovial fluid for crystals should also be carried out as soon as possible. Even though all body fluid specimens should be examined promptly, satisfactory smears for morphologic examination can be made up to 24 hours after collection of pleural, peritoneal, and synovial fluid samples. Fluids containing large numbers of RBCs show more rapid cell deterioration than clear fluids. Leftover fluid should not be discarded because it may be difficult to obtain another specimen. Leftover specimens should be stored in the refrigerator in case additional tests are requested. Microbiologic examination must, however, be performed on fresh, nonrefrigerated specimens, as organisms such as *Neisseria meningitidis* will be destroyed by refrigeration.

The routine analysis of body fluids consists of (1) gross examination, (2) total cell count, (3) differential cell count and search for abnormal cells and crystals, (4) microbiologic examination, (5) chemical analysis, and (6) cytologic examination. Most of the methods used for these laboratory examinations have been mentioned in the main text or referred to in the references. In this appendix, we will describe in detail some of the more commonly used laboratory methods for analysis of body fluids. Seminal fluid analysis will be discussed in Appendix B.

MANUAL CELL COUNT

Diluents

NOTE: Asterisked solutions contain acetic acid, which will clump mucin and fluids that have a high protein content. Such solutions should not be used in analysis of synovial fluids.

1. *Saline* (Both WBCs and RBCs are preserved.)
2. *Gower's solution** for RBCs
   a. Add 12.5 g of sodium sulfate to 33.3 mL of glacial acetic acid and dilute with water to 200 mL.
3. *Türk's solution** for WBCs
   a. Add 3 mL of acetic acid to 1 mL of a 1% gentian violet solution diluted with water to 100 mL.
4. *Hyaluronidase diluent*
   a. Weigh and place the following in a 250-mL flask: 0.1 g of dextrose, 0.02 g of toluidine blue O, and 0.025 g of hyaluronidase (Type 1-S, Sigma Chemical Co.).
   b. Prepare buffer solutions:
      1. Potassium phosphate monobasic buffer (good for three months at room temperature): Dilute 2.279 g of potassium phosphate monobasic (FW 136.09) with distilled water to 250 mL (0.067 M).
      2. Sodium phosphate dibasic buffer (0.067 M): Dilute 9.511 g of sodium phosphate dibasic (FW 141.96) with distilled water to 1,000 mL. The buffer will be good for three months in refrigerator.
   c. Mix diluent by combining 6.5 mL of potassium phosphate monobasic (0.067 M), 43.5 mL of sodium phosphate dibasic (0.067 M), and 6.5 mL of absolute methanol. Add to the solution prepared in 4a and swirl to mix well.
   d. Store counting diluent in refrigerator in a tightly stoppered bottle. Filter before use; the so-

lution is good for one week at room temperature or for three months at 4 °C.

5. *Absolute basophil diluent*

a. Dissolve 0.42 g of toluidine blue O in 40 mL of a 0.85% saline solution.

b. Make a saturated solution of saponin in a 50% methanol solution and allow excess saponin to settle until clear; do not centrifuge or filter.

c. Mix together 40 mL of toluidine blue O solution, 11 mL of absolute methanol, and 1 mL of saponin solution. Store in refrigerator and filter before use with slow-speed paper. (Other methods for lysing RBCs include dilution with a 0.3% saline solution, 0.1 N hydrochloric acid, or a 1% saponin-in-saline solution.)

NOTE: This diluent is particularly useful for grossly bloody specimens. It lyses the RBCs and stains the WBCs.

Comments

Synovial fluids are often highly viscous or mucoid and may be difficult to work with. The addition of hyaluronidase in phosphate buffer (see #4 under "Manual Cell Count") will reduce the viscosity, making the fluid easier to pipette and resulting in a more even cell distribution. Add 1 drop of a 0.05% hyaluronidase-in-phosphate buffer (50 mg of hyaluronidase to 100 mL of buffer; see p 154, step 4b1 for buffer preparation) to each milliliter of synovial fluid, mix, and wait four minutes; then dilute with buffered diluent, as described previously.

Clotting of the fluid invalidates the results of a cell count. If the fluid clots, the clinician should be notified immediately. The specimen, however, should not be discarded. If the clinician insists on having the cell count done, it should be noted on the report that the specimen was clotted. A laboratory procedure to follow in analyzing body fluids is illustrated in Figure 171.

CELL COUNT IN A HEMACYTOMETER

1. The fluid should first be thoroughly mixed. Using an improved Neubauer hemacytometer counting chamber, the fluid is added undiluted and covered with a thick coverslip. Both sides of the hemacytometer should be filled with fluid and counted to ensure accuracy.

FIGURE 171. *Examination of body fluids.*

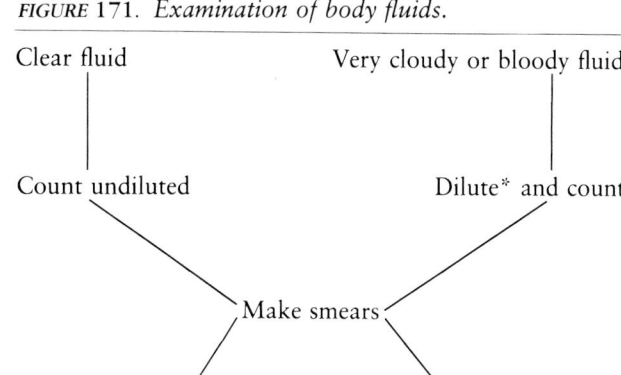

Clear fluid — Count undiluted

Very cloudy or bloody fluid — Dilute* and count

Make smears

Wright's stain

Wright's stain
Gram's stain

*1 : 10 dilution on slightly cloudy fluids
1 : 20 dilution on moderately cloudy fluids
1 : 100 dilution on very cloudy or bloody fluids (lyse RBCs if necessary).

FIGURE 172. *Neubauer hemacytometer for counting RBCs and WBCs.*

HEMACYTOMETER
(Neubauer ruling of chamber)

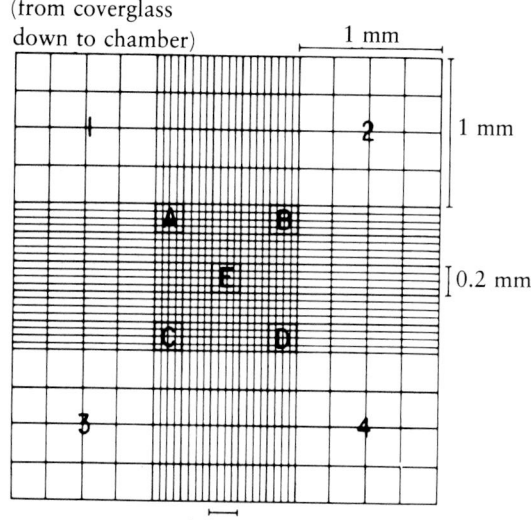

0.1 mm deep
(from coverglass
down to chamber)

Hemacytometer calculations:

$$\frac{\text{no. of cells counted} \times \text{dilution}}{\text{no. of squares counted} \times \text{volume of each square}} = \text{Total cells/μl}$$

1, 2, 3, 4 = WBC counting squares;
each has a volume of 0.1 μl
A, B, C, D, E = RBC counting squares;
each has a volume of 0.004 μl

---

2. If the fluid is not too thick (ie, if there is no overlapping of cells), count the undiluted specimen. Count the RBCs and WBCs on both sides of the chamber and average the two counts.

3. If the cells are too numerous to count, the fluid must be diluted according to the number of cells present, using an RBC or WBC pipette (eg, 1:10, 1:100). Let the dilutions stand in the pipette for five minutes before putting fluid in the chamber.

    a. When counting RBCs, dilute with Gower's solution, saline, or hyaluronidase diluent. These diluents do not remove the WBCs.

    b. When counting WBCs, use Türk's solution or hyaluronidase diluent.

4. With grossly bloody fluids, RBCs may be lysed with absolute basophil diluent prior to the WBC count. For RBC counts, a dilution of 1:100 or 1:200 is made with a cell-counting diluent.

5. The number of cells present determines the area to be counted (Figure 172).

    a. If there are numerous cells, those in the smaller squares in the center of the chamber (RBC area) should be counted. Five RBC squares should be counted.

    b. If the cells are less numerous, the larger four WBC areas of the chamber may be counted.

    c. When only a few cells are present, the entire chamber should be counted.

6. Cells in the hemacytometer appear as follows:

RBCs: Distinct outline with halo and clear centers. If crenated, they have many fine-pointed projections.

WBCs: Granular.

Tissue cells: Usually large granular cells with irregular outlines. Broken cells or tissue cells should not be included in the total count.

NOTE: Cell counts should always be verified by Wright's-stained smears.

7. Calculation of results should be based on the following formula:

Total cells/μL =

$$\frac{\text{No. of cells} \times \text{dilution}}{\text{No. of squares counted} \times \text{volume of each square}}$$

This formula represents only one of the many methods used for calculating results. Examples are as follows:

    a. RBC square volume = 0.004 μL

Thirty RBCs were found in five squares of the RBC-counting area when the fluid was diluted by 1:10.

$$\frac{30 \times 10}{5 \times 0.004} = 15{,}000 \text{ RBCs/}\mu\text{L}$$

b. WBC square volume = 0.1 μL
One hundred twenty WBCs were found in the four WBC-counting areas on an undiluted fluid.

$$\frac{120 \times 1}{4 \times 0.1} = 300 \text{ WBCs/}\mu\text{L}$$

c. Entire chamber volume = 0.9 μL
Twenty-five WBCs were counted in the entire chamber on an undiluted fluid specimen.

$$\frac{25 \times 1}{9 \times 0.1} = 28 \text{ WBCs/}\mu\text{L}$$

ELECTRONIC CELL COUNT

Electronic cell counters should not be used for CSF analysis since the background counts cause poor precision in the normal range. Also, many laboratory scientists recommend that electronic counting equipment not be used for any serous fluid analysis, as cellular debris may cause false elevation of the cell count. Nevertheless, many laboratories use them (eg, Coulter electronic counters, Coulter Electronics Inc.) routinely for pleural, peritoneal, and joint fluids.

In analyzing serous fluids, we have found little disagreement between manual and instrument leukocyte counts, but much disparity between manual and instrument RBC counts. Direct aspiration through the sample valve on a Coulter counter is recommended unless the fluid is viscous or contains fibrin clots. If the fluid is viscous or contains clots or only a small amount of fluid is received, a 1:224 dilution (44.7 μL of fluid plus 1 mL of Isoton) should be used, and the sampling valve should be bypassed by use of the microsampler.

Since most electronic counters (such as Coulter) have a background cell count that ranges from zero to approximately 200/μL, WBC counts should be done manually if the count is less than 300/μL. The amount of background varies with the reagents used and with each instrument. Therefore, the background count should be checked daily and deducted from the cell count obtained. Less than 30,000 RBCs/μL should be counted manually. From a practical standpoint, it is most helpful to estimate the number of cells present by examining a drop of undiluted fluid in a counting chamber. A decision can then be made as to how the cell count should be done and what dilutions, if any, may be necessary. An experienced technologist may also, based on gross examination of the specimen, be able to determine how the specimen should best be handled.

It must be remembered that electronic counters count most cells, including histiocytes, macrophages, mesothelial cells, and tumor cells, if present, and the total cell count may have to be adjusted, depending on the cell types seen on smears. Thus if many mesothelial cells, histiocytes, or macrophages are present, this should be indicated in the differential cell count report. (Depending on the threshold setting of the instrument, some of the large mesothelial cells and macrophages may not be counted by an automated electric counter.) No matter which procedure is used, the clinician must know which counting policy has been followed for the laboratory report.

DIFFERENTIAL CELL COUNT

A differential cell count should be performed on stained smears made from concentrated leukocytes and not in the hemacytometer. Numerous methods have been described for concentrating the cells in body fluids. These include centrifugation with smears made from the resuspended sediment, sedimentation,[1-5] centrifugation,[6-8] and filtration[5] methods.

Ordinary centrifugation with staining of the sediment, the routine of the past, has the advantage of requiring no special equipment. There is, however, a variable recovery of cells with this method, and considerable cellular damage occurs during centrifugation, with resultant difficulty in preparing good-quality smears.

The filter techniques using Millipore (Millipore Corp.), Nucleopore (Nucleopore), or Gelman (Gelman Instrument Co.) filters allow excellent recovery of cells. However, it is more time-consuming than some of the other methods, and considerably more skill is required to prepare a satisfactory specimen. The cytocentrifuge method has many advantages and

FIGURE 173. *Cytocentrifuge instrument.*

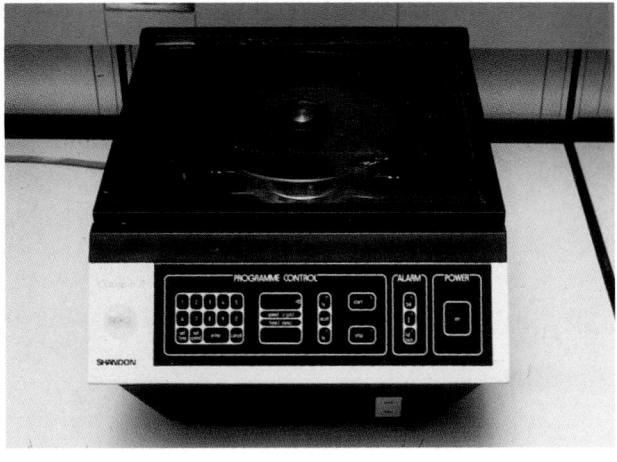

FIGURE 174. *Placement of cytocentrifuge cup with slide and filter paper into centrifuge.*

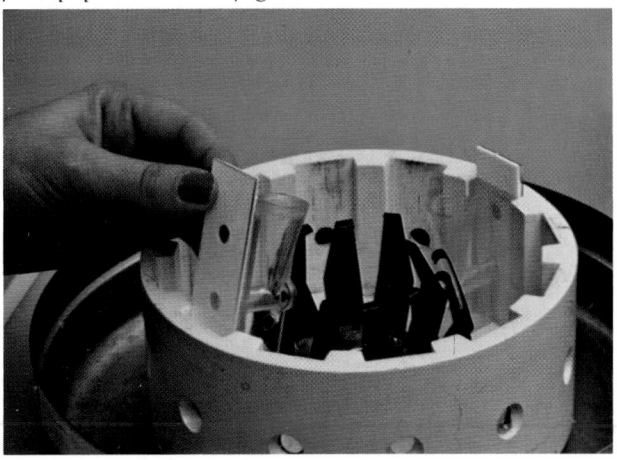

FIGURE 175. *Addition of drops of fluid to cytocentrifuge cup.*

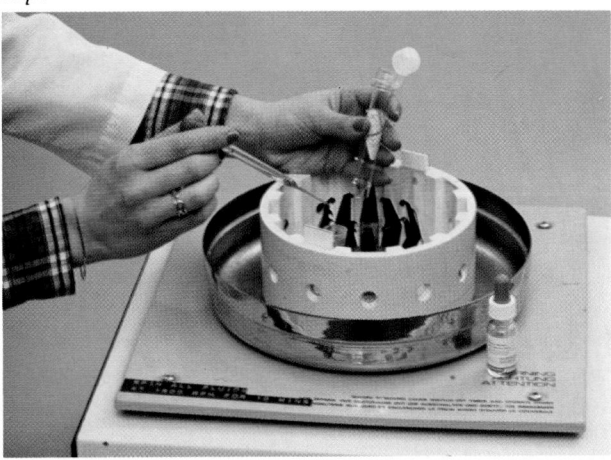

is now widely used. The cell yield is satisfactory, though not as good as that with filter techniques. The centrifugation produces a certain amount of distortion of the cell structure, which will be discussed later.

Several sedimentation methods have been described that provide high-quality smears, but the cell yield is usually not as good, and these methods are more time-consuming than the cytocentrifuge method.

CYTOCENTRIFUGE METHOD

Depending on the appearance and type of fluid, varied amounts may be used: clear fluid, 5 to 10 drops; cloudy fluid, 1 to 3 drops. When the fluid is bloody, a 1:5 dilution with saline is used. When it is grossly bloody, a push smear is recommended. Figure 173 depicts one type of cytocentrifuge instrument.

1. Place the cytocentrifuge cups into the centrifuge (Shandon cytocentrifuge, Shandon Southern Instruments Inc.) opposite each other. Smears should be made in duplicate.

2. Label the slides with patient's name, hospital number, date, and type of fluid.

3. Place special filter paper against a glass slide in back of the cup, making certain the hole in the cup lines up with the hole in the carrier (Figure 174).

4. Put the drops of fluid into the cup with a Pasteur pipette (Figure 175).

5. Add 2 drops of 22% albumin to reduce the cell distortion and to increase the yield.

6. Lock the lid into position, and spin at 1,000 rpm for approximately five minutes.

7. Carefully remove the slides and filter papers together. Mark a circle around the concentrate on the back of the slide with a crayon (Figure 176).

8. Air-dry slides before staining.

9. Stain the slides with Wright's stain, or other stains when indicated, and coverslip (Figure 177). If a malignant disorder, such as leukemia, lymphoma, or carcinoma, is suspected, several extra unstained slides should be made for possible tumor marker studies.

10. Perform a differential cell count. If it is possible, count 100 cells; if not, count all cells present in the concentrate. Mesothelial cells, histiocytes, and macrophages may or may not be included in the differential cell count and may be lumped together into an "others" category, or a percentage of each cell type

may be given. Some laboratorians prefer to indicate the number of mesothelial cells, macrophages, etc, as "few," "moderate," or "many." (In most instances, there is no clinical use in counting the number of mesothelial cells and macrophages.)

11. Cytocentrifuge cups should be soaked in a 5% bleach solution for 15 minutes for decontamination. The cups are then washed in soapy water, rinsed well in tap water and distilled water, and finally air-dried.

Comments

Variable cellular distortion is frequently seen with the cytocentrifuge method. The cells near the center of the circle of cells are often smaller and have less cytoplasm and denser nuclear chromatin than those at the periphery (Figures 178 and 179). Cytoplasmic distortion may be seen, with the formation of irregular cytoplasmic processes (Figure 180). Considerable nuclear distortion, such as clefting or lobulation, may be seen in cytocentrifuge preparations (Figure 181). Other artifacts frequently encountered are the peripheral localization of nuclear lobes in polymorphonuclear leukocytes (Figure 182), the presence of acidophilic or amphophilic paranuclear zones in mononuclear cells, peripheral cytoplasmic vacuolation, localization of cytoplasmic granules, and holes in the nuclei (Figure 183). An acidophilic paranuclear zone and localization of cytoplasmic granules may make it difficult to distinguish lymphocytes from monocytes; and sometimes these cells resemble myelocytes (Figure 184). Nucleoli often appear more prominent in cytocentrifuge preparations than in regular push smears (Figures 179 and 185). A combination of cell transformation occurring in the fluid and centrifuge distortion may make it difficult to recognize the cell line (Figure 186). Clumping together of benign cells, such as mesothelial cells and lymphocytes (Figure 187), is occasionally seen. Such clumps of cells may be mistaken for tumor cells. (See chapters on pleural and peritoneal fluids.) The cellular distortions are not, however, usually troublesome to an experienced observer.

To delay fluid absorption and increase cellular yield, a small amount of immersion oil may be spread around the hole of the filter paper (1 cm in diameter) prior to centrifugation. The speed and time of centrifugation may be varied to ensure maximum cell

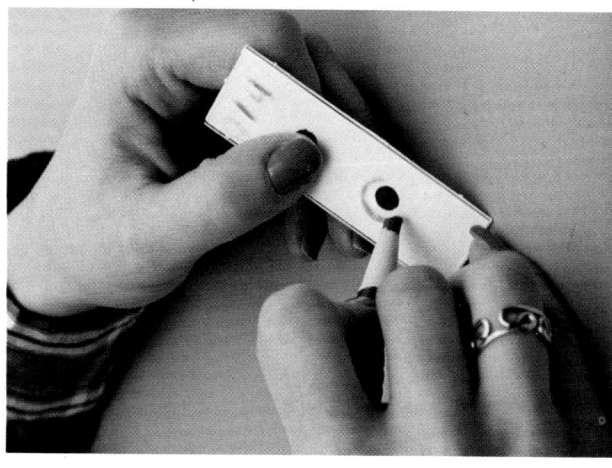

FIGURE 176. *Back of glass slide being marked with crayon to indicate area of cell concentrate.*

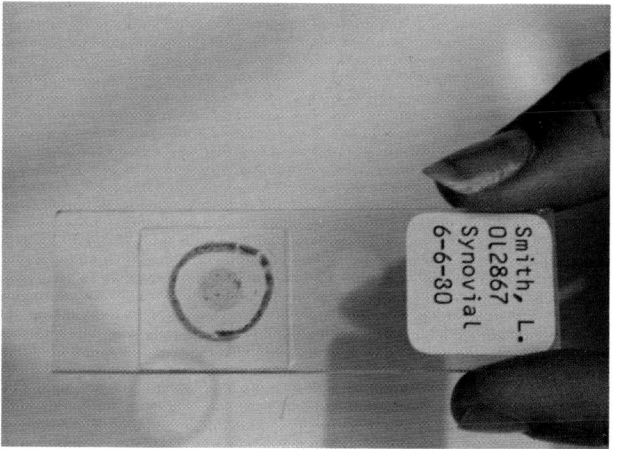

FIGURE 177. *Stained smear made from a cytocentrifuge.*

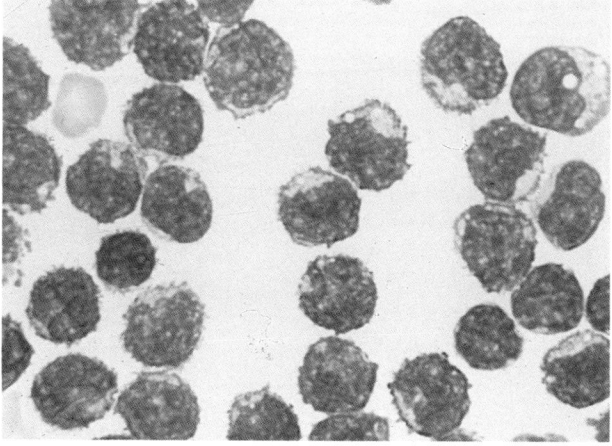

FIGURE 178. *Small lymphocytes present in center of "cell button" made by a cytocentrifuge.*

FIGURE 179. *Appearance of same small lymphocytes seen in Figure 178 but in the periphery of the "cell button." Note how cytoplasm is more abundant, nuclei are more irregular with less clumping of the chromatin, and nucleoli are distinct. The cell appears less mature than in Figure 178.*

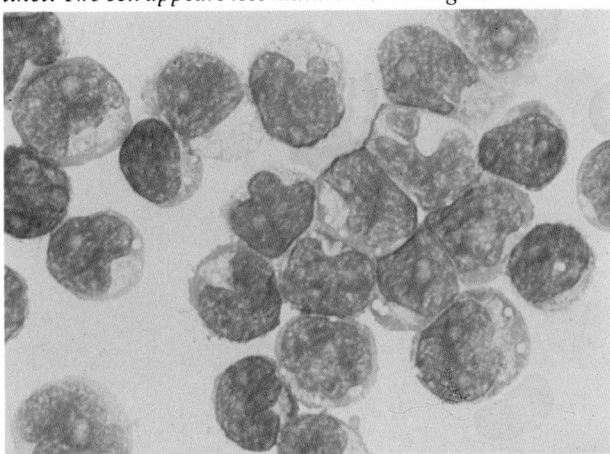

FIGURE 182. *Peripheral localization of nuclear segments in neutrophils, a common cytocentrifuge artifact.*

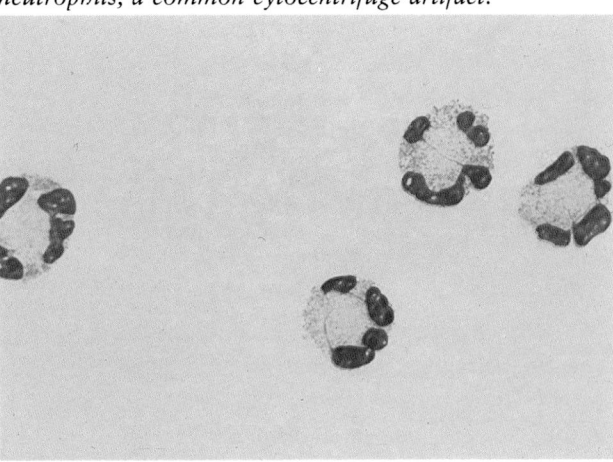

FIGURE 180. *Prominent cytoplasmic processes seen as a result of centrifuge artifact.*

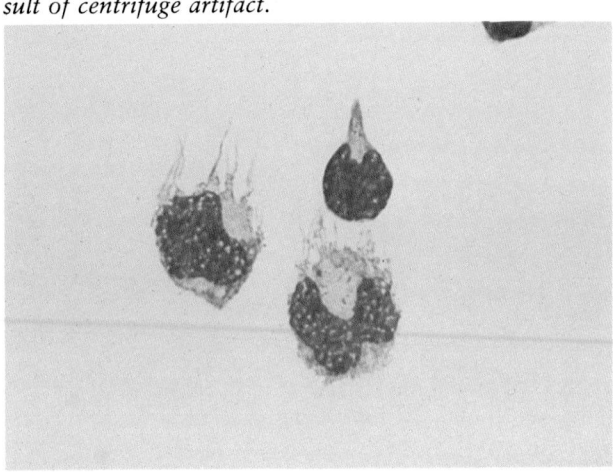

FIGURE 183. *Artifact holes in the nuclei of mononuclear cells in the CSF.*

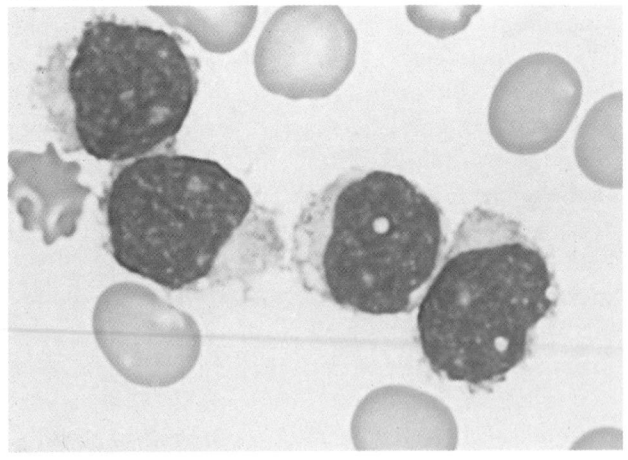

FIGURE 181. *Nuclear irregularities of lymphocytes. Cytocentrifuge artifact.*

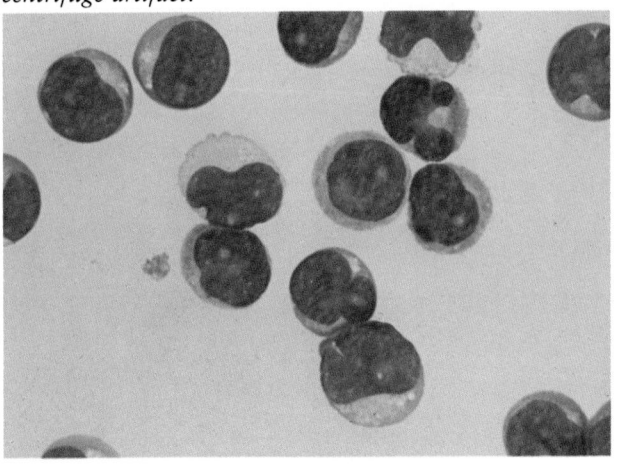

FIGURE 184. *Distortion of lymphocytes, giving them the appearance of monocytes.*

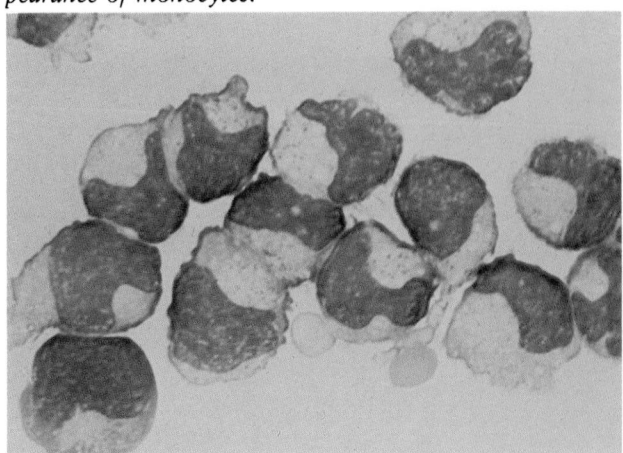

FIGURE 185. *Distinct "nucleoli" in small, mature-appearing lymphocytes.*

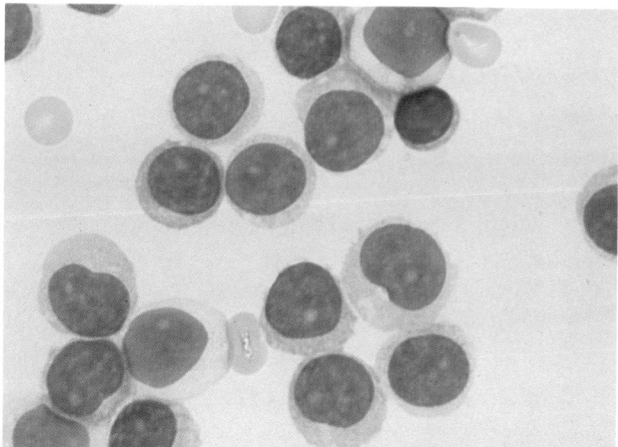

FIGURE 188. *Equipment used for concentrating cells with the sedimentation method.*

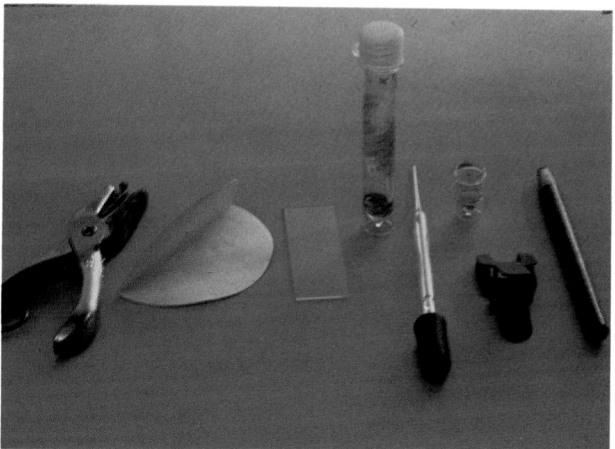

FIGURE 186. *Leukemic cells in pleural fluid sample from a patient with acute myeloblastic leukemia. Notice the large size of the blast cells in comparison with a mesothelial cell and the distortion of the nuclei.*

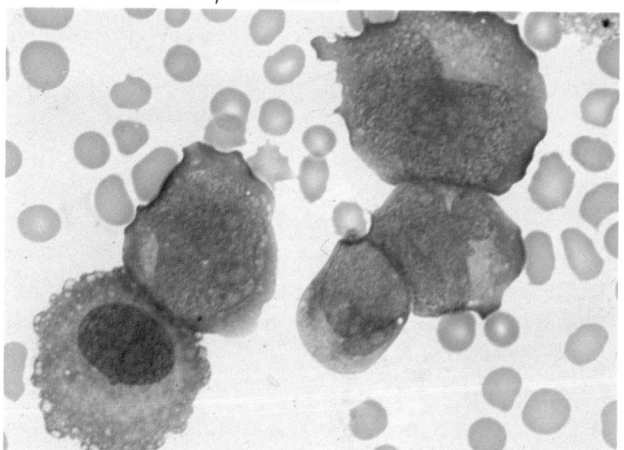

FIGURE 187. *Cluster of lymphocytes resembling malignant cells (oat cell carcinoma). Centrifuge artifact.*

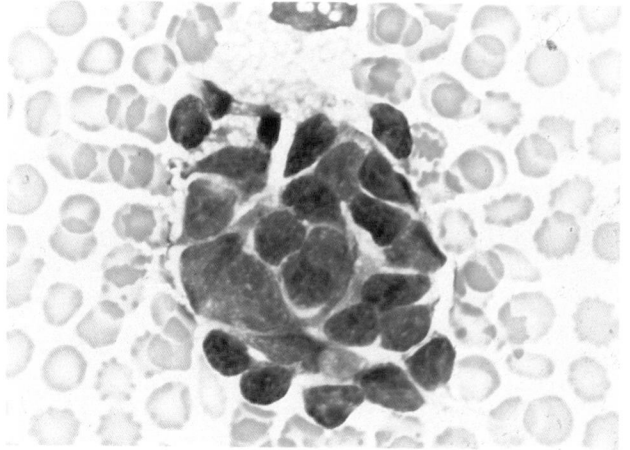

FIGURE 189. *Preparation of the smear using the sedimentation method.*

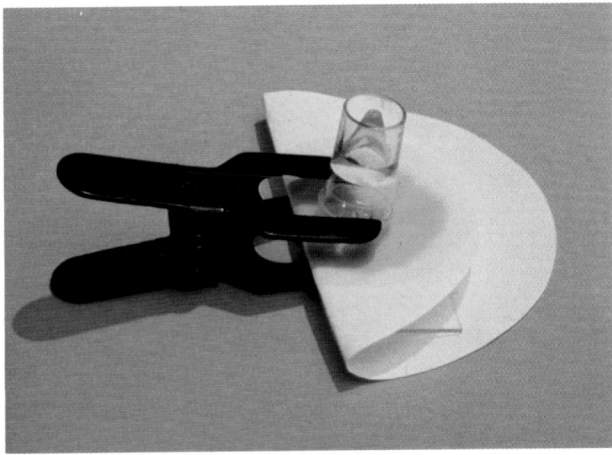

FIGURE 190. *The finished specimen, using the sedimentation method, prior to the staining of the smear.*

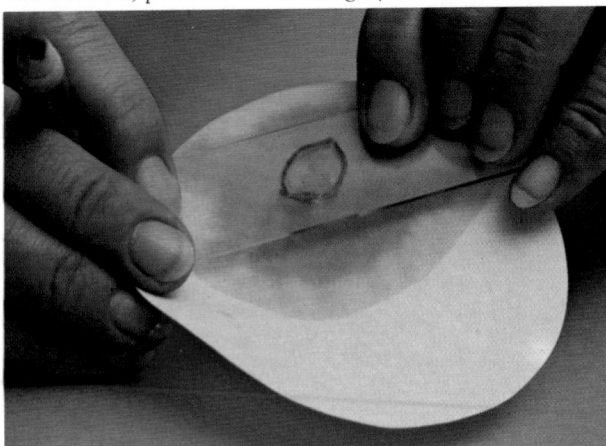

yield and optimum cell preservation. This is best established by each laboratory.

SEDIMENTATION METHOD

Equipment needed for the sedimentation method[1] is featured in Figure 188. The method is carried out as follows:

1. Punch a round hole approximately 1 cm in diameter in the center of a 9-cm (Whatman No. 2, W & R) filter paper.

2. Wrap the filter paper around a microscope slide so that the hole is in the center of the slide.

3. Transfer 0.2 to 1.0 mL of fresh fluid into a shallow, disposable, 1.8-mL plastic cup (Matheson Scientific Co). The amount of fluid used depends on cell concentration.

4. Center the hole on the wrapped slide over the mouth of the cup. The slide should cover the cup mouth completely.

5. Hold the cup and slide together with one hand. With the other hand, slide a No. 18 ball-and-socket joint pinch clamp (Arthur H. Thomas Co.) onto the slide, placing one blade on the clamp above the slide and the other beneath the ledge around the lip of the cup.

6. After the cup and the slide are secured, turn the entire setup over so that the cup is inverted (Figure 189). Allow the fluid to settle for 20 to 30 minutes. The fluid is absorbed by the filter paper, and the cells settle on the exposed surface of the slide. The more fluid there is, the longer it takes to absorb.

7. When the cup is empty, carefully remove the cup and paper and allow the slide to air-dry for a few minutes (Figure 190).

8. Stain the slide.

Comments

Many types of relatively new sedimentation methods have been described, particularly for use in CSF cytologic examination.[1-5]

EXAMINATION OF SYNOVIAL FLUID FOR CRYSTALS

Synovial fluid should be viewed when it is relatively fresh. A small drop is placed on a glass slide, and a coverslip is placed over the top and sealed with petroleum jelly or nail polish to delay drying. The glass slide and coverslip should be cleaned with alcohol and dried with clean gauze prior to placing the specimen on the slide. Crystals may also be seen in stained smears but are more difficult to detect.

The specimens should be examined with a good polarizing microscope (Figure 146), which contains two polarizing lenses and a quartz compensator. In such a microscope, one polarizer is situated below the condenser, and a second polarizing lens is located above the objective and is called the analyzer. A first-order red compensator is placed between the polarizer and the analyzer and separates light into components of slow and fast vibration. This allows visualization of differences in the birefringent properties of monosodium urate and calcium pyrophosphate crystals.

The specimen is first examined with polarized light, without the red compensator. Some examiners prefer to examine the slide initially with compensated polarized light. The specimen is first examined under low power (10× objective). The light intensity is varied, but it should not be too strong, since this may "wash out" the crystals. This is especially true for calcium pyrophosphate crystals. The polarizer or analyzer is rotated until the field is dark. The slide is scanned under low power for WBCs or fibrils to focus on. When crystals have been identified under low power, the crystals should be examined under high dry objective (40×) or under oil using a 100× objective. The number of crystals present is estimated as few, moderate, or many, and the crystals are described as intracellular, extracellular, or both. Sometimes it takes a very careful search of cells to identify calcium pyrophosphate crystals because they are less brilliant than monosodium urate crystals. Clumps of cells and debris where crystals may be trapped should also be examined.

Monosodium urate crystals appear as very bright needles or rods varying from 1 to 30 μm in length. The monosodium urate crystals from a tophus may be particularly large. The crystals may be intracellular or extracellular (Figures 147 and 148) and may occasionally take the form of spherules.

Calcium pyrophosphate crystals measure from 1 to 20 μm in length and up to 4 μm in width. They may be rectangular or rhomboidal or, occasionally, needle-

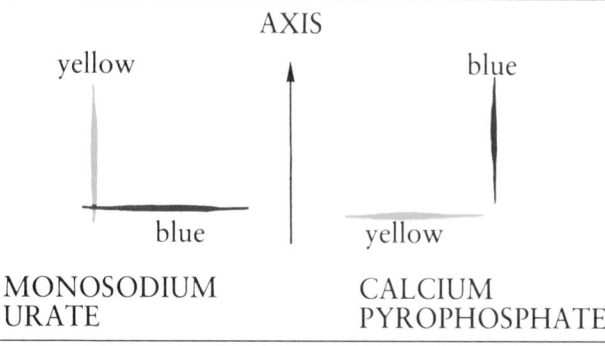

FIGURE 191. *Two-dimensional schematic representation of monosodium urate and calcium pyrophosphate crystals when viewed under polarized light and red compensator.*

shaped (Figures 155 and 156). The calcium pyrophosphate crystals are much less bright than the monosodium urate crystals and may therefore be missed.

When crystals have been identified with polarized light, the separation of urate from calcium pyrophosphate crystals can be carried out by using a first-order red compensator. With the compensator in place, the field background appears red instead of black. The orientation of the crystals to the axis of the compensator determines their color. The long axis of the crystal is lined up parallel to the axis of slow vibration of the compensator (parallel to the compensator) by rotating the stage of the microscope. If the crystal appears blue in this position, the crystal is calcium pyrophosphate and shows positive birefringence. If the crystal appears yellow in this position, it is a monosodium urate crystal, which shows negative birefringence. When the stage is rotated 90° so that the long axis is perpendicular to the axis of the slow vibration of the compensator, monosodium urate crystals turn from yellow to blue, while calcium pyrophosphate crystals turn from blue to yellow (Figure 191).

Crystal identification can also be accomplished without a rotating stage. Some microscopes are arranged so that the compensator rather than the crystal is rotated. This works well for identifying crystals that are parallel or perpendicular to the axis of the compensator. The color of the crystal in one position is noted, then the compensator is rotated 90° while the color change is observed. This type of system, however, does not work when crystals are at an oblique angle to the axis of the compensator. Oblique crystals must be rotated, and this can be done by moving the stage clip back and rotating the slide with the fingers. Moving the slide while observing the crystal with a low-power (10×) objective will help to keep track of the crystal. When many crystals are present, the process is simpler, since one need find only one crystal in the right position.

Optical designs of microscopes vary considerably from manufacturer to manufacturer. Therefore, the color that crystals assume in a particular direction may differ, depending on the type of microscope used. It is important to follow the manufacturer's directions and to use control slides. Also, with multi-headed microscopes, the direction or position of the image may vary from one microscope head to another.

In summary, monosodium urate crystals are needle-shaped and strongly birefringent under polarized light and show a yellow (negative) sign of birefringence when examined with a first-order red compensator. Calcium pyrophosphate crystals may be rod-shaped, needle-shaped, or appear as plates. They are weakly birefringent with polarized light and give a blue (positive) sign of birefringence with a red compensator.

Under polarized light, corticosteroids may appear identical to monosodium urate or calcium pyrophosphate crystals. Therefore, it is essential to know whether a previous intra-articular injection was given. Such crystals may be present in synovial fluid for a month or longer following the injection.

Cholesterol crystals appear as strongly birefringent plates, often with notched margins (Figure 159). Like monosodium urate and calcium pyrophosphate crystals, they may occasionally have the appearance of needles or rhomboids (Figures 162 through 164).

Fragments of cartilage may also appear birefringent under polarized light but have irregular margins, in contrast to the distinct, smooth, parallel margins of monosodium urate or calcium pyrophosphate crystals. Other birefringent materials include dirt from unclean glassware and talcum crystals (Figures 165 through 168). The latter have a Maltese-cross appearance (Figures 166 and 167).

Comments

When several crystals are present, as may occur when a tophus has been aspirated, it is easy to identify the type of crystal present. Frequently, however, the number of crystals is small, and several slides have to be carefully examined. It is recommended that a good polarizing microscope with a rotating stage be available. A satisfactory system can be devised by purchasing a polarizer set that includes a red compensator and adding that to a standard laboratory microscope.

A control or reference slide is extremely useful. A reference slide can be made from a smear of monosodium urate crystal that has been aspirated from a tophus. Such a slide will last for several years. A suspension of betamethasone acetate corticosteroid, which has an appearance similar to that of monosodium urate crystals under compensated polarized light, may also be used as a control slide.[9] The control slides should be rimmed with nail polish or a similar sealing material.

REFERENCES

1. Tang TT, McCreadie SR: A simplified method for the cytologic study of body fluids. *Am J Clin Pathol* 59:113–116, 1973

2. Chu JY, Freiling P, Wassilak S: Simple method for the cytologic examination of cerebrospinal fluid. *J Clin Pathol* 30:486–487, 1977

3. Nishimura K, Hosoya R, Nakajima K: Sedimentation cytology in central nervous system leukaemia with a new simple apparatus. *Br J Haematol* 40:583–586, 1978

4. Kolmel HW: *Atlas of Cerebrospinal Fluid Cells*, ed 2. New York, Springer-Verlag, 1977

5. Oehmichen M: *Cerebrospinal Fluid Cytology: An Introduction and Atlas*. Philadelphia, WB Saunders Co, 1976

6. Hoeltge GA, Furlan A, Hoffman GC: The differential cytology of cerebrospinal fluids prepared by cytocentrifugation. *Cleve Clin Q* 43:237–246, 1976

7. Evans DIK, O'Rourk C, Jones PM: The cerebrospinal fluid in acute leukemia of childhood: Studies with the cytocentrifuge. *J Clin Pathol* 27:226–230, 1974

8. Choi HH, Anderson PJ: Diagnostic cytology of cerebrospinal fluid by the cytocentrifuge method. *Am J Clin Pathol* 72:931–943, 1979

9. Krieg AF: Cerebrospinal fluid and other body fluids, in Henry JB (ed): *Clinical Diagnosis and Management by Laboratory Methods*, ed 16. Philadelphia, WB Saunders Co, 1979, pp 635–679

Analysis of Seminal Fluid

Written by Ronald Urry, PhD
University of Utah School of Medicine

Ideally, the seminal fluid should be analyzed within 30 minutes of collection. If this is not possible, the specimen should be kept warm at approximately 37 °C and examined within one to two hours of collection.

TEST FOR VOLUME OF SEMINAL FLUID

Materials

1. Pasteur pipette
2. Test tube (with lock-on cap)
3. Measuring test tube, same size as test tube, marked out in 0.5-mL intervals

Procedure

1. Approximately 30 minutes after collection of the sample, transfer the semen sample with the pipette from the collection container to the test tube.
2. Place the measuring tube next to the test tube filled with semen and record the approximate volume.

Comments

Normal volume is 2 to 5 mL.

TEST FOR VISCOSITY OF SEMINAL FLUID

After liquefaction, the semen is pipetted into a test tube. With normal viscosity, the semen forms discrete droplets as it is falling into the tube. Increased viscosity varies from progressive stringiness to a jelly-like coagulum that cannot be poured.

TEST FOR VIABILITY OF SPERM

Materials

1. Microscope slides (three per sample)
2. 10% aqueous nigrosin
3. 5% aqueous eosin Y
4. Wooden applicator stick
5. Microscope

Procedure

PREPARATION OF THE SLIDE

1. Label two slides with patient's name and date.
2. Place a drop of semen on one slide.
3. Add 2 drops of a 5% eosin Y solution.
4. Stir with applicator stick for about 30 seconds.
5. Add 3 drops of a 10% nigrosin solution.
6. Transfer about one half the volume of the semen-stain mixture to another slide.
7. Hold a blank slide at a 45° angle to the slide holding the semen-stain mixture, and smear the semen-stain mixture the length of the slide.
8. Dry on a hot plate at about 37 °C until slide is dry. *Remove immediately.*

SPERM VIABILITY

Spermatozoa that are alive will not stain and will appear white (Figure 123). Dead spermatozoa stain pink (Figure 124). With a 40 × objective, count 200 spermatozoa on each slide for a total of 400 spermatozoa. Record the percentage of live and dead spermatozoa present.

Comments

Normally, at least 50% of the spermatozoa should be alive.

SPERM COUNT

Materials

1. Diluting pipettes
2. Hemacytometer
3. Cell counter
4. Sodium bicarbonate
5. Formaldehyde (a 37% solution)

Procedure

1. Estimate the dilution factor, based on an estimate of the number of sperm:

    For 0 to 3 million sperm, dilute 1:10

    For 3 to 20 million sperm, dilute 1:20

    For 20 to 40 million sperm, dilute 1:100

    For 40 million or more sperm, dilute 1:200

2. Vortex sample thoroughly (about half a minute).
3. Diluting solution is made up by mixing the following: 5 g of sodium bicarbonate, 1 mL of formaldehyde, and 100 mL of distilled water.
4. Make an appropriate dilution, depending on the sperm count estimate. Mix for 45 seconds on pipette shaker (longer for specimens in which the spermatozoa agglutinate). Expel the first few drops before loading both sides of the hemacytometer. The hemacytometer is put into a humidified chamber for a couple of minutes to allow the cells to settle.
5. Count all spermatozoa in the four WBC squares and calculate the number of spermatozoa per milliliter.
6. Multiply the sperm count by the ejaculate volume to get the total number of spermatozoa.

Comment

This method is relatively imprecise, and duplicate sperm counts by one technician usually vary by 15% to 25%. When the semen viscosity is greatly increased, counting will be facilitated by diluting the semen 1:1 with a mucolytic agent (such as Alevaire, Breon Laboratories Inc.) or α-amylase prior to the pipette dilution.[1]

TEST FOR MOTILITY OF SPERMATOZOA

Materials

1. Microscope slide
2. Cover slip
3. Pipette
4. Microscope (40× objective)
5. Capped test tube

Procedure

1. About 30 minutes after collection, transfer semen to a capped test tube and gently invert about ten times to ensure mixing.

2. Pipette 1 drop of semen onto a slide and coverslip.

3. Observe the spermatozoa with a 40× objective, and estimate the percentages of spermatozoa moving at the following speeds (identified by grade):

GRADE	TYPE OF SPERM MOTILITY
0	Not moving
1	Moving with no forward progression
2	Moving with slow, meandering movement
3	Moving rapidly in almost straight line
4	Moving with high speed in straight line

4. Obtain a motility score by adding together the products of the percentages at each grade times the grade, as in the following example:

GRADE	PERCENTAGE OF SPERMATOZOA	× GRADE	= MOTILITY
0	30	0	0
1	5	1	5
2	10	2	20
3	25	3	75
4	30	4	120
Total motility score			220

Comment

Using this method, the motility score for spermatozoa in a normal specimen is 150 or higher.

MORPHOLOGIC ANALYSIS OF SPERMATOZOA

Procedure (hematoxylin-eosin stain)

PREPARATION OF SMEAR

1. Vortex the semen sample.

2. Label two slides with patient's name and date.

3. Place 1 drop of semen on the labeled slide.

4. Hold a blank slide at a 45° angle to the labeled slide, and smear the drop of semen the length of the slide.

5. Allow the smear to dry, either by placing it for a minute or two on a hot plate at 37 °C or by letting it dry for five to ten minutes at room temperature.

6. Store the slide in a Coplin jar filled with methanol until ready to stain.

7. Perform a standard hematoxylin-eosin stain.

MORPHOLOGIC COUNT

Under oil immersion, count 200 spermatozoa for each of the two hematoxylin-eosin–stained slides and classify the spermatozoa into the following morphological types (Figures 125 to 133):

TYPE	NORMAL LIMITS, %
Oval heads (normal spermatozoa)	>60
Large heads	<5
Small heads	<5
Tapered heads	<15
Immature spermatozoa (be careful to distinguish these from WBCs)	<15
Duplicate heads	<5
Amorphous spermatozoa	<15

FRUCTOSE TEST

Materials

1. Resorcinol
2. Hydrochloric acid

Preparation of the Resorcinol Reagent

1. Add 33 mL of hydrochloric acid to 50 mg of resorcinol.
2. Then add 67 mL of distilled water and mix.

Procedure

1. Place 0.1 mL of semen in a test tube.
2. Add 1 mL of resorcinol reagent.
3. Boil for five to ten minutes.

Comments

The solution turns reddish brown in the presence of fructose. No change in color indicates that fructose is absent from the semen. Fructose is absent in semen from patients with bilateral aplasia of the vasa deferentia and seminal vesicles and in bilateral obstruction of the ejaculatory ducts.

REFERENCE

1. Amelar R, Dubin L: *Semen Analysis in Male Fertility,* Amelar R, Dubin L, Walsh P (eds). Philadelphia, WB Saunders Co, 1977, pp 105–140

Manufacturers

Breon Laboratories Inc
Division of Sterling Drug
New York, NY 10016

Coulter Electronics Inc
Hialeah, FL 33010

Gelman Instrument Co
Ann Arbor, MI 48106

Hana Biologics, Inc
Berkeley, CA 94710

Matheson Scientific Co
Elk Grove Village, IL 60007

Millipore Corporation
Bedford, MA 01730

Nucleopore
Fairfax, CA 94930

Shandon Southern Instruments Inc
Sewickley, PA 15143

Sigma Chemical Co
St Louis, MO 63178

Arthur H. Thomas Co
Philadelphia, PA 10105

W & R
Balston, England

Key to Optional Slide Set

SLIDE 1

Summary of procedures that may be performed on amniotic fluid. *See Figure 3.*

SLIDE 2

Nile blue stain. Orange-yellow-staining cells are fetal epidermal cells. *See Figure 6.*

SLIDE 3

Barr body (X-chromatin), identified as a small condensation of chromatin (arrow) along the nuclear membrane (Papanicolaou's stain). *See Figure 7.*

SLIDE 4

Hemolytic disease of the newborn. A, Absorbance spectrum of normal amniotic fluid; and B, increased amniotic fluid bilirubin showing absorbance peak at 450 nm. *See Figure 8.*

SLIDE 5

Hemolytic disease of the newborn: prediction of severity. Zones (A, B, and C) indicate varying severity of disease when ΔA_{450} is plotted against gestational age. *See Figure 9.*

SLIDE 6

Hyaline membrane disease. Histologic section of lung showing air spaces lined by pink hyaline membranes with adjacent atelectasis (hematoxylin-eosin stain). *See Figure 10.*

SLIDE 7

α-Fetoprotein levels in amniotic fluid during gestation. (From Johansson et al. [chapter 1, reference 116] Used by permission.) *See Figure 12.*

SLIDE 8

α-Fetoprotein levels in maternal serum during gestation. (From Johansson et al. [chapter 1, reference 116] Used by permission.) *See Figure 13.*

SLIDE 9
Chorioamnionitis. Band of polymorphonuclear leukocytes is seen below the chorionic plate (arrows) (hematoxylin-eosin stain). *See Figure 14.*

SLIDE 10
Chorioamnionitis. The significance of this neutrophilic leukocytosis in the amniotic fluid is controversial. *See Figure 15.*

SLIDE 11
Normal CSF cells with small, normal-appearing lymphocytes. *See Figure 17.*

SLIDE 12
Monocytes in CSF from a newborn. *See Figure 18.*

SLIDE 13
A cluster of choroid plexus cells in CSF. *See Figure 20.*

SLIDE 14
A cluster of ependymal cells in CSF. *See Figure 21.*

SLIDE 15
Normal bone marrow cells in CSF resulting from accidental puncture of a vertebral body. *See Figure 22.*

SLIDE 16
Lymphocytes and plasmacytoid lymphocytes in the CSF from a patient with multiple sclerosis. *See Figure 24.*

SLIDE 17
Transformed (atypical) lymphocyte in CSF. *See Figure 25.*

SLIDE 18
CSF lymphocytosis in a partially treated case of bacterial meningitis. The large mononuclear cell (arrow) is a transformed lymphocyte or an immunoblast. *See Figure 26.*

SLIDE 19
Cluster of blast-like lymphocytes in CSF sample from a newborn. *See Figure 28.*

SLIDE 20
Signet-ring cell macrophage in CSF. *See Figure 30.*

SLIDE 21
Macrophage in CSF with phagocytosed RBCs appearing as empty holes, and hemosiderin pigment. *See Figure 32.*

SLIDE 22
Macrophage in CSF with hemosiderin (bluish-black) pigment and hematoidin pigment (yellow crystals). *See Figure 33.*

SLIDE 23
Several siderophages in CSF sample from a patient with repeated intracerebral hemorrhages. *See Figure 35.*

SLIDE 24
Neutrophils in CSF sample from a patient with bacterial meningitis. Degenerating cells with pyknotic nuclei may be mistaken for nucleated RBCs. *See Figure 37.*

SLIDE 25
Eosinophils and two basophils in CSF sample from a patient with malfunctioning intracranial shunt. *See Figure 39.*

SLIDE 26
Gram's stain showing intracellular gram-negative bacteria in CSF from a patient with *Hemophilus influenzae* meningitis. *See Figure 41.*

SLIDE 27
A spectrum of reactive (transformed) lymphocytes seen in the CSF in viral meningitis. *See Figure 45.*

SLIDE 28
Acute lymphoblastic leukemia in CSF. Note the uniformity of the blast cells. *See Figure 46.*

SLIDE 29
Acute myeloblastic leukemia in CSF. Easily identifiable myeloblasts are seen. *See Figure 47.*

SLIDE 30
Terminal deoxynucleotidyl transferase is seen on nuclei of blast cells from a patient with acute lymphoblastic leukemia (immunofluorescent method). *See Figure 49.*

SLIDE 31
Glioblastoma cells in CSF. *See Figure 51.*

SLIDE 32
Clustering of malignant cells in CSF in a patient with medulloblastoma. *See Figure 52.*

SLIDE 33
Clump of cells in CSF specimen from a patient with metastatic neuroblastoma. *See Figure 53.*

SLIDE 34
Typical "cannonball" formation of metastatic breast carcinoma. *See Figure 55.*

SLIDE 35
High-power view of breast tumor cells seen in Figure 34. *See Figure 56.*

SLIDE 36

Characteristic clumping of cells and molding of nuclei in metastatic oat cell carcinoma of the lung. *See Figure 58.*

SLIDE 37

Lymphoblastic lymphoma involving the CSF. The cells are similar to those seen in acute lymphoblastic leukemia. *See Figure 59.*

SLIDE 38

Burkitt's lymphoma in the CSF. The cells are characterized by deep blue cytoplasm with vacuoles and a slightly clumped chromatin pattern. *See Figure 60.*

SLIDE 39

Agarose gel electrophoresis of serum and CSF. Normal serum (A) and normal CSF (B) are compared with serum (C) and CSF samples (D) from a patient with multiple sclerosis. Arrows identify oligoclonal bands. *See Figure 61.*

SLIDE 40

Cryptococcus neoformans found in CSF sample from a patient receiving therapy for Hodgkin's disease. *See Figure 63.*

SLIDE 41

Summary of approach to laboratory investigation of pleural fluids. LD, lactic dehydrogenase. *See Figure 64.*

SLIDE 42

Two mesothelial cells in pleural fluid. *See Figure 67.*

SLIDE 43

Several mesothelial cells with more basophilic cytoplasm and several binucleated forms. *See Figure 69.*

SLIDE 44

Clump of mesothelial cells. *See Figure 70.*

SLIDE 45

Single and multinucleated mesothelial cells. *See Figure 73.*

SLIDE 46

Very large mesothelial cell with multiple nuclei. *See Figure 74.*

SLIDE 47

Clump of mesothelial cells resembling tumor cells. *See Figure 75.*

SLIDE 48

Clump of hyperchromatic mesothelial cells that could be mistaken for malignant cells. *See Figure 76.*

SLIDE 49

Two degenerating neutrophils with nuclei appearing as dark, spherical fragments. When only one fragment is present, the neutrophil resembles a nucleated RBC. *See Figure 78.*

SLIDE 50

Lymphocytes with irregular nuclear contours and moderately prominent nucleoli in a patient with viral pneumonia. The nuclear irregularities are artifacts of the cytocentrifuge. *See Figure 80.*

SLIDE 51

Two transformed lymphocytes (immunoblasts) in pleural fluid sample from patient with pancreatitis. *See Figure 82.*

SLIDE 52

Pleural effusion in patient with non-Hodgkin's lymphoma, small-lymphocytic type. *See Figure 85.*

SLIDE 53

Immunoenzymatic study using antibodies to heavy and light chains revealing a monoclonal B cell population and confirming that the lymphocytes in Figure 52 were malignant. Immunoalkaline phosphatase stain with antibody to κ light chain shows strong activity (red staining). *See Figure 86.*

SLIDE 54

Pleural fluid eosinophilia in patient with chronic renal failure. Two basophils are also seen. A small number of basophils commonly accompany eosinophils in a variety of conditions. *See Figure 88.*

SLIDE 55

"Signet-ring" macrophages in pleural fluid. *See Figure 91.*

SLIDE 56

Gram's stain of pleural effusion in patient with perforated esophagus. A mixed infection of gram-negative and gram-positive bacteria. *See Figure 94.*

SLIDE 57

Candida and fungal organisms in pleural effusion. *See Figure 95.*

SLIDE 58

Clump of bizarre, vacuolated tumor cells from patient with metastatic adenocarcinoma. *See Figure 97.*

SLIDE 59

Typical molding of nuclei in oat cell carcinoma of the lung. *See Figure 98.*

SLIDE 60

Characteristic appearance of metastatic breast carcinoma in a pleural effusion. *See Figure 99.*

SLIDE 61

Higher-power view of cells in Figure 60. When they occur singly outside the clump, these tumor cells look very similar to mesothelial cells. *See Figure 100.*

SLIDE 62

Malignant mesothelial cells from the pleural fluid in a patient with mesothelioma. *See Figure 106.*

SLIDE 63

Carcinoembryonic antigen (CEA) demonstrated in a clump of adenocarcinoma cells with an immuno-alkaline phosphatase technique (immuno-alkaline phosphatase stain with antibody to CEA). *See Figure 108.*

SLIDE 64

Epithelial membrane antigen (EMA) demonstrated in a clump of metastatic breast carcinoma cells (immuno-alkaline phosphatase stain with antibody to EMA). *See Figure 109.*

SLIDE 65

Epithelial membrane antigen (EMA) present in two tumor cells with a negative mesothelial cell and several negative lymphocytes (immuno-alkaline phosphatase stain with antibody to EMA). *See Figure 110.*

SLIDE 66

An approach to the use and interpretation of tumor cell markers in body fluids containing cells that are suspicious for malignancy. *See Figure 111.*

SLIDE 67

Eosinophils and macrophages in ascitic fluid sample from a patient undergoing long-term peritoneal dialysis. *See Figure 115.*

SLIDE 68

Adenocarcinoma of the colon in a peritoneal effusion. Note several malignant "signet ring" cells. *See Figure 117.*

SLIDE 69

Burkitt's lymphoma cells in peritoneal effusion. Note characteristic cells with blue, vacuolated cytoplasm, moderately clumped chromatin, and often prominent nucleoli. *See Figure 118.*

SLIDE 70

Burkitt's lymphoma cells showing immunofluorescence with antibody to λ light chain. The presence of surface immunoglobulins is characteristic of B cells. The identification of a monoclonal B-cell population is consistent with a diagnosis of malignant lymphoma. *See Figure 119.*

SLIDE 71

Clumps of atypical mesothelial cells resembling malignant cells. *See Figure 122.*

SLIDE 72

Live spermatozoa having white appearance since they did not take up the stain (eosin stain). *See Figure 123.*

SLIDE 73

Dead spermatozoa having orange-red appearance (eosin stain). *See Figure 124.*

SLIDE 74

Spermatozoon with normal, oval-shaped head (hematoxylin-eosin stain). *See Figure 125.*

SLIDE 75

Spermatozoon in the center with large head (hematoxylin-eosin stain). *See Figure 126.*

SLIDE 76

Spermatozoon with small head (hematoxylin-eosin stain). *See Figure 127.*

SLIDE 77

Spermatozoon with tapered or elongated head (hematoxylin-eosin stain). *See Figure 128.*

SLIDE 78

Immature spermatozoon with tail coiled around its head (hematoxylin-eosin stain). *See Figure 129.*

SLIDE 79

Spermatozoon with duplicate heads (hematoxylin-eosin stain). *See Figure 131.*

SLIDE 80

So-called amorphous-shaped spermatozoon (hematoxylin-eosin stain). *See Figure 132.*

SLIDE 81

Amorphous spermatozoa with "acorn"-shaped heads (hematoxylin-eosin stain). *See Figure 133.*

SLIDE 82

Pyknosis and karyorrhexis of neutrophils in synovial fluid sample from a patient with gout. *See Figure 139.*

SLIDE 83

Synovial lining cell. *See Figure 141.*

SLIDE 84

Multinucleated synovial cell. *See Figure 142.*

SLIDE 85

Many typical needle-shaped monosodium urate crystals in gout seen with polarized light. *See Figure 147.*

SLIDE 86

Intracellular monosodium urate crystals seen with polarized light with red compensator. *See Figure 148.*

SLIDE 87

Several monosodium urate crystals as seen with polarized light and red compensator. Color of crystals (blue or yellow) depends on orientation of crystals in relation to axis of compensator. *See Figure 151.*

SLIDE 88

Calcium pyrophosphate crystals in synovial fluid as seen under polarized light of Wright's stained smear. Rhomboid-shaped crystal in center is easily recognized, but other crystals are less distinct. *See Figure 155.*

SLIDE 89

The color of the calcium pyrophosphate crystal, as seen under polarized light with red compensator, depends on the crystal's orientation in relation to the axis of the compensator. *See Figure 156.*

SLIDE 90

Numerous cholesterol plate-like crystals in synovial fluid seen with polarized light. *See Figure 159.*

SLIDE 91

Ring-shaped cholesterol crystals in synovial fluid (polarized light). *See Figure 163.*

SLIDE 92

Plate-like (blue) and needle-shaped (yellow) cholesterol crystals in synovial fluid. The latter may be mistaken for monosodium urate crystals (polarized light with red compensator). *See Figure 164.*

SLIDE 93

Gram's stain of synovial fluid showing *Neisseria gonorrhoeae. See Figure 169.*

SLIDE 94

Small lymphocytes present in center of "cell button" made by a cytocentrifuge. *See Figure 178.*

SLIDE 95

Appearance of same small lymphocytes seen in Slide 93 but in the periphery of the "cell button." Note how cytoplasm is more abundant, nuclei are more irregular with less clumping of the chromatin, and nucleoli are distinct. The cell appears less mature than in Slide 93. *See Figure 179.*

SLIDE 96

Prominent cytoplasmic processes seen as a result of centrifuge artifact. *See Figure 180.*

SLIDE 97

Nuclear irregularities of lymphocytes. Cytocentrifuge artifact. *See Figure 181.*

SLIDE 98

Distortion of lymphocytes, giving them the appearance of monocytes. *See Figure 184.*

SLIDE 99

Distinct "nucleoli" in small, mature-appearing lymphocytes. *See Figure 185.*

SLIDE 100

Cluster of lymphocytes resembling malignant cells (oat cell carcinoma). Centrifuge artifact. *See Figure 187.*

Index

Pages on which color figures and tables appear are included in the page range for the topic; slide numbers refer to slides in the optional slide set